Maritime Psychology

Malcolm MacLachlan

Editor

Maritime Psychology

Research in Organizational & Health
Behavior at Sea

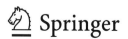
Springer

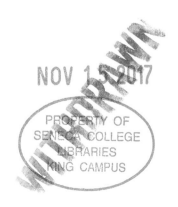

Editor
Malcolm MacLachlan
School of Psychology
Trinity College Dublin
Dublin
Ireland

ISBN 978-3-319-45428-3   ISBN 978-3-319-45430-6   (eBook)
DOI 10.1007/978-3-319-45430-6

Library of Congress Control Number: 2016956822

Printed on acid-free paper

This Springer imprint is published by Springer Nature
The registered company is Springer International Publishing AG
The registered company address is: Gewerbestrasse 11, 6330 Cham, Switzerland

Preface

This is a research volume that brings together organisational, social and health psychology research concerned with the maritime. There is no other volume that attempts to do this and hence this is the first volume of its type in this rapidly developing area. The contributors to the volume cover a range of disciplines, including psychology and maritime science; along with other social, health and physical scientists and practitioners.

The importance of psychosocial factors is being increasingly recognised in the maritime field; by students, lecturers, seafarers, employers, unions, insurance companies and international regulatory bodies. With over 1 million seafarers and English as the required international maritime language, this English-language volume on *Maritime Psychology* is intended to both recognise and give impetus to the further development of this field internationally.

Of course prior to this volume many people have been doing maritime psychology, for many years, and we make no claim for this volume being in any way exhaustive or comprehensive. Rather the idea here was to provide both individual researchers and research teams with an opportunity to evaluate the state of the literature in their own area, and to think through how their area might develop in the near future, identifying key research questions.

The volume is unashamedly applied, with most chapters having a case study to illustrate the topic of the chapter. Most, but not all, of the chapters focus on the commercial maritime transport sector; and while this sector is certainly central to maritime psychology, it is not synonymous with it.

The book will be of interest to practitioners, lectures, researchers and students of occupational and health psychology, of maritime science, occupational medicine and nursing; architecture and design; and of other social, health and physical scientists in the area. I would like to thank the contributors for participating in this volume; Emma Sherry for editorial assistance and Springer editorial team for their patience and support in bringing this volume to fruition.

Dublin, Ireland   Malcolm MacLachlan

Contents

Editor and Contributors

About the Editor

Prof. Malcolm MacLachlan is Professor of Global Health and Director of the Centre for Global Health at Trinity College Dublin where he is a member of the School of Psychology. His research interests are in the application of organisational and health psychology to global health, particularly for vulnerable, marginalised or hard-to-reach populations. He has worked as an academic, clinician, organisational consultant and policy advisor across several sectors in Europe, Africa and Asia; with corporate, civil society, governments and a range of UN agencies. He is a Fellow of the British Psychological Society and the Psychological Society of Ireland; and a member of the International Maritime Health Association and the Institute of Remote Health Care. He has sea time on several types of merchant navy vessels and has been blown off course on most types of sailing vessels.

Contributors

Apsara Abeysiriwardhane is a Ph.D. student at the Australian Maritime College. Her research focuses on increasing the inclusion of Human Factors considerations into Ship Design, where she combines her previous eight years of working experience as a Naval Architect and university lecturer.

Prof. Mike Barnett is Emeritus Professor of Maritime Safety at Warsash Maritime Academy, Southampton Solent University. After a seafaring career to chief officer rank, Mike joined Warsash in 1985 as a lecturer in tanker safety. He was Head of Research at Warsash from 1991 to his retirement in 2015, directing its research strategy and several externally funded research projects relating to maritime human factors, including both HORIZON and MARTHA projects. Mike has attended IMO since 1995 and is now an advisor to the UK delegation on the revision of the fatigue guidelines in 2016 and 2017. In 2012 he was awarded the MN Medal for his contribution to maritime safety and research, and was the winner of the European Transport senior researcher competition in 2016.

Cpt. Roddy Cooke is a Lecturer at the National Maritime College of Ireland, Cork Institute of Technology, and is the course coordinator on the Institute of Chartered Shipbroker's accredited course, the Foundation Diploma in Shipping. He is a member of the Irish Institute of Master Mariners (IIMM) and has had a long and varied career as a ship's captain.

Henriette Cox has worked as a Dual Maritime Officer working onboard oil tankers for Shell Tankers BV. When she came ashore, she focused on HSE, working in the HSE department for the Shell Fleet. Her main interests include safety and environment but lately have been involved in health projects focusing on health fitness, resilience and fatigue and their relationship with safety.

Dr. Sam Cromie is Assistant Professor of Organisational Psychology and Assistant Director of the Centre for Innovative Human Systems in Trinity College Dublin, The University of Dublin. He has over twenty years' experience of action research into human and organisational factors in aviation, process, manufacturing, pharma, rail, maritime and healthcare sectors. Particular research interests are: the implementation of just culture, risk management of human factors, the impact of human factors training, the role of procedures in managing performance, safety and just culture. Sam led the development of the STAMINA training programme which has been a global benchmark of human factors training in aviation maintenance. He is managing director of Trinity Stamina which delivers human factors and safety management training and consulting internationally. Sam's collaborators and clients have included Airbus, Rolls Royce, Pfizer, Cathay Pacific, British Airways, Fiat and EASA.

Dr. Ian de Terte is a senior lecturer in clinical psychology at Massey University, Wellington, New Zealand. His research interests are psychological resilience, posttraumatic stress disorder, high-risk occupations, and at-risk populations. He views psychological resilience from a multidimensional perspective, and investigates it in high-risk occupations or at-risk populations. Dr. de Terte is interested in how to enhance psychological resilience or how psychological resilience may alleviate mental health difficulties in these populations. Dr. de Terte has 27 academic publications and has made 55 academic presentations.

Niamh Doyle completed her undergraduate degree in Psychology in Trinity College Dublin followed by a Masters in Neuropsychology in Maastricht University, the Netherlands. She is currently a Clinical Psychologist in Training in University College Cork.

Dr. Marianne Dyer is a consultant occupational physician and Fellow of the Faculty of Occupational Medicine. She has extensive experience in a wide range of industries including the military, aviation, safety critical industries, rail construction, energy, oil and gas and manufacturing. She won the Faculty of Occupational Medicine 'Wilf Howe Award' for the occupational health services for the construction of London 2012 Olympic Park. She is currently the Health Manager for Shell International covering the UK, Mediterranean and Shipping.

Dr. Alistair Fraser is the Vice President of Health for Royal Dutch Shell plc based in The Hague. His area of interest is the impact of intentionally focusing on care for people and improving human performance as a way to enhance thriving, quality of life and business outcomes. He is a graduate of Aberdeen University Medical School, a Fellow of the Royal College of Physicians of Glasgow, Fellow of the Faculty of Occupational Medicine and was awarded an Honorary Doctorate of Science by Robert Gordon University in Aberdeen.

Prof. John F. Golding is Professor of Applied Psychology at the University of Westminster, London. He originally trained as a biochemist at the University of Oxford, but became interested in psychology, gaining another first degree, in psychology, before completing his D.Phil. there on the physiological and psychological effects of nicotine (smoking), subsequently working as a research fellow at Oxford. He then did research on psychoactive drugs and pain relief in the Pharmacology Department of Newcastle Medical School. This was followed by an extended period in government service doing a wide range of applied research (human factors) including motion sickness, cognitive performance in divers, desensitisation of pilots, and military selection and training, at the Institute of Naval Medicine, RAF Institute of Aviation Medicine and Centre for Human Sciences (DERA). John has been awarded the posts of Professor of Psychology (Honorary), Guys and St Thomas's Hospital, Kings College, London, and Visiting Professor at Imperial College, London. His current research projects are mainly in the fields of motion sickness, vestibular disorders, spatial disorientation and health psychology.

Dr. Jørgen Riis Jepsen graduated as a medical doctor in 1973 and specialised in occupational medicine and community medicine in 1984. Since 1985, he has been working as head and consultant at the Department of Occupational Medicine, Hospital of Southwestern Jutland in Esbjerg, Denmark. From 2009 he has been part-time Associate Professor at the Centre of Maritime Health and Society, Institute of Public

Health, University of Southern Denmark, heading the centre from 2009 to 2012. In addition to clinical and teaching tasks he has conducted and published research in the field of occupational medicine with a particular emphasis on work-related upper limb disorders, return-to-work and rehabilitation issues, and maritime health.

Dr. Maria Kalafati is Laboratory Teaching Staff at the Nursing Faculty of the National and Kapodistrian University of Athens, and the President of Emergency and Critical Care Nurses Sector of the Hellenic Nurses Association. Most of her studies are focused on the management of health departments (related to health professionals or/and patients), evidence-based practice and nursing assessment.

Cpt. Bill Kavanagh is a Lecturer in Nautical Science at the National Maritime College of Ireland, Cork Institute of Technology. He holds the professional qualification of Master Mariner and a Bachelor's degree in Training and Education, and a Master's degree in Adult Learning and Development. He has contributed to a number of publications and conferences on ship simulation and human factors.

Alison Kay is an occupational psychologist based at the Centre for Innovative Human Systems within the School of Psychology at Trinity College Dublin, the University of Dublin. Her core focus is on the human aspects of transport and industrial systems. She has worked on human factors research projects in aviation, process industries, maritime industry, manufacturing and healthcare at EU, commercial and governmental levels for the past 13 years. Her research has addressed decision-making, process modelling and resource management for training, procedure writing and accident investigation. In 2008, Alison was one of the Human Factors Integration Defence Technology Centre team awarded the UK Ergonomics Society President's Medal 'for significant contributions to original research, the development of methodology and the application of knowledge within the field of ergonomics'.

Dr. Paul M. Liston is a Research Fellow at the Centre for Innovative Human Systems within the School of Psychology at Trinity College Dublin, the University of Dublin. Dr. Liston has over 17 years of experience in initiating, coordinating and participating in research and development projects. He is Principal Investigator on the SEAHORSE project that seeks to transfer learning, knowledge and innovation from the aviation sector to the maritime sector. As part of this project he led the development of a systemic and systematic methodology for transferring safety innovation across different industrial sectors. Paul's research interests span the shipping, aviation, process, and healthcare sectors and focus on improving competence and performance of operations and safety. He has previously been involved with research and consultancy projects that have addressed human factors training in the aircraft maintenance industry (AITRAM, ADAMS2, STAMP).

Prof. Cpt. Margareta Lützhöft is a master mariner, trained at Kalmar Maritime Academy in Sweden. After leaving the sea, she studied for a Bachelor's degree in Cognitive science and a Master's in Computer Science. In December 2004 she received a Ph.D. in Human–Machine Interaction. Presently she is Professor of Nautical Studies at the Australian Maritime College. Her research interests include human-centered design and the effects of new technology.

Dr. Nick McDonald is Associate Professor of Psychology and founding Director of the Centre for Innovative Human Systems in Trinity College Dublin, the University of Dublin. His research interests relate to human factors and organisational aspects of safety in risk-sensitive industries including aviation; the analysis and management of risk; innovation and change in organisations; and technology design for operational systems. Nick led the development and implementation of Trinity College Dublin's first fully online Masters course (M.Sc.) in Managing Risk and System Change. This course brings the next generation of safety, risk and change management to students, embedded in their everyday practice with a systemic, proactive and performance focus. Nick led a team that was awarded the *International Ergonomics Association 2011 IEA/Liberty Mutual Medal* for their contribution to safety research.

Joanne McVeigh is a doctoral researcher in the field of positive organisational psychology in the Centre for Global Health and School of Psychology, Trinity College Dublin, Ireland. Her doctoral research focuses on facilitators and barriers of the well-being of seafarers, including onboard positive psychology interventions. Her research interests also include social inclusion, human rights and disability.

Prof. Claire Pekcan is Professor of Maritime Applied Psychology and Senior Lecturer at Warsash Maritime Academy, Southampton Solent University. She has also been a key member of the research team at Warsash for 20 years, and contributed to both HORIZON and MARTHA projects on seafarer fatigue. She is an advisor to the UK delegation to the IMO sessions on the revision of the fatigue guidelines in 2016 and 2017. Claire sits on a number of shipping industry working groups, including the Human Element Working Group (HEWG) of IMarEST, the Human Element Advisory Group (HEAG) of the UK MCA, and she is also the Vice Chair of the Human Element sub-committee of Intertanko.

Dr. Erik Styhr Petersen holds a B.Sc. in Naval Architecture, and was a consulting naval architect for 13 years, subsequent to which he was head of R&D at the Danish Maritime Institute, for a 6-year period. Following this, Petersen went into industrial research with Lyngsø Marine and SAM Electronics, with a focus on maritime electronic systems, maritime usability and human-centred design in the marine domain. Pursuing his academic interests at Chalmers Technical University in parallel, Petersen received his Lic. Eng., in 2010 and his Ph.D. in 2012, the latter in the subject of 'Engineering Usability'. In addition to his industrial post, Petersen is presently also Adjunct Associate Professor at the Australian Maritime College.

Cpt. Dionysios Rassias is a Greek Master Mariner. Following a seagoing career which spanned 19 years, he is presently working as Assistant Professor and Director of Studies at the Merchant Marine Academy of Ionian Islands. He commanded various tanker ships operating around the world. He also holds a B.Sc. in Maritime Studies and an M.Sc. in Shipping from the University of Piraeus.

Dr. Ana Sliškovic is Assistant Professor at Department of Psychology of University of Zadar (Croatia), where she teaches courses related to the methodology in psychological research and occupational stress. Her research interests relate to the field of work/organisational psychology, primarily occupational stress, workplace well-being, and maritime psychology.

Dr. Ralf Stilz is an accredited specialist in occupational medicine, with a background in general hospital medicine. He has advised on health and work in the healthcare sector, government, public services, education and academic sectors, and the oil and gas sector. He has a special interest in maritime medicine and seafarers' health.

Dr. Elspeth Tilley specialises in applied communication teaching and research, particularly using creative, participatory and constructivist methodologies. Since 2013 she has been collaborating with Massey University's Joint Centre for Disaster Research, bringing a qualitative and social sciences orientation to developing understanding of important New Zealand disaster communication challenges such as safety warnings and community preparedness.

Dr. Ernestos Tzannatos is Professor at the Department of Maritime Studies of the University of Piraeus, and the Dean of School of Maritime and Industrial Studies; specialising on the management of ship technology, including its interaction with the human element, for the promotion of productivity, safety (including security) and environmental protection in shipping.

Wessel M.A. van Leeuwen is a researcher in the Sleep and Fatigue unit at SRI working in the field of sleep and fatigue for over 10 years. He has worked on the measurement and analysis of the data from the HORIZON and MARTHA projects. He has given over 20 talks, including invited ones, at a wide variety of scientific conferences on the topics of sleep and fatigue. He is a member of the Dutch Society for Sleep Wake Research (NSWO), the Swedish Society for Sleep Research and

Sleep Medicine (SFSS), the European Sleep Research Society (ESRS), the Swedish Ergonomics and Human Factors Society (EHSS), and the Marie Curie Fellowship Association (MCFA). In addition, he teaches masters courses on psychobiological processes, stress, and health at Stockholm University.

Cpt. Peter Walter (Master Mariner, BA(Hons), MA, MNI MIIMM) has been a Lecturer at the National Maritime College of Ireland, Cork Institute of Technology, for over 15 years and has teaching experience at all levels in both fishing and merchant navy sectors. Currently specialising in shipboard operations and bridge simulator training he has spent 19 years at sea, and has experience on a large variety of vessels ranging from square rig sailing ships to supertankers.

Dr. Zhiwei Zhao is a Lecturer and Director of Seafarers Development International Research Centre at Dalian Maritime University, China. She is working part-time at Centre of Maritime Health and Society based at University of Southern Denmark. She specialises in sociology in maritime human element, and includes occupational health and safety and maritime human resource management among her areas of expertise. She contributed to the TK Foundation funded Martha project, which investigated fatigue on-board ships; the BIMCO/ICS Manpower Report 2015; and the Employment Relationship of Chinese seafarers, funded by Chinese Maritime Safety Administration.

Yannis Zolotas is a psychologist working at Dromokaiteio Mental Health Hospital in Athens, Greece. His interests lie in the areas of psychoanalytic psychotherapy, the psychodynamics of groups and organisations and psychometric assessment.

Maritime Psychology: Definition, Scope and Conceptualization

Malcolm MacLachlan

Introduction

This is a research volume that brings together organizational and health psychology research concerned with the maritime. Such research is undertaken by psychologists, other social scientists and of course by maritime practitioners, lecturers and researchers, but also by engineers, designers and others, as will be seen in this volume. The importance of psychosocial factors is being increasingly recognized in the maritime field—by students, lecturers, seafarers, employers, unions, insurance companies and international regulatory bodies. There is also now increased research funding, training and accreditation relating to areas of maritime psychology, from both international bodies, government and the industry itself.

With over 1 million seafarers and English as the required international maritime language, I hope that this book on *maritime psychology* will both recognize and give impetus to the further development of this important, complex and challenging field. In this chapter I offer a *definition* of maritime psychology, and then sketch the *scope* of the area, identifying different aspects of the interplay between the study of the maritime and the study of psychology. The primary focus of both this chapter and this book is on maritime transport—the "merchant marine" or "merchant navy". Building on this I offer a broader conceptualization of the maritime transport industry, using a systems perspective and drawing on some of our previous work. While the application of psychology may be compartmentalized for purposes of classification, its application in the maritime transport sector requires a systems perspective and I consider a model that summarizes such an approach.

I then preview the chapters within this volume, which offer real insight and expertise on some of the fascinating and varied aspects of maritime psychology.

M. MacLachlan (✉)
Centre for Global Health and School of Psychology, Trinity College, University of Dublin, Dublin, Ireland
e-mail: malcolm.maclachlan@tcd.ie

© Springer International Publishing Switzerland 2017
M. MacLachlan (ed.), *Maritime Psychology*, DOI 10.1007/978-3-319-45430-6_1

1

The chapters in this volume are certainly not intended to offer a comprehensive coverage of maritime psychology, but rather to be illustrative of the range, dynamism and scientific merit of research and practice in the domain.

It is important to acknowledge that many researchers and mariners have been "doing" maritime psychology for years, indeed centuries. Furthermore, much of our most engaging fiction literature has narrative steeped in the psychology of maritime experiences (e.g. Joseph Conrad). This volume is an attempt to recognize and build on the defining and distinctive characteristics of maritime psychology, whilst also upholding its clear interplay with other social, biological, physical and environmental perspectives. In proposing "maritime psychology" as an entity in itself, I am aware that things do not just spring into existence, but are co-created, collectively constructed, by those who practise them. In this sense each chapter in this volume contributes to the definition of maritime psychology, and with growing interest in this area and more perspectives being taken, it is likely that any definition will—and should—be contested and evolve. To provide focus within this volume, as stated, it is primarily concerned with psychological aspects of commercial maritime transport. Yet maritime psychology should have broader concerns than this. Perusal of Table 1 indicates the vast array of ways in which people and the maritime interact and suggests very different sorts of maritime experience. To acknowledge this, the final chapter in this volume also considers what might be described as the psychological benefit of the maritime as a beneficial intervention. This also hints at the vast range of ways in which the interaction between psychology and the maritime may be developed in future.

Definition

Maritime psychology can be broadly defined as *the study and practice of the interplay between human behaviour and the maritime environment.* Mostly research and practice to date has been concerned with human behaviour aboard seagoing vessels, with the major focus being on maritime transport—the merchant navy or merchant marine. However, as noted, this scope can certainly be expanded. On the one hand a walk along the seashore can be an enriching and inspiring experience, for old and young alike, and our aim here is not to analyse away the existential value, or everyday pleasure, of such an experience. On the other hand, the movement of a ship through busy shipping lanes, in confined and dangerous waters, can be very cognitively demanding, require extensive teamwork, astute judgement and considerable manual skill. While these two types of maritime experience may be quite distinct, for some, they are also braided together: the existential with the task-focused, the personal with the movement of immense loads. We now consider what might be thought of as the coordinates of maritime psychology, locating itself across very different aspects of human functioning and experience.

Table 1 Classification of maritime activities that share and have some distinct psychological attributes

Domains	Categories	Examples
Commercial	Transport	Cargo vessels Cruise ships Construction vessels Tugs
	Energy	Oil rigs Wind farms
	Fishing	Trawling
	Farming	Fish farms Shell fish farms
	Diving	Maintenance of equipment
	Navigational	Charting depths Dredging channels
Recreational	Rowing, sailing, motoring activities	Engine and sail powered activities
	Diving	Inland, coastal and deep sea
	Swimming	
Environmental	Disasters	Tsunamis, floods, storms
	Rhythm	Tides, winds
	Lifestyle	Domicile choice Regenerative visits
Intervention	Occupational	Corporate teambuilding
	Developmental	Outward bound adventure
	Therapeutic	Medium to strengthen self-worth and dignity
Military	Non-combatant	Peace keeping/pirate patrol/refugee rescue
	Combatant	Surface operations
		Submarine operations
Safety	Coastguard	Rescue operations
		Raising awareness of danger
		Use of safety equipment and procedures

Scope

Table 1 outlines the different domains of maritime psychology, where domain refers to broad categories of activities that may be considered to have some common features. Such features are categorized in Table 1 with accompanying examples. Again, this table makes no claim to be comprehensive but rather illustrative, and in doing so helps us to consider the reach of maritime psychology.

Commercial transport is the domain of primary concern in this volume. However, clearly there is also great scope for more work on the psychology of maritime leisure activities, or on how tides mark time for many coastal communities and provide rhythm and meaning to daily life for them. The destructive and restorative elements of the maritime have both long been recognized as dramatically affecting our psychology. We will, however, consider in this volume the idea of the maritime as a beneficial intervention, especially regarding sailing, as an example of maritime psychology outside the commercial transport sector. The military aspects of the maritime in terms of surface and submarine craft have been addressed elsewhere and are not covered here but without doubt psychology has much to contribute and indeed to learn from the sometimes very extreme conditions confronted in military operations (Kimhi 2011). Finally, and what should always be an element of the maritime, are safety considerations—ranging from risk perception to attitudes towards safety equipment, to search and rescue activities. The maritime environment is vast and clearly there are differences in how people perceive both opportunities and threats within their own experience of an environment (Walsh-Danishmandi and MacLachlan 2000). However, let us now turn to our major focus of this book, commercial shipping.

Commercial Shipping

Helen Sampson, of the Seafarer's International Research Centre at Cardiff University, began the introduction to the Centre's 2015 Annual Report, thus:

> It isn't just that 'the strange' has become 'familiar' and that there is less to learn, it is more serious than that. For many seafarers, voyages that were once punctuated with moments of fun are frequently mundane, featureless and dull. Only problems seem to break into the routine and tribulations are no replacement for the frivolity that was often associated with sorties ashore, barbecues by the pool, or birthday parties. These events not only provided seafarers with a few stress-free hours … the pleasure of the moment … they also provided a basis for later tales, told and retold – the building blocks for the establishment of camaraderie on board … teambuilding … mental wellbeing (p. 1, reproduced by kind permission).

This quotation illustrates well not just the human face of working at sea, but also how this has changed. With larger ships, greater mechanization and reduced manning levels, more is required from seafarers and there are fewer outlets for the sort of affiliation that sustains both a sense of collective identity and individual worth and support. The requirements regarding how seafarers are treated are specified in a number of important documents that effectively set the policy context for how maritime psychology can contribute to seafaring.

The Compendium of Maritime Labour Instruments, published in its second and revised edition in 2015, summarizes the ways in which the maritime industry should work. The Compendium comprises the Maritime Labour Convention (2006); the Seafarers' Identity Documents (Revised) Convention (2003); and the Work in Fishing Convention and Recommendation (2007). These documents are about the working and living relationships between people in complex, demanding and sometimes extreme conditions that require the highest degree of human interaction, teamwork, problem solving and physical and cognitive skills. It is, therefore, surprising that conventions that seek to address human behaviour in such circumstances omit the word "psychology".

Nonetheless, Resolutions adopted by the International Labour Conference at its 94th (maritime) Session in 2006 include a "Resolution concerning addressing the human element through international cooperation between United Nations specialised agencies" (p. X). It reads:

> The resolution notes the 'significance of issues related to the human element … [seeks] to promote decent working and living conditions. [It also recognises] … that the human element is multifaceted and can only be addressed in a holistic manner' (p. 131). It goes on to request that priority and resources be given to 'promoting the role of the human element in shipping.'

A further Resolution at the same meeting—see Table 2—details not only the importance of the global shipping industry, but also its reliance on people, and in particular the need for better recruiting, training and retaining of seafarers. The "human element" is, therefore, the "marinized" term used to describe at least some of the aspects of psychology which this book seeks to develop further. The

Table 2 Resolution concerning recruitment and retention of seafarers

The General Conference of the International Labour Organization
Having adopted the Maritime Labour Convention, 2006
Mindful that the core mandate of the Organization is to promote decent work
Being aware that shipping is the engine of the globalized economy and carries around 90 % of world trade in terms of tonnage, and that the shipping industry and the smooth transportation of goods are essential to world trade, which will require the availability of a sufficient number of suitably qualified seafarers
Being aware also that ships are crewed by suitably trained seafarers who have a crucial role in achieving safe, secure and efficient shipping on clean oceans and that it is fundamental to the sustainable operation of this strategic sector that it is able to continue to attract an adequate number of quality new entrants
Noting that there is a projected shortage of suitably qualified seafarers, that many essential shore-based shipping positions require trained seafarers and that filling some of these positions with suitably qualified seafarers is essential to overall maritime safety
Noting also that traditional maritime countries are going through a process of industrial change and have lost substantial parts of their maritime skills base
Noting further that there is a need for proper career paths for officers and ratings alike
Considers that, while there is a need to improve the image of the shipping industry, there is also a need to improve the conditions of employment and of work and opportunities for many seafarers
Considers also that issues such as access to shore leave and security from attack by pirates and armed robbers need to be addressed
Considers further that all flag States should encourage operators of ships which fly their flag to provide training berths for new seafarers and for cadets
Recognizes that the recruitment and retention of seafarers in a global labour market is a complex issue, which involves a social, political and economic dimension and, where appropriate, the provision of suitable policies by governments and industry alike … (pp. 131–132)
Adopted on 22 February 2006 by the International Labour Conference at its 94th (maritime) Session

Resolutions described above have made a significant impact on the development of a stronger psychological perspective within the maritime industry, and the ethos of the "human element" has contributed much to this, along with the impetus provided by several important initiatives in the area. There are also many excellent publications on the human element including several that we draw on quite extensively in this book. However, I believe a broader and more inclusive incorporation of psychology and "behaviour" (by the way that is another word that does not appear in the Compendium) can be beneficial for the maritime industry.

The scope of psychology in the commercial transport sector remains quite underdeveloped. So, for instance, Bengt Schager—who describes himself as a "maritime psychologist"—arguing for the role of psychologists in the maritime transport sector, notes that while many psychologists are employed in the aviation and space sectors, few are employed in the maritime sector (www.profilschager. com). He points out that while crewing a Boeing 747 across the Atlantic requires many important leadership and participation skills for a few hours, taking thousands of passengers on a cruise for weeks, with a much larger crew, undoubtedly requires these and additional skills. The very useful and accessible *Alert!* series, subtitled "The International Maritime Human Element Bulletin", and published by the Nautical Institute, has certainly helped to bring psychological thinking to a wider audience of seafarers.

The scope of maritime psychology also overlaps with some complementary fields, so for instance, the "Textbook of Maritime Medicine", now in its second edition (Carter and Schreiner 2013), is freely available to download. It covers a range of issues where psychological factors are of clear importance. These include: specification of work roles, manning hours and manning ratios; piracy and violent crime, and the trauma and reactions associated with these; crisis interventions for response to critical incidents, perhaps associated with work accidents, drowning, suicide or injury to colleagues; a range of environmental health challenges associated not just with the working conditions on board, but often also the transport of dangerous or toxic cargoes requiring careful handling and protection procedures; motion sickness; shipwreck and survival at sea under extreme conditions; coping with fatigue arising from long passages at sea.

We can anticipate the development of a range of specific maritime psychology practices that can address all of these—and many more—challenges as they arise. However, maritime psychology should also be about setting fair working conditions that recognize the needs of seafarers to have leisure time, privacy, opportunities to socialize and indeed sufficient time off work—just as the quote from Sampson illustrates. Recently, on a flight from Panama I met a Philippine man who worked as a barman on cruise ships. He had just finished a 9-month stint working split shifts: scheduled for 6 h on, followed by a break, and then another 5 h on—*every day* of his 9-month voyage. He claimed that it was in fact rare that he did only the 11 scheduled hours a day, often running to 13 or 14, as passengers enjoyed bar services late into the night. This is certainly not an isolated instance, with lower-ranked crew, from low-income settings, usually having the worst terms and conditions of employment.

The notion of "sweat ships" refers to similar exploitation of workers. Indeed, the phenomenon of flag-of-convenience (FOC) ships, where few labour laws or standards need apply, is a considerable challenge. In practice, working conditions and practice in international waters are effectively at the discretion of the ship's Master. The cruise industry is a particular case in point. On some of these enormous ships large numbers of women work long hours below decks in the housekeeping department, reporting to seniors—often men. This is a situation open to psychological, physical and indeed sexual exploitation, especially as crew who complain run the risk of being dismissed and may be put ashore in a port where they lack the means to return to their own country.

So no matter what sort of clever individual psychological interventions maritime psychologists can develop, implementing these in a fundamentally unfair and exploitive working environment can be counterproductive, individualizing a systems problem (McVeigh et al. 2016). As can be seen in other industries (Carr et al. 2010) this can make us complicit in the maintenance of unjust workplaces. These practices, therefore, affect not only the psychological well-being and rights of individuals, but also the sense of organizational justice and expectations for decency that pervade the workplace (MacLachlan 2016). While strong seafarers unions are present in many countries, the reality is that they are often reluctant to address these sorts of issues because they fear that seafarers from their own country will lose employment if they ask for too much: there are always seafarers from other countries who will work for the terms and conditions on offer.

Conceptualization

Figure 1 presents a conceptualization of the commercial maritime sector which illustrates how individuals' own work tasks are embedded in broader teamworking, which is in turn embedded in the organizational culture of the shipping company, which is embedded in the legislation and policies that set the operating context of the industry. These levels continually interact and so a system allows for the possibility to change something at one level by intervening at other levels. For instance, the space allocated to communal living on board merchant ships has been diminishing in recent times (Sampson 2015): the design of living space on board will reflect the legislative environment and the attitude of the company towards social spaces; the use of such space will reflect the sense of teamwork and congeniality on board—and the existence of such an atmosphere will in turn reflect the demand for such space to be built into ships at the design stage. Sampson and Ellis (2015) argue that the welfare of seafarers is "under-considered" by many companies. While the Maritime Labour Convention (MLC) makes important stipulations regarding seafarer living conditions, these are in reality quite low standards and the aim should be to improve on these rather than simply adhere to them.

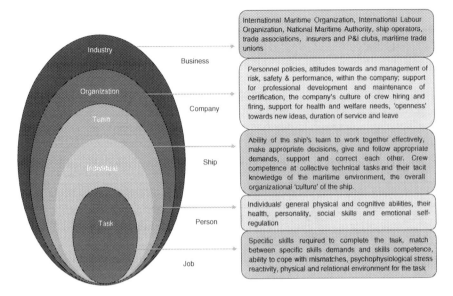

Fig. 1 A nested model of the psychosocial and organisational aspects of maritime work: synthesizing the STAMINA model of human factors with the maritime environment

We have described the operation of this conceptual model elsewhere (MacLachlan et al. 2013). The key point for our discussion here is recognition that while interventions focused on individuals may be of some benefit, such interventions in the absence of systemic change may be ineffective, or, worse, see systems failings as failings within individuals—which may be unfair, inefficient and unsafe.

Some Challenges and Opportunities for Maritime Psychology

Before reviewing the contributions to this volume, I briefly consider some additional features of maritime psychology that are not specifically addressed within the other chapters of this book, but are nonetheless noteworthy in terms of their potential for further research and the development of more psychologically minded practice.

Ship Evacuation

Ship evacuation is an area attracting increasing attention. Boulougouris and Papanikolaou (2002) have sought to model and simulate the process for evacuating a passenger ship. Modelling human behaviour under situations of extreme stress is very complex, and such behaviour may be difficult to predict, but modelling simulations of multiple and varying evacuation scenarios can guide the naval architect to minimize bottlenecks in the ship's layout. Yuan et al. (2014) illustrate, using a neighbourhood particle swarm optimization model, how door sizes, the number of doors, the number of passengers, along with the ship's heel and trim angles, all affect the evacuation time of a given ship design. What these models may not adequately consider is the frailty or mobility of passengers, the range of cognitive or sensory impairments they may have, and so on. With the majority of passengers on some cruise ships being elderly, it seems likely that the evacuation scenarios and times for these passengers are going to be more complex and take longer than for younger or less impaired passengers. Much more work is needed in this area to give greater confidence in the safety of the booming cruising market.

Piracy

The Centre for Seafarers' Rights, of the Seamen's Church Institute, conducted a study of 25 seafarers attacked or held hostage by pirates (Stevenson 2012), which found that most had concerns about returning to work (20), sleep disturbances (12) and diminished energy (10). Some of them also reported increased use of alcohol (7), loss of pleasure from what had been formerly pleasurable activities (6), with fewer reporting a deterioration of significant relationships (5), irritability (5) and sometimes thoughts of suicide (3). Of concern is the finding that less than one-third of them felt that they received adequate follow-up care. Within this small sample there was no relationship between subjective descriptions of stress, and age, rank or length of service at sea, but there was a relationship with the length of time seafarers were held captive—the longer they were held, the more severe the symptoms. Seafarers were concerned with the consequences of any mental health problems for their future eligibility for employment as seafarers, stressing the need for confidentiality in these assessments. The study also recommended that assessment following such events be much broader than assessment for PTSD only, and that the treatment of responses to piracy was a very complex issue. Amongst other suggestions was that there should be development of industry-wide protocols for resilience training; this would comprise preparation for such eventualities that would minimize the likelihood of severe psychological consequences resulting from these traumatic events.

Another study by Aleksandrov et al. (2015) followed up seven Bulgarian seafarers, who had been held captive for 6 months by pirates. They used in-depth assessment interviews, 20 days after their release from being held captive. They compare the impact of such captivity as being psychologically equivalent to exposure to other serious life-threatening events such as terrorist incidents and natural disasters. Participants reported feelings of detachment and alienation from those close to them, being startled by noises, having nightmares and sleep disturbance. Anxiety manifest through apprehension, tension and fear in particular situations, and depressive reactions manifest through low mood, lack of interest and engagement in activities were also noted. Aleksandrov et al. (2015) also emphasize the importance of appropriate supportive care of the victims. Furthermore, they argue; "Stigma discourages many seafarers from seeking consultation or effective therapy … because they fear losing their jobs or not being rehired" (p. 993). This clearly highlights the interaction between individual and systemic factors discussed above.

Organizational Culture

Bergheim et al. (2015) argue that there are "significant differences in the organizational cultures and safety practices onboard ships due to national and/or company specific characteristics" (p. 27). O'Shea (2005) has demonstrated that certain styles of command—generally more democratic styles—are associated with better seafarer well-being. Researching the effects of Work Improvement on Board (WIB) programmes in the Japanese fishing fleet, Shuji and Kazutaka (2015), using participatory action-orientated training, found such interventions to be beneficial, especially when applied in a flexible manner. With modern merchant ships often being crewed by seafarers from a range of nationalities, it is important to take account of differences in matters such as affiliative preferences, risk perception and ideas about health and well-being (MacLachlan 2006). Organizational culture should also cultivate pluralism (MacLachlan and O'Connell 2000) as a diversity of views in the workplace can in fact help solve problems and does not need to be a challenge to one narrow prevailing ethos (Cox and Blake 1991).

Psychological Capital

The concept of "psychological capital", or PsyCap (Luthans et al. 2007), has recently been developed following on from the more established ideas of financial and social capital, as positive reserves of value. The concept of PsyCap combines four somewhat related "good things", these being Hope, Resiliency, Optimism and Self-Efficacy. This motivational state has been shown to be related to organizational effectiveness and positive work outcomes (Newman et al. 2014), and has recently been explored in the maritime environment by Bergheim et al. (2015).

They explored PsyCap in three Norwegian shipping companies across two studies. Their first study found that PsyCap was positively associated with perceptions of safety climate and importantly this effect still held after controlling for socially desirable responding. Of particular interest however was an interaction effect they found: for officers and non-officers who scored relatively low on PsyCap, they perceived the safety climate similarly; however, officers with high levels of PsyCap had a more positive perception of the safety climate, compared to non-officers who also scored high on PsyCap.

In a second study they demonstrated that PsyCap's relationship to safety climate was mediated by its association with job satisfaction. While correlational studies cannot determine causality, this nonetheless suggests that those with high scores on psychological capital felt their ship was safer, at least in part, due to them also having greater job satisfaction. However, as evidence of the complexity of such a relationship, and the importance of cultural differences in health and performance noted above, this indirect effect was evidenced only for European and not for Filipino crew. So while PsyCap may be associated with benefits for some groups, its potential for promoting comprehensive change for all members of a ship's crew has yet to be demonstrated, and its value must therefore be further and very carefully explored so that what works well for one dominant group in the shipping industry is not allowed to determine how all other groups are treated. Taking into account human differences and finding value and benefits in this diversity is perhaps the essence of cultivating pluralism (MacLachlan and O'Connell 2000).

Global Health at Work

The fact that the workplace is also the home of seafarers has meant that a considerable focus of maritime has been through the development of occupational health services, with a particular interest in international health problems. We reviewed publications in the International Maritime Health journal from 2000 to 2010 (MacLachlan et al. 2012) and identified six themes: (1) healthcare access, delivery and integration; (2) tele-health; (3) non-communicable diseases and physical health problems; (4) communicable diseases; (5) psychological functioning and health; and (6) safety-related issues. In that paper we describe these themes in some detail and call on the development of more ambitious and more robust research designs. This should include randomized controlled trials and longitudinal studies, but also more focus on qualitative research, and on research addressing the context of work for non-European seafarers, spouses and family members. This combination of the technical with the contextual, systems and social justice, is also characteristic of the ethos of global health. Indeed strengthening the links between international occupational health in the maritime and global health may contribute to the development of a stronger discipline of *global occupational health*, concerned with the possibilities for and also the threats of global corporations influencing healthcare across vastly different settings and conditions globally. Maritime psychology would have much to contribute to a concern with global health in the workplace.

Chapters in This Volume

In this volume we build on previous work in the area and in this regard special mention should be given to Gregory and Shanahan's (2010) "The Human Element", which was a landmark publication for the maritime transport industry. In addition to its excellent review of psychological factors relevant to maritime transport, it is noteworthy that it was jointly sponsored by the UK's Maritime and Coastguard Agency, British Petroleum, Teekay Marine Services and the Standard P&I Club. The collaboration of these stakeholders constituted a common platform that promoted wide dissemination (with a revision recently completed). One of the motivations for Gregory and Shanahan's publication was to reduce the number of accidents at sea: they note that between 2000 and 2005, on average, *every day*, 18 ships collided, sank, grounded, caught fire or exploded, resulting in an average of two of them actually sinking each day. The cause of these accidents is mostly due to human error. Such accidents cost an average of around 4 million US$ every day and countless human lives. Costs in terms of lost revenue, environmental pollution and human life can all be immense.

Gregory and Shanahan cover a range of psychological factors involved in commercial maritime transport—making decisions and taking risks, getting tired and stressed, how one learns and develops personally and professionally, working and communication with others and how people try to make sense—sometimes in error—of the contexts they find themselves in. Their excellent presentation of this work for seafarers has been a spur to identify, develop and pursue research questions, to more effectively promote satisfying, efficient and safe seafaring. The range of chapters described below illustrates just some of the fascinating ways in which this can be done.

Joanne McVeigh and colleagues review the positive psychology of well-being at sea. While some applications of psychology in the maritime environment are focused on fixing deficits, other aspects are focused on improving performance, living environments, and so on. Positive psychology is concerned with promoting a sense of well-being across all types of contexts, including work contexts. McVeigh et al. provide examples of positive psychology interventions in general, but also such interventions as used in other work contexts. Generally, these studies indicate that relatively modest, or even small-scale, interventions can have quite positive effects, often on well-being and performance, across a range of work environments. Positive psychology is associated with the idea of hardiness and resilience and there is certainly evidence suggesting that greater personal resilience can act as a buffer to stress (Doyle et al. 2015). However, McVeigh et al. (2016) have stressed that such interventions that focus only on the resilience of individuals, while ignoring the broader work context in which those individuals are expected to perform, is not only problematic, but also unethical and likely to cause frustration and disengagement. Positive psychology should be applied much more broadly throughout the shipping industry, not only to individuals, especially if they are working in unjust or obviously stressful situations.

Paul Liston and colleagues explore the challenge of transferring learning across what are referred to as "safety critical industries". They use the frame of Hudson's et al. (2004) levels of safety, moving from organizations with poor practices who simply do not want to be caught doing the wrong thing, to those who react to accidents, to those who actively manage them, to those who plan for and anticipate them, to the preferred level where organizations create an environment pervaded by a concern for quality, health and safety. While the aviation industry is probably the best-practice example in safety critical industries, Liston et al. argue that the maritime industry is somewhat behind it, and therefore the transfer of this learning and ethos is important. One feature that characterizes the aviation sector approach is seeing the different components of safety, quality and health operating as an inter-connected "socio-technical system"; that is, it involves people just as much as it involves technology. Cockpit Resource Management is a crucial part of this in the aviation sector, with Bridge Resource Management being its equivalent in the maritime sector. Liston et al. review some of the challenges of cross-sector learning and outline a model for cross-sector transfer upon which their own SEAHORSE project is based; this will likely produce some very valuable learning for the maritime sector.

Margareta Lützhöft and colleagues have produced a fascinating chapter on the psychology of ship architecture and ship design. Given that a ship is a space at sea that people live in, the characteristics of that space are likely to have significant effects of the behaviour of seafarers. It is one of the very tangible ways in which physical structure shares social structure and so psychological experience. The physical environment also dramatically influences sleep quality, fatigue and opportunities for privacy; and as such can be expected to influence how people like one ship over another, the extent of crew turnover, but perhaps also their attitudes to safety and to caring for one another. The chapter illustrates the potential benefit of combining perspectives on designing living and working spaces at sea with perspectives on living and working behaviour at sea. Interestingly, they also link this to the sort of thinking styles that design engineers generally have and how they may benefit from developing additional thinking styles. They anticipate some very exciting and innovative possibilities for ship design and living in the future.

Ana Slišković then addresses occupational stress in seafarers. She adopts a transactional perspective, reviewing stress at the individual and organizational level. She also considers important individual and organizational characteristics as moderators or mediators between sources of stress and stress as an outcome. Slišković makes the important distinction between occupation-related stressors—such as being away from home for long periods, living separate lives from your partner, or multi-national crewing—and work-related stressors—such as high workloads and difficult work relationships. She also explores the sources of job dissatisfaction among seafarers, finding the living and working conditions on board to be the most significant. This broad-ranging review brings together a greater diversity of stressors, and individual differences in reaction to them, than is conventionally undertaken.

Jørgen Jepsen and colleagues look in depth at fatigue, which may be considered a particular aspect of stress, but is also multifaceted in its own right. They note that fatigue is a common element in marine accidents attributed to human error, which is of course the major reason for such accidents. They review the effects of fatigue, ranging from immediate effects, such as impaired cognition, to longer term autonomic, immunologic and metabolic changes associated with a number of chronic diseases. They question the efficacy of the current legislation on the issues and compliance with it. They call for preventive interventions such as the individual Fatigue Risk Management Systems (FRMS). This chapter therefore nicely complements both the one by Slišković on stress and the one by Liston et al. on safety critical systems.

John Golding's chapter provides a fascinating overview of the management of motion sickness at sea. Many will be familiar with the association of the symptoms of motion sickness with travel by sea, air and land. Fewer will be aware of the presence of the same symptoms in space travel, in simulators, or with wide-screen cinemas; of the ability to induce such symptoms in the laboratory, without the need for motion; and their presence in reactions to toxins, chemotherapy and post-operative recovery. Golding reviews psychological and pharmacological interventions, finding, as often is the case, that some of the traditional sea folklore on managing seasickness has much to commend it. Motion sickness is certainly problematic for maritime work and indeed maritime leisure, but it can also be fatal in survival situations, where the loss of bodily fluids and inability to think clearly can result in loss of life.

Ian de Terte and Elspeth Tilley's chapter on how to communicate risk in a maritime disaster combines psychology and communications science to develop a checklist of things to consider to promote more effective communication. They use the elaboration likelihood model as a framework, where the focus is on how to get people to pay attention to, to focus on—or to elaborate on—certain risk factors and useful protective behaviours. The more deeply people encode information, then the more influential that information is likely to be for them, especially in crisis moments when new information is treated more superficially. They particularly note the importance of a credible source to provide information, and a source that is familiar and liked. In the context of shipping this of course relates to the value of established relationships between a crew who know and respect each other, something which has diminished in some models of crew management for shipping firms.

Yannis Zolotas and colleagues explore the role of psychometric assessment of officers in the Greek merchant fleet, the largest fleet in Europe and one of the largest in the world. They examine the profiles on the Minnesota Multiphasic Personality Inventory—second edition (MMPI-2), one of the most widely used psychometric instruments in the world. This research is important because, at least anecdotally, there are many cases of mariner cadets who complete the shore-based part of their training, only to find that being at sea is not something they can manage. While the aim of the research is not necessarily to identify a "mariner personality profile", it is important to know what sort of people are likely to thrive in the safety critical environments found in the maritime sector. In the case of long passages at sea in confined quarters and little contact with shore-based family or friends, it would indeed be surprising if certain personality types did not do better than others; and so we need to be aware of individual differences. However, as Zolotas et al. stress, the MMPI should not be used as a single measure of psychopathology or to select-out people. Rather, any psychometric instrument offers only one perspective in what needs to be a pattern of different types of information, coming from different sources, and collectively pointing to certain conclusions.

In the final chapter I step outside the confines of maritime transport per se to consider other ways in which maritime psychology may be beneficially developed, focusing on two ways in which sailing can be used as an intervention. First, as an intervention to promote self-development and second sailing as therapy—chiming with the idea of taking therapy outside (Jordan 2013). A fascinating array of studies have used sailing to try and help people experience themselves in new ways, and sometimes as a rehabilitative mechanism, helping people re-experience themselves in old ways—to regain or rekindle aspects of themselves that they may have felt were gone or out of reach. From stroke in older people to sail training for young people with physical disability; to vulnerable and marginalized groups; the idea of embracing the sea with sail, and of finding healing, calmness and invigoration, education and self-development in the maritime environment, is just one of the realms in which maritime psychology may have much to contribute.

Conclusion

Maritime psychology is not new and has been written about, practised and indeed researched for centuries. Yet its recognition as a perspective of value has often been veiled in others terms—such as the "human element'—perhaps hinting that the perceived softness or fuzziness of either the values, methods or aims of psychology are somehow at odds with a traditionally "harder", more macho (Mannov 2015) and individualist industry, one that has thrived and sorrowed over the centuries at great achievements and losses. This book is an attempt to see psychology as central, as about individuals, ships, companies and the maritime industry; as an interrelated system of behaviour, values and practices, ranging from organizational justice to seasickness, from effective communication to designing living spaces, from coping with loneliness to promoting a positive, caring and valued work environment. These differences are all to be found on the same boat. To live and work in a small metal space crossing vast waters is an extra-ordinary type of life. This volume is intended to help make psychology as relevant, important and indeed familiar to the maritime as it is for other areas of transport or other aspects of the environment.

References

Aleksandrov, I., Arnaudova, M., Stoyanov, V., Ivanova, I., & Petrov, P.Y. (2015). On psychological and psychiatric impact of piracy on seafarers. *Journal of IMAB—Annual Proceeding (Scientific Papers) 21*, 991–994.

Bergheim, K., Nielsen, M. B., Mearns, K., & Eid, J. (2015). The relationship between psychological capital, job satisfaction, and safety perceptions in the maritime industry. *Safety Science, 74*, 27–36.

Boulougouris, E. K., & Papanikolaou, A., (2002). Modeling and simulation of the evacuation process of passenger ships. In *Proceedings of 10th International Congress of the International Maritime Association of the Mediterranean (IMAM 2002)*, Crete (Vol. 3).

Carr, S. C., McWha, I., MacLachlan, M., & Furnham, A. (2010). International-local remuneration differences across six countries: Do they undermine poverty reduction work? *International Journal of Psychology, 45*, 321–340.

Carter, T., & Schreiner, A. (Eds.). (2013). *Textbook of maritime medicine* (2nd ed.). Bergen: Norwegian Centre for Maritime Medicine.

Cox, T. H., & Blake, S. (1991). Managing cultural diversity: Implications for organizational competitiveness. *The Executive*, 45–56.

Doyle, N., MacLachlan, M., Fraser, A, Stilz, R., Lismont, K., Cox, H., et al. (2015). Resilience and well-being amongst seafarers: Cross-sectional study of crew across 51 ships. *International Archives of Occupational and Environmental Health*, 1–11.

Gregory, D., & Shanahan, P. (2010). *The human element: A guide to human behaviour in the shipping industry*. UK: TSO for the Maritime and Coastguard Agency.

Hudson, P.T.W., Parker, D., Lawrie, M., v d Graaf, G.C. & Bryden, R. (2004). How to win Hearts and Minds: The theory behind the program. *Proceedings 7th SPE International Conference on Health Safety and Environment in Oil and Gas Exploration and Production*. Richardson TX: Society of Petroleum Engineers.

Jordan, M. (2013). *Taking therapy outside—A narrative inquiry into counselling and psychotherapy in outdoor natural spaces* (Doctoral thesis). University of Brighton, UK.

Kimhi, S. (2011). Understanding good coping: A submarine crew coping with extreme environmental conditions. *Psychology, 2*, 961–967.

Luthans, F., Youssef, C. M., & Avolio, B. J. (2007). *Psychological capital. Developing the human competitive edge*. New York: Oxford University Press.

MacLachlan, M. (2015). Healthy seafarers: Perspectives from maritime psychology. In *13th International Symposium on Maritime Health*, Bergen, Norway, 23–26th June.

MacLachlan, M. (2016). Promoting organisational justice in medicine and health science research and practice. *British Medical Journal, 352*, i1048.

MacLachlan, M., Cromie, S., Liston, P., Kavanagh, B., & Kay, A. (2013). Psychosocial and organisational aspects of work at sea and their implications for health and performance. In T. Carter & A. Schreiner (Eds.), *Textbook of maritime medicine* (2nd ed.). Bergen: Norwegian Centre for Maritime Medicine.

MacLachlan, M., Kavanagh, W., & Kay, A. (2012). Maritime health: A review with suggestions for research. *International Maritime Health, 63*, 1–6.

MacLachlan, M., & O'Connell, M. (2000). *Cultivating pluralism: Psychological, social and cultural perspectives on a changing Ireland*. Cork: Oak Tree Press.

MacLachlan, M. (2006) *Culture & health: a critical perspective towards global health (Second Edition)*. Chichester: Wiley.

Mannov, A. (2015). Masculinity and care among international seafarers. In *13th International Symposium on Maritime Health*, Bergen, Norway, 23–26th June.

McVeigh, J., MacLachlan, M., & Kavanagh, B. (2016). The positive psychology of maritime health. *International Journal of Healthcare in Remote Locations*.

Newman, A., Ucbasaran, D., Zhu, F., & Hirst, G. (2014). Psychological capital: A review and synthesis. *Journal of Organizational Behaviour, 35*, 120–138.

O'Shea, J. (2005). *The organizational culture of a ship: A description and some possible effects it has on accidents and lessons for seafaring leadership* (Doctoral thesis). University of Tasmania, Australia.

Sampson, H. (2015). Healthy shipping. In *13th International Symposium on Maritime Health*, Bergen, Norway, 23–26th June.

Sampson, H., & Ellis, N. (2015). Elusive corporate social responsibility (CSR) in global shipping. *Journal of Global Responsibility, 6*, 80–98.

Shuji, H., & Kazutaka, K. (2015). Effects of the Work Improvement on Board (WIB) program by the Fisheries Agency in Japan. In *Presentation, 13th International Symposium on Maritime Health*, Bergen, Norway, 23–26th June.

Stevenson, D. B. (2012). Update on seafarers' welfare: 2012 report on psychological impact of piracy on seafarers. In *3rd UAE Counter Piracy Conference Briefing Paper*.

Walsh-Danishmandi, A., & MacLachlan, M. (2000). Environmental risk to the self: Factor analysis and development of sub-scales for the Environmental Appraisal Inventory (EAI) with an Irish sample. *Journal of Environmental Psychology, 20*, 141–149.

Yuan, X., Zhao, J., Yang, Y. & Wang, Y. (2014). Hybrid parallel chaos optimization algorithm with harmony search algorithm. *Applied Soft Computing, 17*, 12–22.

Positive Psychology and Well-Being at Sea

Joanne McVeigh, Malcolm MacLachlan, Ralf Stilz, Henriette Cox, Niamh Doyle, Alistair Fraser and Marianne Dyer

Case Study

The Shell Health Resilience Programme was developed to promote thriving of workers on and off shore. It is a voluntary resilience intervention comprising 12 modules based on positive psychology, cognitive behavioural therapy, neuro-linguistic programming, and research on leadership. The programme is delivered to individual teams by lay facilitators who are usually team members. The 12 modules are driven by team interaction, with the facilitator setting the scene and coordinating activities and discussion. The programme can be completed as slowly or as quickly as desired by the team. Prior to trialling at sea, the programme had already been adopted in multiple locations onshore.

Adoption at sea posed some challenges due to circumstances specific to life on a ship. The ships were in remote locations most of the time, limiting the availability of seafarers for training as facilitators. This also meant that more facilitators needed to be trained as each ship required their own facilitator. The working pattern required seafarers to stay on board for several months, followed by a similar length of shore leave, meaning that a sufficient number of facilitators needed to be available on each ship to ensure continuity of the programme. The staggered

J. McVeigh (✉) · M. MacLachlan
Centre for Global Health and School of Psychology, Trinity College Dublin,
7-9 Leinster Street South, Dublin, Ireland
e-mail: jmcveigh@tcd.ie

R. Stilz · A. Fraser · M. Dyer
Shell Health, London, UK

H. Cox
Shell International Trading and Shipping Company Limited, London, UK

N. Doyle
University College Cork, Cork, Ireland

© Springer International Publishing Switzerland 2017
M. MacLachlan (ed.), *Maritime Psychology*, DOI 10.1007/978-3-319-45430-6_2

changeover of crew on each ship resulted in team members participating in a dissimilar combination of modules. In addition, some crew members also changed ship after completing one trip. Furthermore, online information and additional material was available to support facilitators in shore-based locations, but was not routinely accessible at sea.

To overcome some of these obstacles, the programme was adapted and trialled in a pilot with 21 ships. Materials for the modules and supporting information were compiled and tailored to the needs of the seafarers and prepared for offline use. Each ship in the pilot study was equipped with all materials required. A small number of facilitators were trained during a one-hour session at an annual onshore officers' conference. Officers rather than non-officer ranks were selected as they usually deliver routine training on the ships and were thus thought to be more comfortable with the role of a facilitator. Officers were asked to train up a facilitator on board their ship before completing their trip and disembarking. Joint preparation and facilitation of modules by more than one facilitator was encouraged.

A number of innovative examples of module facilitation were shared by the seafarers:

- Several seafarers created presentations for facilitating the programme, shared their personal experiences and reframed the module content in their own words, translating the programme into their cultural and occupational context.
- On one ship, everyone participated in the module preparation and faciliation. This ship chose to complete all of the modules on a single training day, rather than spreading out the delivery over several months.

These examples bear testimony to the seafarers' engagement with, and taking ownership of, the resilience programme. Feedback from the seafarers was positive: "This module brought some lively discussions in the groups" and "Wonderful experience conducting resilience workshop on board. It was indeed amazing to see

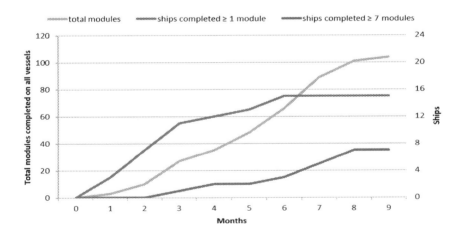

Fig. 1 Completion of the Shell resilience modules across 21 pilot ships

all participate with such enthusiasm and zest. Good to see all appreciating one another. Great fun".

Despite an initially slow uptake, adoption of modules gradually increased over a 9-month period, with a plateau reached after 7 months. At this time, 71 % of the ships had embarked on the programme, with one-third completing more than half of the modules (see Fig. 1). Ships were encouraged to continue with the resilience programme through monthly communications between the onshore office and the ships.

Positive Psychology and Well-Being at Sea

Seafaring has long combined paradoxes, such as social exclusion and continuous social proximity, confinement in open spaces, and multiculturalism, within the single organizational culture of a ship. Consistencies—such as social isolation and confinement with shipmates—are evident in onboard working and living conditions from the earliest seafarers to their contemporaries; nonetheless, substantial social changes are apparent in recent times, including the large-scale introduction of multinational crews, a revolution in information and communication technologies, and faster ship turnaround in ports (Alderton et al. 2004). Moreover, the tasks of ships' officers and crew are increasing, including operating ships' machinery and equipment and ensuring effective functioning of ships' machines and devices (Borodina 2013).

In light of research indicating that mariners are a professional group amongst those at the highest risk for stress (Lipowski et al. 2014) and associated mental health conditions (Jezewska et al. 2006), researchers are calling for the psychological health of seafarers to be adequately investigated, measured, and addressed (Carotenuto et al. 2013). As suggested by Oldenburg and colleagues, there is a substantial need for research to assess the complex life and work situation of seafarers while on board (Oldenburg et al. 2013). In particular, more research on psychosocial aspects of mariners' health is required (MacLachlan et al. 2012). For decades, a collective focus of the fields of psychology, neuroscience and mental health on the long- and short-term consequences of stress is evident, and, more recently, on extreme stress (Southwick et al. 2014). As highlighted by Schager, the shipping industry could gain many benefits by availing of modern scientific psychology (Schager 1997).

This chapter explores positive psychology as an approach to enhancing well-being at sea. To date, the application of positive psychology concepts, interventions and training to the maritime context has been explored only to a limited degree. This chapter commences with a discussion of the seafaring context. The ship as an isolated and confined environment, a safety-critical organization, and as a fusion of maritime-specific stressors is considered. Next, the field of positive psychology—its conception and previous applications—is discussed. Along these lines, the field of positive organizational psychology and the newly emerging field of positive organizational behaviour are explored, with a particular focus on psychological capital, including resilience, as a core construct of positive organizational behaviour. Ensuing these sections is a discussion of the contexts in which positive psychology has previously been applied to promote well-being at sea. To conclude, rationale for future research and key research questions are presented.

Seafaring Environment

Improvements in the life of seafarers are evident, with modern ships frequently being clean and comfortable (Hult 2012a), although it is recognized that accommodation standards vary substantially between ships (Alderton et al. 2004). The living conditions of seafarers have some notable advantages, including long periods of time off, variety, a sense of belonging on board, and a feeling of having acquired good skills (Hult 2012a). As proposed by Leszczynska et al., although there is substantial diversity in standards across national fleets, systematic improvements in the maritime work environment have been occurring for some years, including increased comfort; reduction of exposure to harmful physical, chemical and biological hazards; moderation of noise and vibration; installation of air-conditioning; and increases in living space in the form of single cabins (Leszczynska et al. 2007).

Nonetheless, seafaring continues to be associated with a multitude of mental, psychosocial, and physical stressors, which include authoritative leadership, heavy mental and physical workload, long work hours, lack of exercise and often unhealthy diets (Comperatore et al. 2005), separation from family, loneliness on board, fatigue, sleep deprivation, multi-nationalities, restricted recreation opportunities (Carotenuto et al. 2012), and environmental stressors including ship motion, noise and vibration, perceived as stressful particularly during sleeping times (Oldenburg et al. 2010). In a study conducted by Oldenburg et al. comprising a sample of 134 male seafarers, interviewees reported the most significant stressors on board as separation from their family, time pressure, long working days, heat in workplaces, and insufficient qualifications of subordinate crew (Oldenburg et al. 2009). Indeed, many stressors experienced by mariners may be chronic in nature (Lipowski et al. 2014).

As emphasized by Jezewska and colleagues, people working at sea experience stress related to their specific work conditions, significant job responsibilities and psychosocial factors, which produce health and psychological problems (Jezewska et al. 2006). In a study conducted with seafarers of the Danish merchant fleet, Haka and colleagues found that the majority of job demands and job resources perceived by the seafarers were psychosocial rather than organizational factors, such as interpersonal relationships with crew (Haka et al. 2011). The incidence of seafarer deaths through suicide suggests that the mental health of seafarers continues to be very poor, and there is a call to action to address this by those involved in the maritime shipping industry (Iversen 2012). While mortality studies have provided valid comparisons between the health of seafarers and that of the remainder of the population, a limitation of these studies is their omission of mental health conditions; indeed, the most common form of ill-health at sea on non-passenger vessels is mental health problems (Carter 2011a).

Increasing awareness of mental health problems at sea is apparent, associated with a variety of practical initiatives related to this area; for instance on ships and in docks, leaflets are increasingly made available for the purposes of providing access to mental health information and to address the strong stigma associated with mental health problems that is evident across cultures (MacLachlan et al. 2013). A significant stride forward is the Maritime Labour Convention 2006, widely known as the "Seafarers' Bill of Rights," which provides international seafaring standards, including health on board (International Labour Organization (ILO) 2013). According to the Maritime Labour Convention, consideration should be afforded to investigate "special physiological or psychological problems created by the shipboard environment" [Guideline B4.3.6(c)] and "problems arising from physical stress on board a ship" [Guideline B4.3.6(d)] (ILO 2006). Yet many seafarers may be reluctant to seek medical and psychological assistance as the physical demands and health requirements of seafaring are strict and the job market is seemingly competitive (Oldenburg et al. 2010).

As proposed by Carotenuto and colleagues, in light of the heightened risk of depression and suicide, the psychological ill-health of seafarers should be accurately investigated, measured, followed up and countered as far as possible (Carotenuto et al. 2013). Jezewska and colleagues have called for the training in psychological skills for seafarers as a preventative measure for stress, with the aim of developing interpersonal competence, particularly for the capacity of solving interpersonal conflicts on board, as well as providing and receiving support (Jezewska et al. 2006). In a survey of 78 Royal Australian Navy submariners, psychological distress at sea was found to be moderated by personal resources, including problem-solving skills, social support, involvement in recreational activities, and self-care behaviour (McDougall and Drummond 2010).

When designing interventions to mitigate stress and support seafarers' psychological well-being, it is important to recognize occupational, cultural and demographic factors that may influence how stress may be differentially experienced, expressed, and alleviated on board. For example, in a cross-sectional study of 685 engine room officers in the Swedish merchant fleet, Rydstedt and Lundh found that older engine officers reported significantly higher degrees of perceived stress compared to younger colleagues (Rydstedt and Lundh 2012). In relation to ranks of seafarers, Carotenuto and colleagues found that beyond stressors that represent the most prevalent sources of stress of seafarers, such as loneliness, leisure scarcity and fatigue, a number of specific features differentiate seafarers based on rank and job category. For instance, sleep disturbances are reported by pilots and engineers with higher incidence than by masters/mates and deck crew, although deck crew report the lowest job satisfaction levels (Carotenuto et al. 2012). Oldenburg et al. reported that officers stayed on board for considerably shorter periods than non-officers (4.8 vs. 8.3 months per year) but had significantly more often a substantially higher number of working hours, and Europeans had shorter stays on board in comparison to non-Europeans (4.9 vs. 9.9 months/year) (Oldenburg et al. 2009). As the maritime industry is a global business in which vessels are often manned from several different cultures (ILO 2015; Johnsen et al. 2012), strategies aimed at improving psychological well-being of seafarers require recognition of cultural diversity. For example, Nielsen and colleagues, with a sample of 541 seafarers from two Norwegian shipping companies, found that European and Filipino respondents differed regarding their experience of both the work environment and well-being. The researchers found that Filipino crew members experienced the work environment as more negative, with greater levels of harassment, laissez-faire leadership, and poor safety, although Filipinos also experienced stronger team cohesion and perceived their captains as more authentic (Nielsen et al. 2013).

The Ship as an Isolated, Confined Environment

A ship is an isolated, confined environment—comprising the people, settings, tasks, amenities, and routines to which seafarers may be exposed for weeks and sometimes months at a time. From this perspective, a ship is a "hole" in the water containing the complex work dynamics of a group working on a common task; it is also a "whole" in the water, encapsulating the crew's world occupationally, socially, and personally (MacLachlan et al. 2013). Seafarers are amongst the most isolated demographic occupational groups globally (Oldenburg et al. 2010). Dissimilar to many other occupations, seafarers are periodically at the workplace both during working and non-working hours, 24 hour per day (Hult 2012a).

Opportunities for communication of seafarers with family and friends on shore are frequently highly restricted. In a study conducted by Kahveci, findings indicated that a very small proportion of seafarers had access to the Internet while on board; onboard email access varied substantially with regard to hierarchical structure, quantity, privacy, cost, and freedom of access; restricted access to email facilities on board increased dependence of seafarers on satellite telephone communication, and the most significant barriers to communication on board included access to communication facilities and cost of communication (Kahveci 2011). In a qualitative study of 10 Greek-owned shipping companies, Progoulaki et al. reported that communication was highlighted amongst the most important services, although those services provided were either too limited or expensive for crew. More specifically, while telephone was reported as a highly expensive means of communication, it was also considered as the primary means of communication that connected crew with family and friends on shore. Moreover, although Internet access was present, its use was primarily for business, although seafarers could send a restricted number of emails to family (Progoulaki et al. 2013).

The Ship as a Safety-Critical Organization

The ship may also be conceptualized as a safety-critical organization. Seafaring is a practical and challenging profession that requires fast and correct analyses of situations, as well as rapid, decisive action (Gekara et al. 2011). Safety-critical organizations are complex adaptive systems (Reiman et al. 2015), which operate in high hazard industries, such as aviation, oil and chemical industry organizations (Oedewald and Reiman 2007) and seafaring (Smedley et al. 2013; Wang 2008). Workers in safety-critical organizations such as the offshore oil and gas industry operate in perilous environments, with numerous technological, environmental, and human challenges, which present a significant potential for injuries, accidents, stress, and various adverse health outcomes (Hystad et al. 2014). Almost all jobs at sea are safety critical and therefore declines in performance as a result of any cause, including psychosocial ones, may put seafarers and their vessel at significant risk (Carter 2005). Research and interventions addressing psychosocial factors of seafaring may therefore be astute and important on the basis of seafarers' health, but also, crucially, on performance and safety grounds.

Positive Psychology

Positive psychology is "a science of positive subjective experience, positive individual traits, and positive institutions (which) promises to improve quality of life" and prevent pathologies (Seligman and Csikszentmihalyi 2000, p. 5). As proposed by Gable and Haidt (2005), when defined in these terms, positive psychology has a long history, dating back to James's (1902) writings on what he labelled "healthy mindedness" (James 1902), to Allport's literature on positive human characteristics (Allport 1955), to the advocacy of Maslow for the study of healthy people in 1968 (Maslow 1968). As offered by Maslow (1954):

> The science of psychology has been far more successful on the negative than on the positive side. It has revealed to us much about man's shortcomings, his illnesses, his sins, but little about his potentialities, his virtues, his achievable aspirations, or his full psychological height. It is as if psychology has voluntarily restricted itself to only half its rightful jurisdiction, and that, the darker, meaner half (p. 354).

Indeed, contemporary focus on well-being, and its component attributes such as happiness, subjective appreciation of the values and quality of life, satisfaction and fulfilment, is far from new ground; contemplation of these subjects is traced back as far as ancient Socratic philosophy, and the vast majority of, if not all, religious and spiritual movements express concern and potential insight into the pursuit of happier and more meaningful lives (Gibbs and Burnett 2011). Aristotle believed that happiness (which he named "eudaimonia") was realized through knowing your true self and acting in line with your virtues, while Epicurus and the hedonists believed in achieving happiness through maximizing pleasure and minimizing pain

(Harvard Medical School 2011). From this perspective, positive psychology is thousands of years old, dating back to ancient philosophers and religious leaders who discussed happiness, character values, and the good society (Diener 2009). In such light, positive psychology has a very long past, but (as formally named of 1998) a very short history (Peterson 2006). As proposed by Tugade et al. (2004):

> For centuries, folk wisdom has promoted the idea that positive emotions are good for your health: "A good laugh makes you healthy" (Swedish proverb); "The joyfulness of man prolongeth his days" (Bible, Ecclesiasticus. 30:22); "Mirth and merriment … bars a thousand harms and lengthens life" (Shakespeare). Oftentimes in science, empirical evidence emerges to refute anecdotal wisdom. In the case of positive emotions and health, however, accumulating evidence is providing empirical support for such folk theories (p. 1).

Positive psychology, a novel and influential school of thought, spearheaded by Martin Seligman, President of the American Psychological Association 1998, focuses on promoting the study of well-being, and is disputably considered as foremost and archetypal of positive, well-being-oriented organizational and academic movements (Gibbs and Burnett 2011). This new branch of psychology is primarily concerned with the scientific study of human strengths and happiness, and factors that promote well-being (Carr 2011). Positive psychology is an umbrella term for motivating and organizing research, application, and scholarship on virtues, strengths, excellence, thriving, flourishing, resilience, flow and optimal functioning more generally (Donaldson and Ko 2010).

Contrary to psychology's focus of the past half century on relieving mental disorders, positive psychology seeks to understand positive emotion, build strength and virtue, and support individuals in living what Aristotle termed the "good life" (Seligman 2013). As indicated by Peterson and Park, positive psychologists do not declare to have invented the "good life" or to have propelled it into scientific study; rather, the contribution of positive psychology has been to provide an umbrella term for secluded branches of theory and research, and to assert that the "good life" deserves its own field of inquiry within psychology, at least until all of psychology comprises the study of what is "good" alongside what is "bad" (Peterson and Park 2003). From this perspective, a number of aphorisms underpin positive psychology: first, what is experienced as "good" in life is as genuine as what is experienced as "bad"—not secondary, illusory, or epiphenomenal; second, what is "good" in life is not simply the absence of what is "problematic"; and third, the "good life" necessitates its own explanation, and not simply an oblique or inverted theory of pathology (Peterson 2009). Accordingly, the aim of positive psychology is not to supersede research investigating psychological dysfunction or distress; rather, the aim is to cultivate and integrate knowledge of human resilience, strength, and opportunities to supplement and build on the existing knowledge base (Gable and Haidt 2005; Seligman et al. 2005).

Importantly, as emphasized by MacLachlan and Hand, positive psychology does not seek to eliminate painful emotions, which are frequently an entirely appropriate response to the reality of people's lives, and an integral part of the human experience. So, for example, while the loss of a loved one or personal injury may be justifiably experienced as difficult or painful, at the same time navigating these painful emotions can contribute to increased happiness and possibly reevaluation of one's life (MacLachlan and Hand 2013). As proposed by Seligman, contrary to the idea of positive psychology as a "creature of good times," the strengths that positive psychology seeks to cultivate may serve individuals throughout good times as well as more difficult times, for which the latter may be "uniquely suited to the display of many strengths" (Seligman 2013, p. 12).

In his influential book 'Authentic happiness', Seligman proposes that happiness can be analyzed in relation to three distinct components: first, *positive emotion*— what we feel, such as pleasure, comfort, rapture, and ecstasy, which contribute to the "pleasant life"; second, *engagement*—signifying flow, such as being one with music, the experience of time stopping, and the loss of self-consciousness throughout an absorbing activity, experiences which contribute to the "engaged life"; and third, *meaning*—belonging to and serving something that you believe is bigger than you are, underpinning the "meaningful life" (Seligman 2013). Seligman's views have since shifted, however, from framing positive psychology as a branch of psychological science concerned with happiness and increasing life satisfaction through positive emotion, engagement, and meaning, to a focus on "well-being". According to Seligman, the benchmark for measuring well-being is "flourishing" and the goal of positive psychology is to increase flourishing. As proposed by this new well-being theory, flourishing rests on five pillars: positive emotion, engagement, meaning, accomplishment (or achievement), and relationships (Seligman 2011a).

Relationships, our key to the "connected life," are therefore a cornerstone of flourishing as proposed by Seligman's theory of well-being. As outlined by Seligman, when asked what, in two words or fewer, positive psychology is all about, its cofounder Christopher Peterson responded, "other people" (Seligman 2011b). As declared by Seligman, relationships with other people may be the most effective antidote to the "downs" of life and the single most dependable "up" (Seligman 2011b). As proposed by Haidt, "Happiness comes from between"— some conditions necessary for happiness are within the person, such as coherence among the parts of their personality, while other conditions necessitate relationships to elements beyond the person, so there is a need for love, work, and connection to something larger; if a person gets these relationships right, a sense of purpose and meaning emerges (Haidt 2006). As emphasized by Carr, scientific research indicates three reliable ways to promote happiness: (1) cultivate relationships that comprise deep attachment and commitment; (2) partake in absorbing work and leisure activities in which you avail of your strengths, talents and interests; and (3) cultivate an optimistic, future-oriented perspective on life in which you expect the best to happen (Carr 2011).

In many ways, the core work of positive psychology is focused on the efficacy of psychological interventions to increase individual happiness (Seligman et al. 2005). Positive psychology interventions may be elucidated as intentional activities based on (a) cultivation of positive subjective experiences; (b) building of positive individual traits; or (c) building of civic virtue and positive institutions (Meyers et al. 2013).

Examples comprise keeping a gratitude diary, counting acts of kindness towards others, and focusing on the good aspects of life (Thompson et al. 2014). Approximately 40 interventions purporting to increase long-term happiness have been collected and condensed into replicable and manualizable form by Seligman and colleagues, including "you at your best," whereby participants are asked to write about a time when they were at their best, to reflect on the personal strengths displayed in the story, and to review and reflect on the story once every day for 1 week; and "using signature strengths in a new way," whereby individuals are asked to avail of the inventory of character strengths online and to use one of their identified top strengths in a new way every day for 1 week (Seligman et al. 2005).

The application of positive psychology interventions has been explored across many diverse settings, including *education* (Shoshani and Steinmetz 2014; Waters 2011), such as the PENN Resiliency Program, a group intervention for school children (Penn Positive Psychology Center 2007); *organizations* (Bono et al. 2013; Meyers et al. 2013), including safety-critical organizations, such as the offshore oil industry (Hystad et al. 2014) and U.S. Army (Azar 2011); and *clinical*, including group interventions for breast cancer patients (Cerezo et al. 2014), interventions to reduce stress in people newly diagnosed with HIV (Tedlie Moskowitz et al. 2014), interventions to promote positive states and strengths of character for patients with or at risk of cardiac disease (Dubois et al. 2012), and psychotherapy (Schrank et al. 2014; Seligman et al. 2006).

A growing literature on such positive psychology interventions indicates that the "good life"—positive emotion, engagement, relationships, meaning, and accomplishment—can be strengthened (Seligman 2010). For example, in a meta-analytical study of the effectiveness of positive psychology interventions, Bolier and colleagues reported that positive psychology interventions significantly enhanced subjective and psychological well-being and reduced depressive symptoms (Bolier et al. 2013). In a six-group, randomized placebo-controlled Internet study, Seligman et al. found that two interventions—writing about three good things that happened each day and why they happened, and using signature strengths of character in a new way—made people happier (and less depressed) up to 6 months later (Seligman et al. 2005). As emphasized by Fredrickson, diverse interventions—including finding positive meaning, relaxation training, and invoking empathy or amusement—share the capacity to evoke positive emotions while lessening negative emotions (Fredrickson 2000). Importantly, evidence is accumulating that positive emotions are associated with beneficial psychological and physical health effects; positive emotions can be an important factor that safeguards individuals against maladaptive health outcomes (Tugade et al. 2004).

Contrary to studies such as those outlined above, there is research indicating that under certain circumstances overvaluing happiness may be less conducive to well-being. For example, Mauss et al. (2011) conducted two studies to explore paradoxical effects of valuing happiness. In their first study, female participants who valued happiness more reported lower happiness under conditions of low, but not high, life stress. In their second study, female participants who were induced experimentally to value happiness reacted less positively to a happy, but not a sad, emotion induction, when compared to a control group. Participants' disappointment by their own feelings mediated the effect. The researchers propose that valuing happiness may lead people to feel less happy in positive contexts when expectations for happiness are high (Mauss et al. 2011). As proposed by Ford and Mauss, first, as individuals pursue happiness, they typically set high standards for their happiness, which may create discontent and decrease happiness when their current state falls below such standards; second, individuals are not constantly accurate regarding what will assist them to achieve happiness, and may consequently engage in activities that are ineffective for increasing their happiness; and third, as individuals pursue happiness, they typically monitor their accomplishment of this goal, and such monitoring may reduce their ability to achieve happiness (Ford and Mauss 2014). Accordingly, activities to promote well-being may be more effective when aimed to direct participants' efforts on the specific activity, such as practicing acts of kindness, rather than on the sole value of increasing happiness (Nelson and Lyubomirsky 2012). Indeed, current perspectives of positive psychology assume a focus less on "positive" targets at shallow level, and more on what factors may lead to healthy well-being; in some cases, positive emotion and psychological strengths lead to suboptimal living, while emotions such as anxiety and confrontational behaviours may result in the best possible outcomes (Ciarrochi et al. 2013).

For whom, in what circumstances, and through which mechanisms positive psychology interventions work are largely person, activity, and context dependent. Importantly, positive psychology interventions therefore are required to consider individual differences (Azar 2011). Because individuals have diverse strengths, interests, values, and inclinations that allow them to benefit more from some strategies than others, no one particular activity will help all individuals to become happier (Lyubomirsky et al. 2005). In a study conducted by Brunstein et al. (1998), the researchers found that progress towards motive-congruent goals, in contrast to progress towards motive-incongruent goals, accounted for a sample of students' daily experiences of emotional well-being. Similarly, Fordyce (1977), in relation to a self-study programme designed to increase personal happiness and life satisfaction, reported that the particular components of the programme considered most happiness producing greatly varied between subjects, seemingly determined by individuals' needs and areas of particular weaknesses. In a study conducted by Wood and colleagues, among participants with low self-esteem, those who repeated a positive self-statement ("I'm a lovable person") felt worse than those with low self-esteem who did not repeat the statement; among participants with high self-esteem, those who repeated the statement felt better than those who did not, but only to a limited degree (Wood et al. 2009).

Similarly, Thompson and colleagues investigated how gender may affect self-reported person-activity fit across three positive psychology interventions: gratitude journal; acts of kindness; and savouring life's joys. The results indicated that gender influenced person-activity fit regarding the above interventions, with females in all cases reporting a higher fit than males (Thompson et al. 2014). Lyubomirsky and Layous have proposed the person-activity fit model, which presents: (a) an overview of the activity features and person features that render a positive activity optimally effective; and (b) the mechanisms that underlie the positive activity's successful improvement of well-being. The researchers propose that the degree to which an activity feature affects a positive activity's success is determined by the fit between the person, such as personality or culture, and that activity feature, such as dosage or social support (Lyubomirsky and Layous 2013).

Positive Organizational Psychology

Positive organizational psychology can be interpreted as the scientific study of positive subjective experiences and traits in the workplace and positive institutions (Donaldson and Ko 2010). Positive organizational psychology may be considered as an overarching term comprising the newly emerging fields of *positive organizational scholarship* (POS) and *positive organizational behaviour* (POB) (Donaldson and Ko 2010). POS focuses on the study of positive outcomes, processes, and attributes of organizations and their members (Cameron et al. 2003). Along similar lines, POB is concerned with the study of individual positive psychological conditions and human resource strengths that are related to employee well-being or performance improvement (Bakker and Schaufeli 2008), and such positive psychological conditions and human resource strengths that are "state-like" (Luthans et al. 2008), signifying that they are not fixed and are more easily changed than "trait-like" constructs.

While both POS and POB share the common origins of positive psychology, and are underpinned by the scientific process in the development of knowledge, POB differs from POS in a number of respects: POB primarily focuses on individual psychological qualities and their impact on performance improvement; its studies have been conducted chiefly at the micro and meso levels of analysis using survey research; and POB has tended to develop in an inductive way (i.e. from individual to group to organizational levels of analysis) (Donaldson and Ko 2010). Due to its principal focus on individual psychological qualities that are state-like and therefore more amenable to change, which aligns with the topic of this chapter, POB is discussed below in more detail.

Positive organizational behaviour. The recently developing field of POB follows the lead of positive psychology (Bakker and Schaufeli 2008; Youssef and Luthans 2007). POB is defined as "the study and application of positively oriented human resource strengths and psychological capacities that can be measured, developed, and effectively managed for performance improvement in today's workplace" (Luthans and Church 2002, p. 59). As suggested by this definition, the specific criteria to determine positive capacities include being based on theory and research with valid measurement, and also that such capacities are state-like, signifying, as outlined above, that the capacity must be malleable and open to change (Luthans et al. 2008).

An example of a recent POB study is one conducted by Youssef and Luthans, who tested the impact that positive psychological resource capacities of hope, optimism, and resilience had on work-related employee outcomes, including performance, job satisfaction, work happiness, and organizational commitment. Their findings generally supported their hypotheses that employees' positive psychological resource capacities related to, and contributed equal variance to, the outcomes (Youssef and Luthans 2007). Numerous other studies have shown that positive organizational phenomena can make a distinct contribution to explaining variance in organizational outcomes (Bakker and Schaufeli 2008). For example, Losada's observational study among 60 business teams tested the effect of positive versus negative speech on performance. Specifically, performance was evaluated using three indicators: profitability, customer satisfaction, and assessments of the team by their superiors, peers and subordinates. A speech act was coded as positive if the participant showed support, encouragement, or appreciation, and was coded as negative if the participant speaking showed sarcasm, disapproval or cynicism. Findings indicated that high-performance teams showed more positive speech, providing empirical support for positive speech among team members as distinguishing high-performance teams from less successfully performing teams (Losada 1999).

Psychological capital. Psychological capital is a core construct of POB (Luthans et al. 2006). Luthans et al. (2007a, b) define psychological capital as:

> an individual's positive psychological state of development and is characterized by: (1) having confidence (self-efficacy) to take on and put in the necessary effort to succeed at challenging tasks; (2) making a positive attribution (optimism) about succeeding now and in the future; (3) persevering towards goals and, when necessary, redirecting paths to goals (hope) in order to succeed; and (4) when beset by problems and adversity, sustaining and bouncing back and even beyond (resiliency) to attain success (p. 3).

The term "psychological capital" in this sense signifies individual motivational propensities that accumulate through positive psychological constructs, including efficacy, optimism, hope and resilience (Luthans et al. 2007a, b). Psychological capital constructs are posited as being "state-like," although not momentary states (Luthans et al. 2007a, b).

Psychological capital may be an important factor concerning seafarers' safety climate. From a sample of seafarers working on oil platform supply ships, empirical support is provided by Hystad et al. for psychological capital as an important factor of safety climate (Hystad et al. 2014). Along similar lines, in two studies investigating the potential relationship between psychological capital and perceptions of safety climate among maritime workers from three Norwegian shipping companies, Bergheim et al. reported that psychological capital, including resiliency, was positively associated with perceptions of safety climate (Bergheim et al. 2015).

Resilience. Resilience may be defined as the ability to "bounce back" from adversity (Luthans et al. 2006). Resilience has been conceptualized as the capacity to maintain healthy functioning despite increased stressors, and to recover to full functioning following a demanding period (Stanley et al. 2011). The American Psychological Association (APA) outlines ten ways to build resilience: (1) Make connections; (2) Avoid seeing crises as insurmountable problems; (3) Accept that change is a part of living; (4) Move towards your goals; (5) Take decisive actions; (6) Look for opportunities for self-discovery; (7) Nurture a positive view of yourself; (8) Keep things in perspective; (9) Maintain a hopeful outlook; and (10) Take care of yourself (American Psychological Association 2015).

Research shows that resilience has a positive relationship with recovery from daily stressors. Ong et al. found that psychological resilience accounted for meaningful differences in emotional responses to daily stressors. Their findings indicated that, over time, the experience of positive emotions may function to assist high-resilient individuals in their capacity to recover effectively from daily stress (Ong et al. 2006). This link between positive emotions and resilience is supported by empirical research (Cohn et al. 2009). The Broaden-and-Build theory (Fredrickson 2001) postulates that experiences of positive emotions serve to build enduring personal resources—including physical, intellectual, social and psychological resources—and are a resource that can be used when individuals undergo stressful experiences. As proposed by Fredrickson, positive emotions, when effectively employed, can optimize psychological resilience, health, and subjective well-being (Fredrickson 2000). Positive emotions boost resilience, which in turn stimulates more positive feelings; in other words, positive emotions and resilience mutually reinforce each other (Smith and Hollinger-Smith 2015).

One possible path to resilience is personality hardiness, a characteristic sense that life is meaningful, that we choose our futures, and that change is interesting and valuable (Bartone 2006). Hardy attitudes and strategies may facilitate resilience under stress. Hardy attitudes are: (1) *commitment*, signifying the belief that no matter how difficult life gets, it is important to stay involved with whatever is happening rather than detaching and becoming alienated; (2) *control*, indicating the belief that no matter how difficult life becomes, there is a need to continue trying to turn the stresses from potential disasters into growth opportunities, rather than sinking into powerlessness and passivity; and (3) *challenge*, the view that stressful changes are opportunities to grow in wisdom and capability (Maddi 2013). Alongside commitment, control and challenge, the hardy-resilient style individual shows a strong future orientation—an inclination to look optimistically towards the future while learning from the past (Bartone et al. 2012).

According to Bartone, while the underlying mechanisms of how hardiness may increase resilience regarding stress are not yet fully understood, a significant aspect of the hardiness-resilience mechanism may involve the meaning that individuals attach to events. From this perspective, individuals high in hardiness characteristically interpret experiences as largely interesting and worthwhile; over which they can exert control; as challenging; and as presenting opportunities to learn and grow (Bartone 2010). It is through this "shaping" of stressful experiences that leaders may foster hardy-resilient response patterns in a group setting, whereby a leader high in hardiness communicates a positive construction of shared stressful experiences, which may influence the entire group in the direction of a more positive interpretation of the experience (Bartone 2010, 2012).

Resilience from this standpoint may be fostered. As alluded to above, resilience is posited as not being trait-like in that individuals either have it or do not; rather, it comprises behaviours, thoughts and actions that can be learned and developed (APA 2015). Accordingly, training programmes that aim to develop or enhance resilience may be effective in improving health, well-being and quality of life (Leppin et al. 2014). As proposed by Hystad and Bye, a central aspect of hardiness training may be to assist people to change their mental models so that they may develop a broader perspective of life's circumstances and find alternative ways of understanding themselves and their experiences (Hystad and Bye 2013). Accordingly, resilience training may be conceptualized as providing techniques and a setting to reflect on one's way of thinking and to allow people to initiate changes to their thinking. According to a report of an International Maritime Health Association workshop (Carter 2005), research needs to focus on the resilience and coping strategies of seafarers, with interventions to modify these factors, and additional support and counselling in the early stages of identified distress.

Positive Psychology and Well-Being at Sea

MacLachlan and colleagues have called for the application of positive psychology in the maritime sector for the purposes of developing unique occupational health and performance programmes suitable to life on board. The researchers call on health and occupational practitioners in the maritime industry to more effectively utilize the characteristics of maritime work to develop intervention programmes that stimulate strengths, health and good performance of seafarers (MacLachlan et al. 2013). As proposed by organizational psychologists Gregory and Shanahan in their influential maritime guide 'The human element: A guide to human behaviour in the shipping industry', there are many practical things that can be done to ensure people work to their strengths (Gregory and Shanahan 2010). Table 1 outlines examples of commonly used interventions in positive psychology and their potential relevance to maritime health.

The familiar expression of "happy ship" suggests that job satisfaction may be a crucial element in maritime organizations (Bergheim et al. 2015). Yet, the application of positive psychology to the maritime context has been restricted primarily to resilience and "mindfulness" training. However, Van Wijk and Waters present a case study of the implementation of an interview model that focuses on strengths and positive health aspects, for the purposes of the annual psychological assessment of a group of naval specialists. In contrast to the traditional approach of a medical diagnostic interview, a significant difference was found in relation to post-assessment referrals for counselling, suggesting that this innovative positive psychology interview approach may have contributed to preventing later distress (van Wijk and Waters 2008).

Programmes aiming to enhance resilience of mariners are evident. For example, the U.S. Navy Operational Stress Control Programme aims to assist sailors to avoid stress injuries, recover from adverse situations and build resilience—to strengthen

Table 1 Examples of commonly used positive psychology interventions

Study	Intervention	Outcomes	Relevance to Maritime Health
1. Seligman et al. (2005)	*Three good things in life* —Participants were asked to write down three things that went well each day and their causes every night for 1 week	At the 1-month follow up, participants were happier and less depressed than they had been at baseline, and stayed happier and less depressed at 3-month and 6-month follow-ups	Maritime workers may be at heightened risk of depression and suicide. Positive psychology interventions such as "Three good things in life" for seafarers may facilitate increases in happiness and decreases in depressive symptoms for up to 6 months
2. Luthans et al. (2008)	*Developing psychological capital*—A highly focused, 2-hour web-based training intervention to develop psychological capital, including efficacy, hope, optimism, and resilience. A pretest, posttest experimental design was used ($n = 187$ were randomly assigned to the treatment group and $n = 177$ to the control group)	The treatment group experienced a significant increase in psychological capital, while the control group that participated in a different but relevant intervention did not show a significant increase in their psychological capital	Computer-based training for seafarers on board and on shore may provide an effective approach for programmes aiming to enhance psychological capital and well-being of seafarers on a wider and cost-effective scale
3. Zeidan et al. (2010)	*Brief meditation training* —A study with a sample of 49 university students examining if the effects of brief meditation training can be found on cognitive tasks with varying demands on working memory, sustained attention, visual coding, and verbal fluency	Brief training significantly increased mindfulness scores in comparison to a control group. The training protocol had significant effects on several cognitive tasks that require sustained attention and executive processing efficiency, e.g. processing speed, executive attention and verbal fluency	Mindfulness meditation training may enhance cognitive capacity of maritime workers, such as improved sustained attention, the effect of which may be enhanced performance and safety in maritime organizations
4. King (2001)	*Writing about life goals* —A sample of 81 undergraduates wrote for 20 min each day for 4 days. Participants were randomly assigned to	Writing about life goals was significantly less upsetting than writing about trauma and was associated with a significant increase in	Writing about life goals may generate health benefits for maritime workers such as increased subjective well-being and decreased illness.

(continued)

Table 1 (continued)

Study	Intervention	Outcomes	Relevance to Maritime Health
	write about their most traumatic life event, their best possible future self, both of these topics, or a non-emotional control topic	subjective well-being. Five months after writing, a significant interaction emerged such that writing about trauma, one's best possible self, or both were associated with decreased illness compared with controls	Mental health is an essential component of productivity (WHO Europe 2005). Psychological interventions that increase subjective well-being of maritime workers may also increase productivity of maritime organizations
5. Peterson et al. (2005)	*Using signature strengths in a new way—* Participants were asked to take an inventory of character strengths online and received individualized feedback about their top five ("signature") strengths. They were then asked to use one of these top strengths in a new and different way every day for 1 week	Participants showed increased happiness and decreased depressive symptoms for 6 months	Positive psychology interventions such as identifying and using one's signature strengths may be an effective approach to increasing happiness and decreasing depressive symptoms of maritime workers

preparation to perform when confronting new challenges (U.S. Navy 2015). In non-military seafaring contexts, resiliency programmes are also apparent. As proposed by Greenberg, "Equipping mariners with the right psychologically focused skills and regular psychological monitoring can be effective methods of improving psychological resilience, detecting problems at an early stage, ensuring timely support and where necessary signposting to evidence based medical interventions" (March on Stress 2013). For example, as outlined above, peer-to-peer resilience training is currently being piloted by Shell Health (Jacobs 2013). Along similar lines, the SEAHORSE project comprises a consortium of 13 organizations from air and maritime transport sectors, with the overall aim of addressing "human factors and shipping safety." A primary goal of this project is to develop a multilevel resilience approach involving individuals, teams, multi-teams and organisations to ensure that interventions to strengthen resilience at one level have a positive effect on resilience at other levels (SEAHORSE project 2014).

Research is evident on the training of marines to cultivate the state-like quality of "mindfulness"—a moment-to-moment awareness of one's experiences, which has been shown to increase positive affect and decrease negative affect (Davis and Hayes 2012). Mindfulness fosters human characteristics that are central to positive psychology, including character strengths and virtues and psychological well-being, although it does so through acceptance-based rather than change-based approaches (Baer and Lykins 2011). In a study by Johnson and colleagues, marines who received Mindfulness-Based Mind Fitness Training (MMFT) showed *inter alia* enhanced recovery including heart rate and breathing rate after stressful training, signifying that mechanisms relating to stress recovery can be altered in healthy individuals prior to stress exposure (Johnson et al. 2014). Similarly, Stanley and colleagues found that marines who engaged more in MMFT practice showed greater self-reported mindfulness, associated with decreases in perceived stress (Stanley et al. 2011). Advantageous health effects of "mindfulness" training may also extend to mariners in the non-military context. Outlined in Table 2 are examples of interventions used in positive organizational psychology and their potential relevance to maritime health.

Rationale for Future Research in the Area

Due to the isolated and dispersed nature of the maritime context, online or computer-based positive psychology interventions and training may be a viable and important avenue of future research. Online positive psychology interventions have the capacity to empower people to manage their own well-being, while being highly accessible, low-cost, and scalable, reaching diverse types of populations (Bolier et al. 2014; Drozd et al. 2014; Redzic et al. 2014). Empirical support for the efficacy of online positive psychology interventions is provided by current research. For example, while Layous and colleagues found that a positive activity intervention significantly increased positive affect, no differences were found between participants who completed the positive activity online versus in person (Layous et al. 2013). Similarly, Luthans et al. found that the treatment group in a web-based training intervention to develop positive psychological capital, but not the control group, experienced a significant increase in their psychological capital (Luthans et al. 2008).

As proposed by Bergheim and colleagues, captains on board vessels are an important yet difficult group to include in a traditional management training programme, due to their prolonged time at sea, frequently in isolated environments, so that structured web-based or computer-based training programmes may be a valuable and cost-effective way to provide training opportunities during their off-duty hours on board (Bergheim et al. 2015). Of course, such interventions and training would need to be designed and administered with due cognizance of highly restricted Internet access of a large proportion of seafarers (Kahveci 2011; Progoulaki et al. 2013). However, positive psychology computer-based interventions and training, by which such programmes are readily accessible on computers

Table 2 Examples of positive organizational psychology interventions

Study	Intervention	Outcomes	Relevance to Maritime Health
1. Hulsheger et al. (2013)	*Mindfulness self-training—*Participants (*n* = 64) were randomly assigned to a self-training mindfulness intervention group/control group. The sample comprised various job types, e.g. teachers, social workers and bankers	Participants in the mindfulness intervention group experienced significantly more job satisfaction than participants in the control group	Job satisfaction is considered a crucial element in maritime organizations (Bergheim et al. 2015). Employees who are more satisfied with their work care about the quality and safety of their work, are more committed to the organization and more productive (Håvold 2007; Hult 2012b)
2. Lambert et al. (2012)	*Gratitude intervention—*Eight studies (*n* = 2973) testing the theory that gratitude is related to fewer depressive symptoms through positive reframing and positive emotion	Results from these studies indicate that gratitude is related to fewer depressive symptoms, with positive reframing and positive emotion serving as mechanisms that account for this relationship	The most common form of ill-health at sea on non-passenger vessels is mental health problems. Positive psychology training such as the "Gratitude" intervention may decrease depressive symptoms of maritime workers
3. Andersson et al. (2007)	*Hope and gratitude intervention—*A longitudinal study of 308 white-collar U.S. employees to assess effects of feelings of hope and gratitude on self-reported concern for corporate social responsibility	Employees with stronger hope and gratitude were found to have a greater sense of responsibility towards employee and societal issues, such as social justice	Interventions for maritime workers to increase feelings of gratitude and hope may increase sense of responsibility toward employee and societal issues
4. Fredrickson et al. (2008)	*Meditation practice—*A field experiment with working adults (*n* = 139), half of whom were randomly assigned to begin a practice of loving-kindness meditation	The meditation practice produced increases over time in daily experiences of positive emotions, which produced increases in personal resources (e.g. purpose in life, social support, and decreased illness symptoms). These increases in personal resources predicted increased life satisfaction and reduced depressive symptoms	The incidence of seafarer deaths through suicide suggests that the mental health of seafarers continues to be very poor. Meditation training of seafarers could increase personal resources, such as purpose in life, which may generate increased life satisfaction and decreased depressive symptoms

(continued)

Table 2 (continued)

Study	Intervention	Outcomes	Relevance to Maritime Health
5. Millear et al. (2008)	*Resilience-building programme*—A pilot trial of the Promoting Adult Resilience (PAR) programme, a strengths-based resilience-building programme that integrates interpersonal and cognitive-behaviour therapy. Pre, post and follow-up measures on 20 PAR participants from a resource-sector company were compared with a non-intervention-matched comparison group	The PAR group maintained significant post-test improvements in coping self-efficacy and lower levels of stress and depression. Process evaluations of the PAR programme showed that skills were rated highly and widely used in everyday life at both post and follow-up measurement times	People working at sea may experience a multitude of stressors. Strengths-based resilience-building programmes may enhance coping self-efficacy and decrease levels of stress and depression of maritime workers. As mental health is an essential component of social cohesion (WHO Europe 2005), interventions to enhance psychological well-being of seafarers may also strengthen social cohesiveness of employees of maritime organizations

on board, may be a viable and judicious option for those aiming to increase positive psychological affect and capital of seafarers.

Effect duration and effect maintenance of positive psychology interventions are also pertinent areas of inquiry. As proposed by Seligman and Csikszentmihalyi, one fundamental gap of positive psychology relates to the relationship between momentary experiences of happiness and longer-lasting well-being (Seligman and Csikszentmihalyi 2000). However, studies indicating longer-term positive effects on well-being of positive psychology interventions are evident. For example, Cohn and Fredrickson found that many participants of a meditation intervention continued to meditate, to experience boosted positive emotions, and to maintain increased personal resources, more than one year after the end of training, signifying that skills-based positive psychology interventions may show longer-term effectiveness (Cohn and Fredrickson 2010). In relation to a self-administered "Three funny things" intervention in an online setting, Proyer et al. found that the intervention led to an increase in happiness and an amelioration of depressive symptoms at 6-months follow-up (Proyer et al. 2014). Similarly, Seligman and Steen reported two exercises—"Using signature strengths in a new way" and "Three good things"—that were found to increase happiness and decrease depressive symptoms of participants for 6 months (Seligman et al. 2005).

A further promising line of inquiry relates to maritime health at the systems level. As emphasized by Carter, while the collection and analysis of information on seafarers' health is mostly addressed by health professionals, the use of such information is important for all areas of the maritime sector, and this introduces a variety of social, political, economic, regulatory, and ethical factors into all parts of the advancement of a knowledge base (Carter 2011b). Similarly, MacLachlan et al. propose that environmental, organizational, operational, safety, and cultural aspects all have an impact on maritime health; accordingly, the authors recommend a systems-based approach to research to facilitate the targeting and implementation of integrated health care interventions in the maritime environment (MacLachlan et al. 2012). A systems approach to managing stressors is the basis of the Crew Endurance Management System, extensively used in more recent times for implementing practices to control shipboard stressors (Comperatore et al. 2005; United States Coast Guard 2014). Along these lines, Comperatore and colleagues suggest that managing the complexity of shipboard stressors necessitates a systems approach that identifies individual elements in the complex system and determines how these elements are individually and collectively impacting on seafarers' endurance (Comperatore et al. 2005).

Key Research Questions

While recognizing that a range of questions may be proposed on the topic of positive psychology and well-being at sea, a number of selected research questions are presented below:

1. Do positive psychology interventions and training enhance well-being, performance and safety in the workplace, and through what mechanisms do these interventions and training operate? Are these mechanisms transferable to the maritime environment?
2. What are the facilitators and barriers to the effective implementation of positive psychology interventions that are specific to the maritime context?
3. Do positive psychology interventions show signs of effect maintenance in the maritime context?
4. Do positive psychology interventions present any advantages or disadvantages relative to other forms of psychological intervention in the maritime context?
5. How can positive psychology interventions and training be designed and administered to be accessible across ranks, sexes, ages, cultures and ethnicities on board?
6. Are positive psychology computer-based interventions and training an effective and viable option in the maritime context?
7. How can a systems-based approach to research and implementation be designed to facilitate integrated health care interventions in the maritime environment?

Conclusion

While for centuries folk theory has promoted the concept that positive emotions are good for your health, accumulating empirical evidence is offering support for this anecdotal knowledge, indicating that positive emotions are associated with beneficial psychological and physical health effects (Tugade et al. 2004). Furthermore, a growing literature on positive psychology interventions suggests that the "good life"—positive emotion, engagement, relationships, meaning, and accomplishment—can be strengthened (Seligman 2010). The seafaring environment offers a unique context in which positive psychology interventions and training may be applied and tested. The isolated, confined, and safety-critical environment of the ship exposes seafarers to a very particular assortment of stressors. Conversely, as proposed by MacLachlan et al., this environment also offers unique opportunities to develop occupational health and performance programmes suitable to life on board, and the field of positive psychology may contribute in this respect due to its focus on facilitating positive health, attitudes and work behaviour, rather than on correcting for a "lack of," "failures," "errors" or "dysfunctions" (MacLachlan et al. 2013). Robust research is essential that shows scientifically the effects on well-being of positive psychology interventions administered on board. As proposed by Seligman, interventions that work are required, and a systematic programme of interventions that is scientifically proven to raise the level of human well-being (Seligman 2003).

Of course, as previously outlined, for whom, in what circumstances, and through which mechanisms positive psychology interventions work are largely dependent on the individual, activity, and context. As individuals have diverse strengths, interests, values, and inclinations that allow them to benefit more from some strategies than others, no one particular activity will help all individuals to become happier (Lyubomirsky et al. 2005). Moreover, interventions to mitigate stress and support seafarers' well-being should recognize the occupational, cultural and demographic factors that may influence how stress may be differentially experienced, expressed and alleviated on board.

To date, the application of positive psychology interventions and training to the maritime context has been examined only marginally—although research on "mindfulness" techniques and resilience training is evident in the navy and broader seafaring setting. As proposed by Progoulaki and colleagues, shipping companies are seemingly willing to invest in the well-being of seafarers as it is considered a primary source of productivity (Progoulaki et al. 2013). Whether the emergent focus of maritime organizations on supporting seafarers' well-being is health or productivity motivated, or both, an increasing awareness of mental health problems at sea is evident, associated with a variety of practical initiatives in this area. Importantly, however, as proposed by MacLachlan et al. (2012), a systems-based perspective that addresses safety, cultural, environmental, operational and organizational aspects can ensure a more comprehensive approach to maritime health.

References

Alderton, T., Bloor, M., Kahveci, E., Lane, T., Sampson, H., Thomas, M. ... Zhao, M. (2004). *The global seafarer: Living and working conditions in a globalized industry.* Geneva: International Labour Office, Cardiff, UK: Seafarers International Research Centre.

Allport, G. W. (1955). *Becoming: Basic considerations for a psychology of personality.* New Haven: Yale University Press.

American Psychological Assocation. (2015). *The road to resilience.* Retrieved from http://www.apa.org/helpcenter/road-resilience.aspx

Andersson, L., Giacalone, R., & Jurkiewicz, C. (2007). On the relationship of hope and gratitude to corporate social responsibility. *Journal of Business Ethics, 70*(4), 401–409. doi:10.1007/s10551-006-9118-1

Azar, B. (2011). *Positive psychology advances, with growing pains.* Retrieved from http://www.apa.org/monitor/2011/04/positive-psychology.aspx

Baer, R. A., & Lykins, E. L. B. (2011). Mindfulness and positive psychological functioning. In K. M. Sheldon, T. B. Kashdan, & M. F. Steger (Eds.), *Designing positive psychology: Taking stock and moving forward* (pp. 335–348). New York: Oxford University Press Inc.

Bakker, A. B., & Schaufeli, W. B. (2008). Positive organizational behavior: Engaged employees in flourishing organizations. *Journal of Organizational Behavior, 29*(2), 147–154. doi:10.1002/job.515

Bartone, P. T. (2006). Resilience under military operational stress: Can leaders influence hardiness? *Military Psychology, 18*(Suppl), S131–S148. doi:10.1207/s15327876mp1803s_10.

Bartone, P. (2010). Forging stress resilience: Building psychological hardiness. In R. E. Armstrong, M. D. Drapeau, C. A. Loeb, & J. J. Valdes (Eds.), *Bio-inspired innovation and national security* (pp. 243–255). Washington, D. C.: NDU Press.

Bartone, P. T. (2012). Social and organizational influences on psychological hardiness: How leaders can increase stress resilience. *Security Informatics, 1*(21), 1–10. doi:10.1186/2190-8532-1-21

Bartone, P. T., Hystad, S. W., Eid, J., & Brevik, J. I. (2012). Psychological hardiness and coping style as risk/resilience factors for alcohol abuse. *Military Medicine, 177*(5), 517–524.

Bergheim, K., Nielsen, M. B., Mearns, K., & Eid, J. (2015). The relationship between psychological capital, job satisfaction, and safety perceptions in the maritime industry. *Safety Science, 74*, 27–36. doi:10.1016/j.ssci.2014.11.024

Bolier, L., Haverman, M., Westerhof, G. J., Riper, H., Smit, F., & Bohlmeijer, E. (2013). Positive psychology interventions: A meta-analysis of randomized controlled studies. *BMC Public Health, 13*(119), 1–20. doi:10.1186/1471-2458-13-119

Bolier, L., Majo, C., Smit, F., Westerhof, G. J., Haverman, M., Walburg, J. A., et al. (2014). Cost-effectiveness of online positive psychology: Randomized controlled trial. *The Journal of Positive Psychology, 9*(5), 460–471. doi:10.1080/17439760.2014.910829

Bono, J. E., Glomb, T. M., Shen, W., Kim, E., & Koch, A. J. (2013). Building positive resources: Effects of positive events and positive reflection on work stress and health. *Academy of Management Journal, 56*(6), 1601–1627. doi:10.5465/amj.2011.0272

Borodina, N. V. (2013). Use of sail training ship in seafarers' professional education. *Asia-Pacific Journal of Marine Science & Education, 3*(1), 87–96.

Brunstein, J. C., Schultheiss, O. C., & Grassmann, R. (1998). Personal goals and emotional well-being: The moderating role of motive dispositions. *Journal of Personality and Social Psychology, 75*(2), 494–508.

Cameron, K. S., Dutton, J. E., & Quinn, R. E. (2003). Foundations of positive organizational scholarship. In K. S. Cameron, J. E. Dutton, & R. E. Quinn (Eds.), *Positive organizational scholarship: Foundations of a new discipline* (pp. 3–13). San Francisco, California: Berrett-Koehler Publishers Inc.

Carotenuto, A., Fasanaro, A. M., Molino, I., Sibilio, F., Saturnino, A., Traini, E., et al. (2013). The Psychological General Well-Being Index (PGWBI) for assessing stress of seafarers on board merchant ships. *International Maritime Health, 64*(4), 215–220.

Carotenuto, A., Molino, I., Fasanaro, A. M., & Amenta, F. (2012). Psychological stress in seafarers: A review. *International Maritime Health, 63*(4), 188–194.

Carr, A. (2011). *Positive psychology: The science of happiness and human strengths* (2nd ed.). East Sussex, UK: Routledge.

Carter, T. (2005). Working at sea and psychosocial health problems: Report of an International Maritime Health Association Workshop. *Travel Medicine and Infectious Disease, 3*(2), 61–65. doi:10.1016/j.tmaid.2004.09.005

Carter, T. (2011a). Mapping the knowledge base for maritime health: 3 illness and injury in seafarers. *International Maritime Health, 62*(4), 224–240.

Carter, T. (2011b). Mapping the knowledge base for maritime health: 2. a framework for analysis. *International Maritime Health, 62*(4), 217–223.

Cerezo, M. V., Ortiz-Tallo, M., Cardenal, V., & De La Torre-Luque, A. (2014). Positive psychology group intervention for breast cancer patients: A randomised trial. *Psychological Reports, 115*(1), 44–64. doi:10.2466/15.20.PR0.115c17z7

Ciarrochi, J., Kashdan, T. B., & Harris, R. (2013). The foundations of flourishing. In T. B. Kashdan & J. Ciarrochi (Eds.), *Mindfulness, acceptance, and positive psychology* (pp. 1–29). Oakland, CA.: Context Press.

Cohn, M. A., & Fredrickson, B. L. (2010). In search of durable positive psychology interventions: Predictors and consequences of long-term positive behavior change. *The Journal of Positive Psychology, 5*(5), 355–366. doi:10.1080/17439760.2010.508883

Cohn, M. A., Fredrickson, B. L., Brown, S. L., Mikels, J. A., & Conway, A. M. (2009). Happiness unpacked: Positive emotions increase life satisfaction by building resilience. *Emotion, 9*(3), 361–368. doi:10.1037/a0015952

Comperatore, C. A., Rivera, P. K., & Kingsley, L. (2005). Enduring the shipboard stressor complex: A systems approach. *Aviation, Space and Environmental Medicine, 76*(6 Suppl), B108–B118.

Davis, D. M., & Hayes, J. A. (2012). *What are the benefits of mindfulness*. Retrieved from http://www.apa.org/monitor/2012/07-08/ce-corner.aspx

Diener, E. (2009). Positive psychology: Past, present and future. In S. J. Lopez & C. R. Snyder (Eds.), *The Oxford handbook of positive psychology* (2nd ed.). New York: Oxford University Press Inc.

Donaldson, S. I., & Ko, L. (2010). Positive organizational psychology, behavior, and scholarship: A review of the emerging literature and evidence base. *The Journal of Positive Psychology, 5* (3), 177–191. doi:10.1080/17439761003790930

Drozd, F., Mork, L., Nielsen, B., Raeder, S., & Bjørkli, C. A. (2014). Better Days—A randomized controlled trial of an internet-based positive psychology intervention. *The Journal of Positive Psychology, 9*(5), 377–388. doi:10.1080/17439760.2014.910822

Dubois, C. M., Beach, S. R., Kashdan, T. B., Nyer, M. B., Park, E. R., Celano, C. M., et al. (2012). Positive psychological attributes and cardiac outcomes: Associations, mechanisms, and interventions. *Psychosomatics, 53*(4), 303–318. doi:10.1016/j.psym.2012.04.004

Ford, B. Q., & Mauss, I. B. (2014). The paradoxical effects of pursuing positive emotion: When and why wanting to feel happy backfires. In J. Gruber & J. Moskowitz (Eds.), *Positive emotion: Integrating the light sides and dark sides* (pp. 363–381). New York: Oxford University Press.

Fordyce, M. W. (1977). Development of a program to increase personal happiness. *Journal of Counseling Psychology, 24*(6), 511–521. doi:10.1037/0022-0167.24.6.511

Fredrickson, B. L. (2000). Cultivating positive emotions to optimize health and well-being. *Prevention & Treatment, 3*(Article 0001a).

Fredrickson, B. L. (2001). The role of positive emotions in positive psychology. The broaden-and-build theory of positive emotions. *American Psychologist, 56*(3), 218–226.

Fredrickson, B. L., Cohn, M. A., Coffey, K. A., Pek, J., & Finkel, S. M. (2008). Open hearts build lives: Positive emotions, induced through loving-kindness meditation, build consequential personal resources. *Journal of Personality and Social Psychology, 95*(5), 1045–1062. doi:10.1037/a0013262

Gable, S. L., & Haidt, J. (2005). What (and why) is positive psychology? *Review of General Psychology, 9*(2), 103–110. doi:10.1037/1089-2680.9.2.103

Gekara, V. O., Bloor, M., & Sampson, H. (2011). Computer-based assessment in safety-critical industries: The case of shipping. *Journal of Vocational Education & Training, 63*(1), 87–100. doi:10.1080/13636820.2010.536850

Gibbs, P. C., & Burnett, S. B. (2011). Well-being at work, a new way of doing things? A journey through yesterday, today and tomorrow. In A. S. Antoniou & C. Cooper (Eds.), *New directions in organizational psychology and behavioral medicine* (pp. 25–42). Surrey, UK: Gower Publishing Ltd.

Gregory, D., & Shanahan, P. (2010). *The human element: A guide to human behaviour in the shipping industry*. London: The Stationary Office (TSO).

Haidt, J. (2006). *The happiness hypothesis: Putting ancient wisdom and philosophy to the test of modern science*. London, UK: Arrow Books.

Haka, M., Borch, D. F., Jensen, C., & Leppin, A. (2011). Should I stay or should I go? Motivational profiles of Danish seafaring officers and non-officers. *International Maritime Health, 62*(1), 20–30.

Harvard Medical School. (2011). *Positive psychology special health report*. Boston, MA, U. S.: Harvard Health Publications, Harvard Medical School.

Håvold, J. I. (2007). *From safety culture to safety orientation: Developing a tool to measure safety in shipping* (Doctoral thesis). Norwegian University of Science and Technology, Norway. Retrieved from http://brage.bibsys.no/xmlui/handle/11250/265609

Hulsheger, U. R., Alberts, H. J., Feinholdt, A., & Lang, J. W. (2013). Benefits of mindfulness at work: The role of mindfulness in emotion regulation, emotional exhaustion, and job satisfaction. *Journal of Applied Psychology, 98*(2), 310–325. doi:10.1037/a0031313

Hult, C. (2012a). Swedish seafaring life in 2009-2010. In C. Hult (Ed.), *Swedish seafarers and seafaring occupation 2010: A study of work-related attitudes during different stages of life at sea* (pp. 9–22). Kalmar, Sweden: Kalmar Maritime Acadamy.

Hult, C. (2012b). Work, motivation, and commitment. In C. Hult (Ed.), *Swedish seafarers and seafaring occupation 2010: A study of work-related attitudes during different stages of life at sea* (pp. 31–50). Kalmar, Sweden: Kalmar Maritime Academy.

Hystad, S. W., Bartone, P. T., & Eid, J. (2014). Positive organizational behavior and safety in the offshore oil industry: Exploring the determinants of positive safety climate. *Journal of Positive Psychology, 9*(1), 42–53. doi:10.1080/17439760.2013.831467

Hystad, S. W., & Bye, H. H. (2013). Safety behaviours at sea: The role of personal values and personality hardiness. *Safety Science, 57*, 19–26. doi:10.1016/j.ssci.2013.01.018

International Labour Organization. (2006). *Maritime Labour Convention*. Retrieved from http://www.ilo.org/wcmsp5/groups/public/@ed_norm/@normes/documents/normativeinstrument/wcms_090250.pdf

International Labour Organization. (2013). *Basic facts on the Maritime Labour Convention 2006*. Retrieved from http://www.ilo.org/global/standards/maritime-labour-convention/what-it-does/WCMS_219665/lang–en/index.htm

International Labour Organization. (2015). *International Labour Standards on Seafarers*. Retrieved from http://ilo.org/global/standards/subjects-covered-by-international-labour-standards/seafarers/lang–en/index.htm

Iversen, R. T. (2012). The mental health of seafarers. *International Maritime Health, 63*(2), 78–89.

Jacobs, K. (2013). *Focus on 'resilience' to improve wellbeing, says Shell's health chief*. Retrieved from http://www.hrmagazine.co.uk/hro/news/1140491/focus-resilience-improve-wellbeing-shells-health-chief

James, W. (1902). *The varieties of religious experience: A study in human nature*. New York: Longmans, Green & Co.

Jezewska, M., Leszczynska, I., & Jaremin, B. (2006). Work-related stress at sea self estimation by maritime students and officers. *International Maritime Health, 57*(1–4), 66–75.

Johnsen, B. H., Meeus, P., Meling, J., Rogde, T., Eid, J., Esepevik, R., et al. (2012). Cultural differences in emotional intelligence among top officers on board merchant ships. *International Maritime Health, 63*(2), 90–95.

Johnson, D. C., Thom, N. J., Stanley, E. A., Haase, L., Simmons, A. N., Shih, P. B., et al. (2014). Modifying resilience mechanisms in at-risk individuals: A controlled study of mindfulness training in marines preparing for deployment. *American Journal of Psychiatry, 171*(8), 844–853. doi:10.1176/appi.ajp.2014.13040502

Kahveci, E. (2011). *Seafarers and communication*. London, UK: ITF Seafarers' Trust. Retrieved from http://workinglives.org/fms/MRSite/Research/wlri/WORKS/Seafarers%20and%20Communication%20Report.pdf

King, L. A. (2001). The health benefits of writing about life goals. *Personality and Social Psychology Bulletin, 27*(7). doi:10.1177/0146167201277003

Lambert, N. M., Fincham, F. D., & Stillman, T. F. (2012). Gratitude and depressive symptoms: The role of positive reframing and positive emotion. *Cognition & Emotion, 26*(4), 615–633. doi:10.1080/02699931.2011.595393

Layous, K., Nelson, S. K., & Lyubomirsky, S. (2013). What is the optimal way to deliver a positive activity intervention? The case of writing about one's best possible selves. *Journal of Happiness Studies, 14*(2), 635–654. doi:10.1007/s10902-012-9346-2

Leppin, A. L., Gionfriddo, M. R., Sood, A., Montori, V. M., Erwin, P. J., Zeballos-Palacios, C. … Tilburt, J. C. (2014). The efficacy of resilience training programs: A systematic review protocol. *Systematic Reviews, 3*(20). doi:10.1186/2046-4053-3-20

Leszczynska, I., Jaremin, B., & Jezewska, M. (2007). Strategies towards health protection in maritime work environment involving the role of health promotion—Invitation to join in discussion. *International Maritime Health, 58*(1–4), 185–194.

Lipowski, M., Lipowska, M., Peplinska, A., & Jezewska, M. (2014). Personality determinants of health behaviours of merchant navy officers. *International Maritime Health, 65*(3), 158–165. doi:10.5603/imh.2014.0030

Losada, M. (1999). The complex dynamics of high performance teams. *Mathematical and Computer Modelling, 30*(9–10), 179–192. doi:10.1016/S0895-7177(99)00189-2

Luthans, F., Avey, J. B., & Patera, J. L. (2008). Experimental analysis of a web-based training intervention to develop positive psychological capital. *Academy of Management Learning & Education, 7*(2), 209–221. doi:10.5465/AMLE.2008.32712618

Luthans, F., Avolio, B. J., Avey, J. B., & Norman, S. M. (2007a). Positive psychological capital: Measurement and relationship with performance and satisfaction. *Personnel Psychology, 60* (3), 541–572. doi:10.1111/j.1744-6570.2007.00083

Luthans, F., & Church, A. H. (2002). Positive organizational behavior: Developing and managing psychological strengths [and executive commentary]. *The Academy of Management Executive, 16*(1), 57–75.

Luthans, F., Vogelgesang, G. R., & Lester, P. B. (2006). Developing the psychological capital of resiliency. *Human Resource Development Review, 5*(1), 25–44. doi:10.1177/1534484305285335

Luthans, F., Youssef, C. M., & Avolio, B. J. (2007b). *Psychological capital: Developing the human competitive edge*. New York: Oxford University Press.

Lyubomirsky, S., & Layous, K. (2013). How do simple positive activities increase well-being? *Current Directions in Psychological Science, 22*(1), 57–62. doi:10.1177/0963721412469809

Lyubomirsky, S., Sheldon, K. M., & Schkade, D. (2005). Pursuing happiness: The architecture of sustainable change. *Review of General Psychology, 9*(2), 111–131. doi:10.1037/1089-2680.9.2.111

MacLachlan, M., Cromie, S., Liston, P., Kavanagh, B., & Kay, A. (2013). Psychosocial and organisational aspects. In A. Schreiner (Ed.), *Textbook of maritime medicine*. Retrieved from: http://textbook.ncmm.no/

MacLachlan, M., & Hand, K. (2013). *Happy nation? Prospects for psychological prosperity in Ireland*. Dublin, Ireland: The Liffey Press Ltd.

MacLachlan, M., Kavanagh, B., & Kay, A. (2012). Maritime health: A review with suggestions for research. *International Maritime Health, 63*(1), 1–6.

Maddi, S. R. (2013). *Hardiness: Turning stressful circumstances into resilient growth*. New York: Springer.

March on Stress. (2013). *March on stress news: Supporting occupational mental health in the shipping industry*. Retrieved from http://www.marchonstress.com/index.php/news/article/73

Maslow, A. H. (1954). *Motivation and personality*. New York: Harper.

Maslow, A. H. (1968). *Toward a psychology of being*. New York: D. Van Nostrand Company.

Mauss, I. B., Tamir, M., Anderson, C. L., & Savino, N. S. (2011). Can seeking happiness make people happy? Paradoxical effects of valuing happiness. *Emotion, 11*(4), 807–815. doi:10.1037/a0022010

McDougall, L., & Drummond, P. D. (2010). Personal resources moderate the relationship between work stress and psychological strain of submariners. *Military Psychology (Taylor & Francis Ltd), 22*(4), 385–398. doi:10.1080/08995605.2010.513231

Meyers, M. C., van Woerkom, M., & Bakker, A. B. (2013). The added value of the positive: A literature review of positive psychology interventions in organizations. *European Journal of Work and Organizational Psychology, 22*(5), 618–632. doi:10.1080/1359432X.2012.694689

Millear, P., Liossis, P., Shochet, I. M., Biggs, H., & Donald, M. (2008). Being on PAR: Outcomes of a pilot trial to improve mental health and wellbeing in the workplace with the Promoting Adult Resilience (PAR) program. *Behaviour Change, 25*(4), 215–228. doi:10.1375/bech.25.4.215

Nelson, S. K., & Lyubomirsky, S. (2012). Finding happiness: Tailoring positive activities for optimal well-being benefits. In M. Tugade, M. Shiota, & L. Kirby (Eds.), *Handbook of positive emotions* (pp. 275–293). New York: Guilford.

Nielsen, M. B., Bergheim, K., & Eid, J. (2013). Relationships between work environment factors and workers' well-being in the maritime industry. *International Maritime Health, 64*(2), 80–88.

Oedewald, P., & Reiman, T. (2007). *Special characteristics of safety critical organizations: Work psychological perspective (VTT Publications 633)*. Finland: VTT Technical Research Centre of Finland. Retrieved from http://www2.vtt.fi/inf/pdf/publications/2007/P633.pdf

Oldenburg, M., Baur, X., & Schlaich, C. (2010). Occupational risks and challenges of seafaring. *Journal of Occupational Health, 52*(5), 249–256.

Oldenburg, M., Hogan, B., & Jensen, H. J. (2013). Systematic review of maritime field studies about stress and strain in seafaring. *International Archives of Occupational and Environmental Health, 86*(1), 1–15. doi:10.1007/s00420-012-0801-5

Oldenburg, M., Jensen, H. J., Latza, U., & Baur, X. (2009). Seafaring stressors aboard merchant and passenger ships. *International Journal of Public Health, 54*(2), 96–105. doi:10.1007/s00038-009-7067-z

Ong, A. D., Bergeman, C. S., Bisconti, T. L., & Wallace, K. A. (2006). Psychological resilience, positive emotions, and successful adaptation to stress in later life. *Journal of Personality and Social Psychology, 91*(4), 730–749. doi:10.1037/0022-3514.91.4.730

Penn Positive Psychology Center. (2007). *Resilience in children*. Retrieved from http://www.ppc.sas.upenn.edu/prpsum.htm

Peterson, C. (2006). *A primer in positive psychology*. New York: Oxford University Press Inc.

Peterson, C. (2009). Foreword. In C. R. Snyder & S. J. Lopez (Eds.), *Oxford handbook of positive psychology* (2nd ed.). New York: Oxford University Press Inc.

Peterson, C., & Park, N. (2003). Positive psychology as the evenhanded positive psychologist views it. *Psychological Inquiry, 14*(2), 143–147. doi:10.2307/1449822

Peterson, C., Park, N., & Seligman, M. E. P. (2005). Assessment of character strengths. In G. P. Koocher, J. C. Norcross, & S. S. Hill III (Eds.), *Psychologists' desk reference* (2nd ed., pp. 93–98). New York: Oxford University Press.

Progoulaki, M., Katradi, A., & Theotokas, I. (2013). Developing and promoting seafarers' welfare under the Maritime Labour Convention: A research agenda. *SPOUDAI Journal of Economics and Business, 63*(3–4), 75–82.

Proyer, R. T., Gander, F., Wellenzohn, S., & Ruch, W. (2014). Positive psychology interventions in people aged 50–79 years: Long-term effects of placebo-controlled online interventions on well-being and depression. *Aging & Mental Health, 18*(8), 997–1005. doi:10.1080/13607863.2014.899978

Redzic, N. M., Taylor, K., Chang, V., Trockel, M., Shorter, A., & Taylor, C. B. (2014). An Internet-based positive psychology program: Strategies to improve effectiveness and engagement. *The Journal of Positive Psychology, 9*(6), 494–501. doi:10.1080/17439760.2014.936966

Reiman, T., Rollenhagen, C., Pietikäinen, E., & Heikkilä, J. (2015). Principles of adaptive management in complex safety-critical organizations. *Safety Science, 71*, Part B(0), 80–92. doi:10.1016/j.ssci.2014.07.021

Rydstedt, L. W., & Lundh, M. (2012). Work demands are related to mental health problems for older engine room officers. *International Maritime Health, 63*(4), 176–180.

Schager, B. (1997). *Advantages of psychological assessment prior to employment and promotion.* Halmstad, Sweden: Marine Profile. Retrieved from http://www.marine-profile.com/Articles.html

Schrank, B., Brownell, T., Tylee, A., & Slade, M. (2014). Positive psychology: An approach to supporting recovery in mental illness. *East Asian Archives of Psychiatry, 24*(3), 95–103.

SEAHORSE project. (2014). *SEAHORSE: The project.* Retrieved from http://www.seahorseproject.eu/TheProject/tabid/4193/Default.aspx

Seligman, M. E. P. (2003). *Authentic happiness: Testing positive interventions.* Retrieved from https://www.authentichappiness.sas.upenn.edu/newsletters/authentichappiness/testinginterventions

Seligman, M. E. P. (2010). *Flourish: Positive psychology and positive interventions* (Tanner lectures on human values, delivered at the University of Michigan). Retrieved from http://tannerlectures.utah.edu/_documents/a-to-z/s/Seligman_10.pdf

Seligman, M. E. P. (2011a). *Flourish: A visionary new understanding of happiness and well-being.* New York: Free Press.

Seligman, M. E. P. (2011b). *Authentic happiness: Flourish: A new theory of positive psychology* (Archived newsletter). Retrieved from https://www.authentichappiness.sas.upenn.edu/newsletters/flourishnewsletters/newtheory

Seligman, M. E. P. (2013). *Authentic happiness: Using the new positive psychology to realize your potential for lasting fulfillment.* New York: Atria Books.

Seligman, M. E. P., & Csikszentmihalyi, M. (2000). Positive psychology. An introduction. *American Psychologist, 55*(1), 5–14.

Seligman, M. E. P., Rashid, T., & Parks, A. C. (2006). Positive psychotherapy. *American Psychologist, 61*(8), 774–788. doi:10.1037/0003-066X.61.8.774

Seligman, M. E., Steen, T. A., Park, N., & Peterson, C. (2005). Positive psychology progress: Empirical validation of interventions. *American Psychologist, 60*(5), 410–421. doi:10.1037/0003-066X.60.5.410

Shoshani, A., & Steinmetz, S. (2014). Positive psychology at school: A school-based intervention to promote adolescents' mental health and well-being. *Journal of Happiness Studies, 15*(6), 1289–1311. doi:10.1007/s10902-013-9476-1

Smedley, J., Dick, F., & Sadhra, S. (2013). Clinical tasks and procedures. In J. Smedley, F. Dick, & S. Sadhra (Eds.), *Oxford handbook of occupational health* (pp. 747–770). Oxford, UK: Oxford University Press.

Smith, J. L., & Hollinger-Smith, L. (2015). Savoring, resilience, and psychological well-being in older adults. *Aging & Mental Health, 19*(3), 192–200. doi:10.1080/13607863.2014.986647

Southwick, S. M., Bonanno, G. A., Masten, A. S., Panter-Brick, C., & Yehuda, R. (2014). Resilience definitions, theory, and challenges: Interdisciplinary perspectives. *European Journal of Psychotraumatology, 5*. doi:10.3402/ejpt.v5.25338

Stanley, E. A., Schaldach, J. M., Kiyonaga, A., & Jha, A. P. (2011). Mindfulness-based mind fitness training: A case study of a high-stress predeployment military cohort. *Cognitive and Behavioral Practice, 18*(4), 566–576. doi:10.1016/j.cbpra.2010.08.002

Tedlie Moskowitz, J., Carrico, A. W., Cohn, M. A., Duncan, L. G., Bussolari, C., Layous, K., et al. (2014). Randomized controlled trial of a positive affect intervention to reduce stress in people newly diagnosed with HIV; protocol and design for the IRISS study. *Open Access Journal of Clinical Trials, 6*, 85–100. doi:10.2147/OAJCT.S64645

Thompson, R. B., Peura, C., & Gayton, W. F. (2014). Gender differences in the person-activity fit for positive psychology interventions. *The Journal of Positive Psychology, 10*(2), 179–183. doi:10.1080/17439760.2014.927908

Tugade, M. M., Fredrickson, B. L., & Barrett, L. F. (2004). Psychological resilience and positive emotional granularity: Examining the benefits of positive emotions on coping and health. *Journal of Personality, 72*(6), 1161–1190. doi:10.1111/j.1467-6494.2004.00294.x

United States Coast Guard. (2014). *Crew endurance management.* Retrieved from http://www.uscg.mil/hq/cg5/cg5211/cems.asp

U.S. Navy. (2015). *Plan of the day announcements: Operational stress control.* Retrieved from http://www.navy.mil/planOfDay.asp

van Wijk, C. H., & Waters, A. H. (2008). Positive psychology made practical: A case study with naval specialists. *Military Medicine, 173*(5), 488–492.

Wang, H. (2008). *Safety factors and leading indicators in shipping organizations: Tanker and container operations* (A thesis submitted to the Graduate Faculty of Rensselaer Polytechnic Institute in partial fulfillment of the requirements for the degree of Doctor of Philosophy). Rensselaer Polytechnic Institute, Troy, New York. Retrieved from http://search.proquest.com/docview/304531513

Waters, L. (2011). A review of school-based positive psychology interventions. *The Australian Educational and Developmental Psychologist, 28*(2), 75–90. doi:10.1375/aedp.28.2.75

WHO Europe. (2005). *Mental health: Facing the challenges, building solutions; Report from the WHO European Ministerial Conference.* Copenhagen, Denmark.: World Health Organization, Regional Office for Europe. Retrieved from http://www.euro.who.int/en/health-topics/noncommunicable-diseases/mental-health/publications/2005/mental-health-facing-the-challenges,-building-solutions

Wood, J. V., Perunovic, W. Q. E., & Lee, J. W. (2009). Positive self-statements: Power for some, peril for others. *Psychological Science, 20*(7), 860–866. doi:10.1111/j.1467-9280.2009.02370.x

Youssef, C. M., & Luthans, F. (2007). Positive organizational behavior in the workplace: The impact of hope, optimism, and resilience. *Journal of Management, 33*(5), 774–800. doi:10.1177/0149206307305562

Zeidan, F., Johnson, S. K., Diamond, B. J., David, Z., & Goolkasian, P. (2010). Mindfulness meditation improves cognition: Evidence of brief mental training. *Consciousness and Cognition, 19*(2), 597–605. doi:10.1016/j.concog.2010.03.014

Transferring Learning Across Safety-Critical Industries

Paul M. Liston, Alison Kay, Sam Cromie, Nick McDonald, Bill Kavanagh, Roddy Cooke and Peter Walter

Case Study

Let's consider two practical examples of transferring learning across safety-critical industries. Shane is a safety manager at a small shipping company. His company recently had a serious incident where company procedures were not followed. This resulted in damage to equipment and significant delays and cost overruns, but there were no injuries. He is struggling to put in place measures to prevent a future reoccurrence and thinks aviation may have something to offer as this sector has many standard operating procedures (SOPs); the nuclear sector might also has innovation and learning to transfer. Contrast this example with that of Yvonne, the head of safety at a large shipbuilding company. Her budget has been increased considerably for the coming year, and she wants to develop her company's human factors capacity and profile by implementing human factors training in the whole company—training everyone in the company, from the boardroom to the shop floor, just like in aviation. The approaches of Shane and Yvonne are not aligned but represent two common "arrival points" or motivations for transferring innovation and learning across safety-critical industries. This chapter will explore both approaches and outline a new, more structured approach to transfer.

P.M. Liston (✉) · A. Kay · S. Cromie · N. McDonald
Centre for Innovative Human Systems, School of Psychology, Trinity College Dublin,
The University of Dublin, Dublin, Ireland
e-mail: pliston@tcd.ie

B. Kavanagh · R. Cooke · P. Walter
National Maritime College of Ireland, Cork, Ireland

© Springer International Publishing Switzerland 2017
M. MacLachlan (ed.), *Maritime Psychology*, DOI 10.1007/978-3-319-45430-6_3

Introduction

Safety-critical industries, by their very nature, are characterized by a desire to manage risk and produce consistently safe outputs. Safety is critical to their operation and the dual goals of safety and efficiency must be optimally managed. This necessitates a strong commitment to continuous improvement, and oftentimes a source of change and improvement can be found in other sectors facing similar existing, or future, challenges. As maritime operators step up their efforts to meet the safety management system (SMS) requirements enshrined in the International Safety Management (ISM) Code, they are increasingly looking to other transport sectors and safety-critical industries for opportunities to learn and improve the safety of their operation. This chapter reviews the state of the art of innovation and learning transfer across safety-critical industries and focuses in particular on how aviation innovations that have been transferred to maritime and other sectors. The drivers for transfer are discussed and the two dominant existing approaches to transfer are detailed. Through the use of two case studies, a number of general principles about these approaches to transfer are delineated. The discussion then moves to a new, systematic approach to transfer that is being pioneered in a European research project, before concluding with possible future directions for transferring learning to the maritime sector.

What Drives Transfer of Learning?

Safety-critical industries value safety more than other sectors, and the relationship between safety and efficiency is not easy to categorize. It is not a compromise—that is to say—when you improve safety you compromise on efficiency or vice versa. For many companies, embracing safety, and investing in safety, can reap efficiency rewards. Obviously regulatory requirements drive compliance, but the idea that safety and efficiency (or cost) are competitors is losing traction. Ward et al. (2010) demonstrated this dynamic in a safety-oriented performance improvement exercise in an aircraft maintenance company over a period of 8 months. By using an operationally valid model of the system (representing the formal system and how this system is interpreted in normal everyday operations) and a "Blocker Resolution Process" to overcome the problems identified, the company was able to deliver 20 aircraft "early" or "on-time", saving 22 days for the customer and resulting in a substantial bonus payment for the maintenance company. It might seem rather counter-intuitive in the context of the current economic environment—that by spending money on safety you can save money. This may be about safety research finally finding a way of demonstrating impact (as exemplified by Ward et al.'s (2010) work) or it may be about a growing recognition that safety goals can help achieve economic ones too.

If safety, or more broadly conceived QHSE (quality, health, safety, environment), is a driver for the transfer of learning and knowledge, then safety culture must be part of the discussion (Parker et al. 2006). An agreed definition of safety culture is still elusive (cf. Guldenmund 2000; Schein 1992), but a useful way of thinking about it is as follows: safety culture is how people behave when no one is looking. The International Maritime Organization (IMO 2003) offers a practicable working definition:

> A safety culture can be defined as a culture in which there is considerable informed endeavor to reduce risks to the individual, ships and the marine environment to a level that is as low as is reasonably practicable. Specifically, for an organisation making efforts to attain such a goal, economic and social benefits will be forthcoming, as a sound balance between safety and commerce will be maintained [IMO, MSC 77/17].

Safety culture, therefore, is about the values that people, and by extension the organization, have in relation to safety. High-profile accidents such as the Costa Concordia, the MV Sewol in South Korea or Air France Flight 447 inevitably highlight safety failures and operational shortcomings. The focus of the subsequent accident investigations is a retrospective analysis of the factors that led to the accident and a typical output would be a list of recommendations to improve safety and reduce risk. In these situations, these recommendations act as drivers for safety improvement for the company involved, and for the industry generally, but they are "reactive" drivers for safety. However, safety culture can act as a proactive driver for safety improvement—pushing organizations to better manage risk.

Hudson (2007) described a model of safety culture maturity which offers an explanation of the relationship between the desire to improve safety and the transfer of learning across safety-critical industries. This model arose from a need to resolve the inherently dichotomous nature of safety culture definitions (i.e. if your organization has this characteristic you have safety culture, if your organization does not have this characteristic you do not have safety culture) (Hudson 2007). The model has the following five progressive levels of safety culture:

1. Pathological—who cares about safety as long as we are not caught?
2. Reactive—safety is important: we do a lot every time we have an accident.
3. Calculative—we have systems in place to manage all hazards.
4. Proactive—we try to anticipate safety problems before they arise.
5. Generative—QHSE is how we do business round here.

The framework posits that as an organization's culture develops and becomes more mature it progresses upwards through the levels. In so doing, there is an increase in trust and accountability—people within the organization view the changes positively—and there is a concomitant increase in organizational informedness based on free and open reporting (Reason 1997; Weick and Sutcliffe 2001).

The Maritime Case

So where might the maritime sector fit in this framework? In 1989, the IMO first developed SMS guidelines (A.647(16), Guidelines on Management for the Safe Operation of Ships and for Pollution Prevention). These guidelines informed the International Management Code for the Safe Operation of Ships and for Pollution Prevention (the ISM Code), which the IMO adopted in 1993. In 1998, the ISM Code became mandatory under an amendment to the International Convention for the Safety of Life at Sea (SOLAS). The ISM code states that the

> safety management system should ensure compliance with mandatory rules and regulations; and that applicable codes, guidelines and standards recommended by the Organization, Administrations, classification societies and maritime industry organizations are taken into account (ISM Code 1.2.3).

The IMO's development of SMS guidelines and their subsequent adoption as part of the SOLAS convention represents a clear progression in safety culture for the maritime industry from the reactive level (2) to the calculative level (3) of Hudson's (2007) model of safety culture. The ISM code, in real terms, requires the development, implementation and maintenance of the following:

A safety and environmental protection policy
Instructions and procedures to ensure safe operation of ships and protection of the environment in compliance with relevant international and flag State legislation
Defined levels of authority and lines of communication between, and amongst, shore and shipboard personnel
Procedures for reporting accidents and nonconformities with the provisions of this Code
Procedures to prepare for and respond to emergency situations, and
Procedures for internal audits and management reviews.

[ISM Code 1.4]

The putting in place of policies, instructions and procedures, as represented in the ISM code, clearly places the maritime sector at the calculative level of safety culture maturity. The implementation of a mandated SMS in the maritime sector represents a move away from a reactionary approach to investigating and retrospectively understanding accidents as a way of preventing reoccurrences to one where identified hazards are managed through systems, policies and processes. But is that sufficient? How does the maritime sector compare to the aviation sector (the "teacher's pet" of safety-critical sectors)?

The Aviation Case

SMS in the aviation sector relates to more than just systems and policies—or at least the systems and policies which are mandated in the aviation sector go above and beyond those mandated by the ISM code. One of the mandated components of European aviation SMS is "safety assurance"—all planned and systematic actions necessary to afford adequate *confidence* that a product, a service, an organization or a functional system achieves acceptable or tolerable safety (Commission Regulation (EU) 1035/2011). According to the International Civil Aviation Organization (ICAO 2013), safety assurance includes the following activities:

1. Safety performance monitoring and measurement
2. Management of change
3. Continuous improvement of the SMS.

It is clear from this focus on managing risk and change that the mandated SMS in the aviation sector would position the aviation sector at the proactive level (4) of Hudson's (2007) model of safety culture: trying to anticipate safety problems before they arise. There is of course a lack of clarity or agreement about the elements of an effective SMS (in any safety-critical system) and their relationship to safety outputs (cf. Pedersen et al. 2012; Thomas 2012), and there are issues associated with the oversight of the maritime sector's transition to SMS use as noted by Padova (2013). However, it would seem that the maritime sector, as it increasingly looks to other sectors for solutions to existing and anticipated problems, is slowly reaching a proactive level of safety culture. Learning from other sectors and adopting new techniques is necessary in order for the maritime sector to progress to the proactive step of safety culture, but it is insufficient on its own. There also needs to be a different approach to managing safety—one where there is clear safety leadership and a focus on continuous improvement, not merely the managing of hazards.

From Whom/Whence to Learn?

It is fair to say that a lot of learning and knowledge has been transferred from aviation to other sectors. The medical field in particular has looked to aviation for established ways of dealing with risk and safety (cf. Wilf-Miron et al. 2003; Kosnik et al. 2007; Stahel 2008; Wauben et al. 2012). The assumption seems to be that aviation does safety better, so if a sector is trying to improve its management of safety and risk it automatically looks to aviation. But is aviation "doing" safety better than other sectors? Maybe this is not the way to look at things. Clearly, in the aviation sector safety has a commercial value—passengers will choose to fly an airline that is perceived to be safe over one that does not have the same safety image.

One only needs to look at the finances of Malaysian Airlines after it lost two wide-bodied aircraft in 6 months (MH370, MH17) to understand why aviation companies invest so much time, effort and money in safety. The Financial Times reported that passenger bookings fell by a third following the MH17 disaster and the quarterly losses had almost doubled compared to the previous year (Grant 2014).

So maybe it is not a question of aviation being better at safety. Perhaps the aviation sector merely puts more resources into managing safety. Perhaps, the aviation sector just perseveres more in their efforts to tackle entrenched issues. Perhaps, this is the key to the aviation sector's contribution to learning and knowledge transfer.

This is not to say that aviation cannot learn from sectors to which it "feeds" learning and knowledge. Take the case of the automotive sector. We know that car design has been benefiting from innovation transferred from airplane cockpits for some time (e.g. Young et al. 2007), but now EU-funded research projects are attempting to introduce into the aviation sector technologies which have been pioneered in the automotive sector. Driver monitoring technologies monitor the operator's attentiveness and will alert in case of dangerous lack of attention. The ACROSS[1] (Advanced Cockpit for Reduction Of Stress and workload) project is currently developing a new cockpit for commercial aviation which will reduce stress and workload for flight crew, and technology and knowledge developed in the automotive sector presents a key input for the aviation technology developers.

It is also worth considering that learning and knowledge transfer can happen within industrial sectors also, not just between them. The trajectory of safety initiatives within aviation is well established, moving from a focus on technical factors, through human factors, then organizational factors to a point today where all are considered together as a complex socio-technical system. This "system of systems" perspective which dominates current thinking acknowledges that all constituent parts of the aviation system (Air Traffic Management (ATM), maintenance, flight operations, design, etc.) are very different from one another and can operate independently but when they interact they expose emergent properties of the system. In complex systems, those problems in one distinct part of the system which have an impact on another operation will undoubtedly drive safety and quality departments to find a solution or a way of understanding things better. This can offer an explanation for why within the aviation system there has been much transfer of knowledge and learning from the flight deck to maintenance and air traffic control.

Case Studies of Transfers

Case Study 1: Aviation to maritime—Crew Resource Management

In March 1977, a major air disaster occurred when two planes collided on a runway in Tenerife, resulting in 583 fatalities. Investigators concluded that the management style of the captain of one of the aircraft engendered a steep authority gradient in the cockpit aspect and this may have contributed to the collision. The management

---

[1]ACROSS is a Large-Scale Integrating Project funded by the European Commission under the Seventh Framework Programme (FP7/2007-2013). Grant Agreement n° ACP2-GA-2012-314501.

culture that prevailed in that airline prevented the co-pilot from challenging the decisions of the captain, even though they were considered to be incorrect. Investigative reports recommended several changes to aviation operational procedures, including the need to change interpersonal cultural and organizational behaviour in aircraft cockpits. This accident was the impetus for the introduction of Cockpit Resource Management (CRM) training across the airline industry.

CRM course syllabi typically include the topic of advocacy, which is also known as "challenge and response". This refers to the empowerment of junior pilots to question the decisions of more senior pilots as a cross-check before actions are taken as it is linked to good management and effective teamwork. Updated CRM training now includes role play and simulation exercises whereby various scenarios are re-enacted to emphasise differences in seniority, cultures and genders which can lead to conflicts. These conflicts can result in the development of steep authority gradients. In this way pilots are trained to speak up and question decisions by challenging senior personnel in a variety of operational contexts, the objective being to increase the transfer of training from the classroom to the cockpit.

CRM training for the airline industry was adapted for use in the shipping industry almost 20 years ago and in its current incarnation is known as Bridge Resource Management (BRM) (Hetherington et al. 2006). In the maritime sector, unlike in aviation, BRM is not mandated but there are non-technical skills requirements as set out in the International Maritime Organization's Seafarer's Training, Certification and Watchkeeping Code (IMO 1995). In meeting these requirements, resource management training has established itself as a central part of maritime training syllabi, but BRM can take many forms (Barnett et al. 2003).

Typically, simulators are involved in BRM and this affords the opportunity to practise the technique of advocacy ("challenge and response"). During this part of the training, the course coordinator selects a team consisting of appropriate members that reflect varying degrees of authority. For example, a mature, experienced ship's officer will lead a team of junior officers. A problem-based scenario is executed using a simulator with visuals and technical equipment and specific objectives are given to the team pre-exercise. The exercise is designed to be sufficiently complex to create high workload and induce mild stress in the participants. A successful outcome would be good communication, a team approach, listening to junior officers and for junior officers to be comfortable in asking questions and offering advice. If the instructor is unable to select a suitable senior officer due to the lack of senior personnel, the role of senior officer or ship's port pilot may be acted by instructors.

The exercise is recorded on video (ethical permission is obtained beforehand) and re-played during debriefing. Debriefing includes asking each participant how they felt during the exercise in terms of pressure and ability to speak up. The video is analysed in detail in terms of advocacy, communication skills, leadership and management. Learning points are highlighted and reinforced for use in future exercises.

Challenges in Transferring CRM to the Maritime Sector

Advocacy is sometimes considered the most challenging part of BRM training (Kavanagh 2008). It is particularly difficult with mature, experienced officers and with personnel from cultures where power distance is strong. Power distance describes the ability of personnel in senior and junior roles to communicate freely and effectively. This difference in role or rank is also known as an authority gradient. The gradient is directly related to difference in seniority. When power distance is strong, junior officers are reluctant to question the actions of senior officers, even though they are part of the same team (Hofstede et al. 2010). For those reasons, the techniques have not always worked, either during training or in practice, in some industry sectors. The technique of advocacy is most successfully executed in sections of the shipping industry that are considered to be highly safety critical, such as cruise liners and vessels in the oil/gas trades. However, not all sections have embraced the technique due to lack of training, cultural differences and management styles.

The differences between the sectors presented a few challenges also. The commercial aviation sector has two main manufacturers and within one manufacturer's product range there is a degree of standardization of cockpit. This results in a simplified simulation layout. The maritime industry does not have a standard navigating bridge layout and, therefore, innovative and creative BRM exercise design is required. Nevertheless, the overriding principles can be implemented during exercises by modifying the learning outcomes. Human–machine interface learning cannot be easily included in the course because of the ubiquity of non-standard equipment. Therefore, training can only be given to enable students to carry out basic ship manoeuvres. Similarly, the aviation industry is highly regulated, with oversight on a regular and continuous basis, whereas the shipping industry, although regulated, includes many vessels that spend long periods on passage, trading worldwide, often in places where regulations cannot be easily enforced. This results in some students attending BRM courses who are not familiar with the importance and need for checklists, pre- and post-planning briefings, and record keeping.

The most challenging aspect of BRM is to impart the ethos that it is an "attitude" course rather than a "technical skills" training course. Some students complete the course not accepting this premise. Seafaring is a traditional occupation which has developed a strong hierarchical ethos over many years. BRM students initially adopt power-centred management styles, and the change from such a culture to a team-based approach presents a strong challenge for BRM lecturers to overcome in a course that is of 4–5 days' duration. Transfer of learning to the workplace is thus jeopardised.

Regarding cultural differences, in aviation, there is a relatively long history of pilots taking recurrent CRM training on an annual or 6-monthly basis. Pilots expect to be presented with situations and simulations that they find challenging. They consider this to be part of a learning process that will increase their competence and enable them to make better decisions as an individual and as part of a team when faced with challenges on the flight deck, both in their daily operations and in emergency situations. They are also aware that all pilots are required to undergo similar challenging training situations in which they will not always succeed. In short, their recurrent CRM training is viewed as part of what makes them better pilots. In the maritime industry, there is not yet a comparable history of recurrent BRM training and trainees may not be as used to being in the classroom or simulator environments as pilots are. The design and delivery of BRM courses should reflect this if training is to be effectively transferred. Trainees should be able to trust in the process of learning. The learning environment should not be viewed as a "test" or "performance measure" aligned with potential structural changes within an organization. Taking part in the learning process should not be equated with risk or threat to job roles or level of seniority. There needs to be a culture shift away from trainees viewing the learning process as a "testing" one which tests and blames individuals for making errors to trainees viewing BRM training to be the "norm" for improving seamanship, just as CRM training is viewed as improving airmanship in aviation. Only then will learning successfully make its way out of the classroom and into the workplace. Only then will trainees be inclined to apply ownership for their sense of responsibility in the safety process in maritime operations as the teaching process intended.

Case Study 2: Aviation to the Process Sector—Human Factors Training

Human factors (HF) training has been mandated in aviation maintenance in Europe since the early 2000s, with all Joint Aviation Authority countries mandated to have implemented regulations by 2005 (Civil Aviation Authority (CAA) 2003). The STAMINA[2] training programme, launched in 2000, was developed to meet the requirement using training developed out of targeted research in aviation maintenance to ensure that the training addressed the key human factors of the sector. STAMINA has been successfully delivered to the industry ever since and has been recognised as an industry benchmark for human factors training.

The STAMINA BPM project[3] was tasked with translating the STAMINA innovation from aviation to the bio-pharmaceutical manufacturing (BPM) sector (Koumadatis et al. 2011). The challenge was not to lose the benefit of the research and development work carried out in the original project, while at the same time ensuring that the new programme effectively addressed the context of the new sector. The project initially carried out an in-depth study of the BPM sector. This comprised interviews, focus groups, surveys, analysis of incident data and reviews

---

[2]Funded under the EC Leonardo Da Vinci programme. See for more details: https://www.tcd.ie/cihs/trainingconsultancy/training/.

[3]Funded under the EC Leonardo Da Vinci programme LLP/LV/TOI/2009/IRL-512.

of documentation and regulations. Only when this research was completed was the BPM version of the training developed. An exhaustive analysis of the differences between the sectors is not possible here. But we can highlight a few of the critical differences and their impact.

Challenges in Transferring HF Training to the Bio-pharmaceutical Sector

The regulatory regimes in the two sectors are very different. In aviation, there are relatively harmonised international regulations explicitly addressing human factors—e.g. more than 10 different requirements cover topics such as human factors training, shift-handover procedures, etc. In the bio-pharmaceutical sector, the regulations are not effectively harmonized internationally and contain little or no reference to human factors. One of the key implications is that the two sectors have a fundamentally different reaction to the concept of deviation from procedures. Within aviation it has long been recognised, and has been established by research, that deviations from operating procedures occur and that they generally happen with good intentions—to solve operational problems such as limited resources or competing requirements of concurrent tasks. The sector has adopted a relatively open approach to deviation, where reporting of deviations is encouraged to enable the underlying operational problems to be addressed. By contrast, the regulatory regime in the bio-pharmaceutical sector is much more punitive on deviations, and companies are very reluctant to discuss deviations, much less admit them and share data on them.

A clear implication from this for training was that non-conformance with procedures had to be much more sensitively addressed in the BPM training, with a reduced expectation of open interaction from trainees (including trainees offering any examples from their daily work). There was also an implication for training targeted at regulators to make them aware of the implications of their approach on human factor practice. This, however, was beyond the scope of the project.

A second implication of the lack of a human factors mandate in the regulation was that a different approach to promoting the training was required. In aviation, companies know they have to invest in human factors training (it is mandated); the challenge is to persuade them of the merits of investing in one training product over another. In the pharmaceutical sector, the promotion needed to be more directly on the value of the training itself in helping the organization meet its quality and safety goals. Since there is no industry-standard format or duration, there was much more focus on the length and methodology of the course—with pressure to shorten it and deliver it online.

A final noteworthy difference between the sectors is the nature of the core activity, and the role of humans within it. Aviation maintenance is a human-driven activity; much technology is used but it is humans who generally control the scheduling of the activity. Tasks can be scheduled and paced to suit shift patterns, tool availability etc. Pharmaceutical manufacturing, by contrast, is a process-driven activity. The timing, pattern and duration of tasks are determined by the nature of the chemical process and the design and programming of the processing equipment. With increased automation, the role of the human is increasingly restricted to a passive one of monitoring. This has implications for the relevant human factors to be focused on in the training. Increased emphasis needed to be given to the challenges of monitoring and maintaining situational awareness of the chemical process as much as the operational process.

From the two case studies (above), we can clearly see what motivates the transfer of safety and knowledge across sectors and how this transfer comes about. However, what about how to approach the transfer and what can current research initiatives on transferring innovation and learning contribute?

How to Approach Transferring Innovation and Learning

The impetus to transfer innovation and learning from one sector to another may come from the *bottom up* ("We need something to help us tackle this problem we are experiencing, let's look to other sectors to see how they are handling it") or it may be *top-down* ("*x* tool or method works well in *y* sector, we should transfer it to our sector"). Going back to the practical examples at the beginning of the chapter, the *bottom-up* approach is represented in Shane's impetus to transfer innovation. His is a problem focuses where he wants to solve a challenge by transferring learning and innovation from another sector. The *top-down* approach aligns with Yvonne's impetus. Hers is an opportunity focuses—looking for an opportunity to transfer a tool or an approach that has been effective in another sector. Either way, Shane and Yvonne will typically have to engage in one of two activities at the outset of their efforts to transfer innovation and learning across sectors, irrespective of their approach. These activities are sector profiling and challenge identification.

Sector Profiling

The EXCROSS[4] (Exploiting safety results a CROSS transportation modes) project was an EU-funded project to enhance cross-fertilization and synergy between safety research initiatives in various transportation modes (maritime, road, rail, aviation). The project was focused on addressing the fragmentation of safety initiatives in the different transportation modes, with little cross-domain learning and sharing of experience. The project, in seeking to identify opportunities for synergy in terms of

---

[4]EXCROSS was a Supporting Action funded by the European Commission under the Seventh Framework Programme (FP7/2007-2013). Grant Agreement n° TCS1-GA-2011-284895.

incident/accident reporting and analysis, noted stark contrasts in the way adverse events are viewed or categorized—e.g. what is considered a reportable event in one sector is not in another. The authors of the project's final report (EXCROSS 2014) state that the potential to transfer a tool or technique from one domain to another for incident/accident reporting and analysis is "strictly related to the domain structural characteristics" (p. 45), and they identified four dimensions upon which a sector can be plotted. Their proposition is that if the "departure" sector differs too widely from the "arrival" sector on these dimensions the transfer of the tool or technique will not be successful or possible. These four dimensions to define the structural characteristics of a domain are:

Degree of centralization as determined by the way the domains are regulated and managed; highly centralized domains are regulated by international agencies and bodies that oversee the whole industry, while in less centralized domains standards and rules can differ from nation to nation or from industry to industry.

Degree of standardization this reflects the regulatory framework and the standards existing in the domain. Technical requirements, infrastructure and organizational processes are strictly defined and regulated in highly standardized sectors.

Safety indicators relates to the presence of reliable and consistent ways to evaluate and monitor the safety performance. Transport modes can then be differentiated on the basis of the availability of a shared set of safety indicators (consistent definition vs. highly differentiated), quality of indicators (trustworthy vs. untrustworthy), and quality of the measurement tools (trustworthy vs. untrustworthy; harmonised vs. heterogeneous).

Safety culture maturity reflects the approach that each organization/domain has with respect to safety, from a pathological level to a generative level (Hudson 2007). High safety culture maturity is associated to "just culture"—an atmosphere of trust in which people are encouraged to provide essential safety-related information, but in which they are also clear about where the line must be drawn between acceptable and unacceptable behaviour.

[adapted from EXCROSS 2014]

The tenet of this approach is that in order for transfer to be successful you must first properly, and fully, understand the characteristics of the two sectors implicated.

Identifying the Challenges

The examination of the structural characteristics of the "departure" and "arrival" sectors as detailed above is necessary to understand the high-level challenges of the transfer project. However, the transfer project itself will need a more detailed profiling of the types of challenges that the "departure" sector is facing. If a tool or solution is being transferred from one sector to another it is important to identify the challenges that it should address. MacLachlan et al. (2014) proposed a "nested" model of organizational issues in the maritime domain which builds upon the

STAMINA model (Koumaditis et al. 2011) developed in the aviation sector. This is a useful framework for this analysis and posits five levels of sector analysis to identify challenges:

1. The task
2. The individual
3. The team
4. The organization
5. The industry.

The fundamental level of analysis is that of the task. A thorough understanding of transfer challenges needs a thorough understanding of the key task(s) in the target sector—their duration and complexity, their physical, cognitive, information and coordination requirements, the critical decision points and bottlenecks in the process. There are many methodologies for task and process analysis. Generally they focus on particular dimensions of the task (e.g. training requirements or interface design) and have limited usefulness outside of that. Some approaches to task/process modelling are being developed that facilitate a much richer account of the psychological, social and organizational dimensions of the task (e.g. Leva et al. 2009).

The second level of analysis is the individual. This level focuses on the demands placed on the individual in a particular sector as well as the challenges that individual limitations place on performance of key tasks. The relevance of fatigue, stress, distraction, perceptual ability, boredom, etc. needs to be established. A distinctive feature of the maritime sector is the extended periods of time spent at sea, away from family and friends. This is present in a few other sectors (save perhaps offshore oil).

The third level of analysis is the team. The structure and functioning of teams differ greatly across sectors and a thorough analysis of team structure is needed to appreciate the specific challenges it presents. In aviation flight operations, the flight crew form a coherent team who interact with cabin crew and air traffic control teams for the duration of a flight or shift and then disband to re-form in the next shift, perhaps, with a different configuration. Communication and coordination within these teams is critical. In aviation maintenance teams are often less stable across shifts, forming and dispersing as the work requires. The major coordination challenges are often between rather than within teams (Baranzini and Cromie 2002).

The fourth level of analysis is the organization. At this level, it is important to get an appreciation both of the "hard" elements of the organization—the structure of the organization, its policies and procedures, and the "soft" elements—the culture of the organization, how things really work on the ground. In this way, a comprehensive picture of the normal operational practices of the organization can be produced—detailing the official way of doing things as prescribed in policies and the actual way things normally happen.

The fifth level of analysis is the industry. This deals with the way in which a sector is composed at a national and international level. The composition and remit of national and international regulatory bodies can radically change how an industry functions and how individual organizations are held to account. This is the final element of the systems model of analysis that can assist in identifying challenges.

A Structured Methodology

Sector profiling, it could be argued, relates most closely to a bottom-up approach to transfer, where a desire to resolve an operational problem drives a search for solutions in other sectors with similar characteristics. Identifying challenges, similarly, could be viewed as being more closely aligned with a top-down approach to transfer, where the desire to transfer a tool necessitates an investigation of the challenges it might address. Irrespective, these two main approaches to transferring innovation and learning, outlined above, constitute the "lessons learned" from years of applied research on transferring innovation from one sector to another. Building on this wealth of experience the SEAHORSE[5] project has advanced a structured methodology for transferring learning and innovation (Liston et al. 2016). The SEAHORSE project is a research and development project funded by the EU which aims to transfer safety technology from the aviation sector to the maritime sector. This project will finish in late 2016 and is currently finalizing the implementation plan for the transfer of aviation solutions such as Mandatory Occurrence Reports (MOR) to meet identified needs regarding standardization, transnational regulation, reporting culture and command conflict. These needs were specified in a scenario highlighting the lack of a common system to help operators learn from risk and hazard reports within their own fleet or from incidents within the wider maritime community.

The project has developed a theoretical approach to transferring learning/innovation across sectors which has a systemic basis. This approach has three broad steps:

1. *Comparison*: Comprehensively comparing the sectors involved to establish a common database of safety dimensions and sector characteristics—this looks at the entire socio-technical system, not solely those parts of the system in which problems are currently presenting.
2. *Match*: The comparison provides information on the needs of the "destination" sector and the potential offering of the "departure" sector. This is the input to matching the safety needs of one domain with the successful solutions implemented in the other domain. The identification of successful solutions in the departure destination is comprehensive and not limited a priori. Part of this process involves the specification of scenarios which are practical instantiations of a particular need.

---

[5]SEAHORSE is a research project funded by the European Community's Seventh Framework Programme (FP7-SST-2013-RTD-1). Grant Agreement n° SCP-GA-2013-605639.

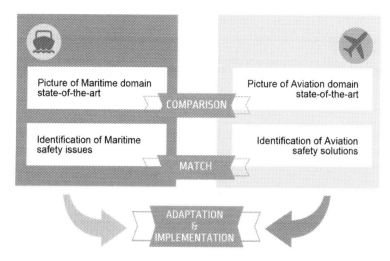

Fig. 1 A theoretical approach to cross-sector transfer from aviation to maritime. Adapted from Liston et al. (2016)

3. ***Adaptation and Implementation***: Those solutions which match the identified needs are then adapted and implemented in a systematic manner, taking into account the impact on other parts of the system also.

A cross-sector transfer of learning has to begin with a common overview of the characteristics of both sectors (a comprehensive overview of operational demands, sector characteristics and safety needs). This systematic comparison (like for like) can then act as the framework to inform the matching of safety needs from one sector with the successfully implemented solutions (targeting the same safety needs) of the other sector. This results in solutions from another sector being mapped onto the safety needs of the targeted sector. The final step then is to perform a principled adaptation and implementation based on the information gathered in the previous two stages. Figure 1 represents the approach.

While the adaptation and implementation of the SEAHORSE solution transfer is not yet complete, it is clear that this project has adopted a bottom-up and top-down approach (identifying problems and needs to be satisfied, while simultaneously identifying a comprehensive database of solutions which could be transferred) as part of a systematic approach to transferring learning across sectors. In practice, this approach has many more sub-steps—reflecting the complexity of seeking to comprehensively understand two distinct socio-technical systems. The mapping of potential candidate solutions from one sector to address safety needs in another sector is, especially, challenging as it involves an atypical gap analysis. Usually gap analyses are performed on a single process or system and the gaps represent the difference between how the system currently performs or operates and how it might operate in the future following the introduction of a new tool or process. In this instance, however, it is necessary to perform a gap analysis comparing one sector's sectorial characteristics or its handling of an issue with another sector. These are challenges of performing a principled analysis of two domains and their safety needs, and while they should not be underestimated, the final task, adaptation and implementation, is key to the success of any transfer project.

Discussion

There is clearly a strong demand for cross-sector learning in safety-critical industries—sometimes this demand can be met within the sector (aviation has many examples of innovation transferring from one part of the sector to another). This chapter interrogated the two dominant existing approaches to transfer—sector profiling and identifying the challenges—and it has also examined a number of case studies of tools and techniques that have been transferred across sectors. In addition, a new, systematic and systemic approach to transfer has been described. This approach, based on the research being carried out in the SEAHORSE project, advocates the use of both sector profiling and identification of challenges (conducted at a systemic level, in a principled, systematic manner) in addition to a comprehensive adaptation and implementation phase. The key message from this twin-pronged approach is borne out by two case studies. While BRM might have been developed as a response to shortcomings in the competence of maritime personnel to manage resources and crises situations (Barnett et al. 2003), it does not necessarily follow that the transfer from CRM has been successful. Indeed, recent research by O'Connor (2011) on the effectiveness of BRM in the US Navy has suggested that the training was not achieving impact in relation to knowledge and skills (when compared to impacts achieved for similar courses in aviation), possibly because a formal sector needs assessment had not been carried out prior to the training and what the US Navy required in terms of training was not what BRM could provide. This is a stark reminder of the importance of interrogating both the requirements of the sector and the challenges being faced. Just because the challenges faced by two sectors are similar does not mean that what they need as an intervention or solution should be the same. The sector characteristics have a mediating role on the effectiveness of a transfer, even when the sectors share the same challenges. Just because aviation and maritime share a problem with workarounds and procedural deviations does not mean that the intervention to solve the problem should be the same. The characteristics of the sector have too strong a role to be sidelined in any transfer project.

This is borne out by the experience of transferring HF training from the aviation maintenance sector to the bio-pharmaceutical sector. Part of the transfer process of STAMINA involved understanding the requirements of the bio-pharmaceutical sector. Only when this was complete was the adaptation and customization work undertaken. While there is no extensive evaluation data of the transfer of STAMINA-BPM, trainee feedback data suggest the course is perceived positively by both staff and management (Ross 2012). It should be noted that the effectiveness of the adaptation and customization activities was influenced positively by the fact that the training developers had extensive experience of developing (and performing); the training in the aviation sector and, armed with the newfound information about the needs of the "arrival" sector, was able to systematically tailor the training.

The contrast between how these two transfer projects (BRM and STAMINA-BPM) were approached reflects not just the departure points of the two approaches but how, in the absence of a standardized methodology, an ad hoc approach can bring about mixed results. Sector profiling relates to bottom-up approaches to transfer—those instances in which operational problems drive a search for solutions in other sectors with similar characteristics. Starting from the task of identifying challenges relates most closely to top-down approaches to transfer—those instances in which the attractiveness of the tool itself drives an investigation of the challenges it might address.

The approach being developed by Liston et al. (2016) following the work in the SEAHORSE project provides a new focal point for best practice in learning and knowledge transfer. This new approach posits that only by examining both needs and challenges can the prerequisites for performing a comprehensive adaptation and customization be provided. Armed with this data, and a comprehensive methodology, it is hoped that the effectiveness of future transfer projects will be assured.

Future Directions

A key area for overlap between future operations in both the maritime and aviation industries is that of collaborative decision making. In aviation, there is a move towards Airport Collaborative Decision Making (A-CDM) so that the movement of aircraft in European airspace is more efficient and predictable. This allows for optimum levels of planning and anticipation of where aircraft are now and where they are likely to be in the future. This is especially important with the growth of air travel and the scarcity of airport resources for time slots, runways, terminal gates etc. Corrigan et al. (2014) highlight a number of the key challenges involved in implementing and evaluating the relative success of A-CDM. A-CDM is a plan to get all relevant stakeholders involved in managing the throughput of aircraft through airports talking to one another, working towards common goals (i.e. getting the aircraft in and out of the airports as efficiently and as safely as possible). This plan has been driven by the industry regulators EUROCONTROL, IATA (International Airport Transport System) and CANSO (Civil Aviation Navigation Services Organisation). Corrigan et al. (2014) highlight the importance of the common goal. In A-CDM, this was viewed as the turnaround process. This is also where the potential for improved efficiency and safety could be applied to maritime operations.

In particular, Corrigan et al. discuss how critical the "take off blocks time" (TOBT) is for stakeholders. This is the time when the aircraft is ready (with doors closed) to leave the terminal gate for push back to the runway. All stakeholders stated that the TOBT was the main reference point that everyone was working towards. This was also the time that they measured their own performance against and how they anticipated their future interaction with other stakeholders. The turnaround process in port can be a very busy time (especially for the captain) and is also the time that some of the crew often look forwards to catching up on rest. It would be much more feasible for crew to plan for separation of rest/active duty in port. If the interaction with stakeholders for port logistics (such as customs, harbour master, refuelling, cargo loading and unloading, ship supply deliveries, shipping companies, staff changeovers etc.) could be coordinated so that everyone is working towards the same "ship-out-of-port-time", potential benefits of a safer, more efficient turnaround process could be achieved as well as a reduction in workload and stress, and an increase in rest time for crew could potentially be realized. Corrigan et al. (2014) outline the necessary investment in infrastructure for stakeholders to be able to communicate with one another. They also stress that appropriate training on communication and on the operational process needs to be addressed in the learning process for all stakeholders. Stakeholders placed huge emphasis on the benefits of immersing themselves in other stakeholders' shoes, e.g. for ground handling crew to realize what was important for air traffic control, pilots and airports to be able to do their job and contribute to the TOBT. Feedback on this training highlighted the benefit of "operationalizing" the classroom content and making it relevant to their own role within a larger systems perspective. This implementation of A-CDM was successful for competitors working alongside one another, which would also be relevant for maritime port operations. Due consideration should be given to who would regulate such port collaborative decision making and how it could be implemented for the benefit of all relevant stakeholders.

References

Baranzini, D., & Cromie, S. (2002, September 16–29). *Team systems in aviation maintenance: Interaction and co-ordination across work teams*. 25th European Association for Aviation Psychology (EAAP) Conference, Warsaw, Poland.

Barnett, M., Gatfield, D., & Pekcan, C. (2003 October). *A research agenda in maritime crew resource management*. Proceedings of the International Conference on Team Resource Management in the 21st Century, Daytona Beach, Florida.

Civil Aviation Authority (CAA) (2003) *CAP 716 Aviation maintenance human factors (EASA/JAR145 approved organisations). Guidance material on the UK CAA interpretation of Part-145 Human Factors and Error Management Requirements*. UK: CAA.

Corrigan, S., Mårtensson, L., Kay, A., Okwir, S., Ulfvengren, P., & McDonald, N. (2014). Preparing for Airport Collaborative Decision Making (A-CDM) implementation: An evaluation and recommendations. *Journal of Cognition, Technology & Work, 17*(2), 207–218.

EXCROSS. (2014). *D4.3 Final report on synergies and opportunities*. Report to the European Commission under the Seventh Framework Programme (FP7/2007-2013). TCS1-GA-2011-284895. Retrieved from http://www.excross.eu/pdf/EXCROSS_D4.3_Final_Report_on_Synergies_Opportunities_v6.pdf

Grant, J. (2014, August 28). *Malaysia Airlines cleared for radical restructuring*. Financial Times. Retrieved from: http://www.ft.com/intl/cms/s/0/6d0b6c6c-2e68-11e4-b330-00144feabdc0. html#axzz3U0ZawoJq

Guldenmund, F. W. (2000). The nature of safety culture: A review of theory and research. *Safety Science, 34*(1), 215–257.

Hetherington, C., Flin, R., & Mearns, K. (2006). Safety in shipping: The human element. *Journal of Safety Research, 37*(4), 401–411.

Hofstede, G., Hofstede, G. J., & Minkov, M. (2010). *Cultures and organizations: Software of the mind* (3rd ed.). New York: McGraw-Hill.

Hudson, P. (2007). Implementing safety culture in a major multi-national. *Safety Science, 45*, 697–722.

International Civil Aviation Organisation. (2013). *Doc 9859—safety management manual*. Retrieved from http://www.skybrary.aero/index.php/ICAO_Safety_Management_Manual_Doc_9859

International Maritime Organisation. (1995). *Seafarer's training, certification and watchkeeping code (STCW Code)*. London: IMO.

International Maritime Organisation. (2003). *MSC 77/17—role of the human element*. London: IMO.

Kavanagh, W. (2008, March 27–30). *Bridge resource management for pilots*. Proceedings: International Simulator Lecturer's Conference, St. John's, Newfoundland, Canada.

Kosnik, L. K., Brown, J., & Maund, T. (2007). Patient safety: Learning from the aviation industry. *Nursing Management, 38*(1), 25–30.

Koumaditis K., Themistocleous, M., Byrne, P., Ross, D., Cromie, S., & Corrigan, S. (2011). Investigating human factors in biotechnology and pharmaceutical manufacturing industries. In *European, Mediterranean & Middle Eastern Conference on Information Systems* (pp. 294–305). Retrieved from: http://www.tara.tcd.ie/handle/2262/56902

Leva, M. C., Kay, A. M., Mattei, F., Kontogiannis, T., Ambroggi, M., & Cromie, S. (2009). A dynamic task representation method for a virtual reality application. In *Engineering psychology and cognitive ergonomics*, Berlin Heidelberg: Springer. Retrieved from: http://dl. acm.org/citation.cfm?id=1611181.1611186

Liston, P. M., Silvagni, S., & Ducci, M. (2016). *Safety transfer methodology (STEM)—a structured methodology for transferring safety innovation across sectors*. Manuscript in preparation.

MacLachlan, M., Cromie, S., Liston, P., Kavanagh, B. & Kay, A. (2014) Psychosocial and organisational aspects. In T. Carter & A. Schreiner (Eds.). *Textbook of maritime medicine* (2nd ed., pp. 178–194). Bergen: Norwegian Centre for Maritime Medicine.

O'Connor, P. (2011). An evaluation of the effectiveness of bridge resource management training. *International Journal of Aviation Psychology, 21*(4), 357–374.

Padova, A. (2013). *Safety management systems: A better approach for transportation?* Canadian Parliamentary Information and Research Service. Retrieved from http://www.lop.parl.gc.ca/content/lop/ResearchPublications/2013-77-e.htm

Parker, D., Lawrie, M., & Hudson, P. (2006). A framework for understanding the development of organisational safety culture. *Safety Science, 44*, 551–562.

Pedersen, L. M., Nielsen, K. J., & Kines, P. (2012). Realistic evaluation as a new way to design and evaluate occupational safety interventions. *Safety Science, 50*(1), 48–54.

Reason, J. (1997). *Managing the risks of organizational accidents*. Aldershot: Ashgate. ISBN 1840141042.

Ross, D. (2012). *Deliverable report into design, development, delivery and evaluation of the training course human factors in biotechnology and pharmaceutical manufacturing*. Unpublished report, TCD.

Schein, E. H. (1992). *Organizational culture and leadership*. San Francisco: Jossey-Bass.

Stahel, P. F. (2008). Learning from aviation safety: a call for formal "readbacks" in surgery. *Patient Safety in Surgery, 2*, 21.

Thomas, M. J. W. (2012). *A systematic review of the effectiveness of safety management systems.* Australian Transport Safety Bureau, Report No. AR-2011-148, ISBN 978-1-74251-303-4. Australia: ATSB.

Ward, M., McDonald, N., Morrison, R., Gaynor, D., & Nugent, A. (2010). A performance improvement case study in aircraft maintenance and its implications for hazard identification. *Ergonomics, 53*(2), 247–267.

Wauben, L. S., Lange, J. F., & Goossens, R. H. (2012). Learning from aviation to improve safety in the operating room: A systematic literature review. *Journal of Healthcare Engineering, 3*(3), 373–390.

Weick, K. E., & Sutcliffe, K. M. (2001). *Managing the unexpected: Assuring high performance in an age of complexity.* San Francisco, CA: Jossey-Bass.

Wilf-Miron, R., Lewenhoff, I., Benyamini, Z., & Aviram, A. (2003). From aviation to medicine: Applying concepts of aviation safety to risk management in ambulatory care. *Quality and Safety in Health Care, 12*(1), 35–39.

Young, M. S., Stanton, N. A., & Harris, D. (2007). Driving automation: Learning from aviation about design philosophies. *International Journal of Vehicle Design, 45*(3), 323–338.

The Psychology of Ship Architecture and Design

Margareta Lützhöft, Erik Styhr Petersen
and Apsara Abeysiriwardhane

Introduction

Early studies into the effects of design on behaviour were conducted on Norwegian ships in the 1970s, when *M/S Hoegh Mistral* and *M/S Hoegh Multina* were subject to action research (1970–1975) and *M/S Balao* was designed in cooperation between social researchers, architects and naval engineers (Johansen 1978; Lezaun 2011). On the two Hoegh ships, the aim was to develop a stimulating working situation by increasing autonomy and changing roles on board—including reducing status differences between officers and ratings. The aim of the *M/S Balao* was similar, but included the physical domain: to construct a physical artefact (the ship as a home and workplace) that would support a democratic mini society on board. There was in those days low morale on board the fleets of Northern Europe, allegedly due to hierarchically organized work, intense work schedules and tensions between crew members—leading to stress symptoms, injuries, high crew turnover and low effectiveness. The results of these interventions were positive, but no more studies followed, as we will discuss later.

State of the Practice: Ship Design and Ship Designers

Modern ship design is complex; the bill of materials of a ship counts in the millions of parts. For this reason alone, the process of designing a ship necessarily must involve a large team of diverse specialists; the complexity is, however, not only in the numbers, but also in the particular disciplines which contribute.

M. Lützhöft (✉) · E.S. Petersen · A. Abeysiriwardhane
Australian Maritime College, University of Tasmania, Launceston TAS 7250,
Tasmania, Australia
e-mail: margareta.lutzhoft@utas.edu.au

© Springer International Publishing Switzerland 2017   69
M. MacLachlan (ed.), *Maritime Psychology*, DOI 10.1007/978-3-319-45430-6_4

Consider, as a starting point, the discipline of naval architecture. In a sense comparable to the architects working on land, the primary undertaking of the naval architect is to be responsible for the main characteristics of a ship, i.e. the size, speed, stability, manoeuvrability, cargo carrying properties, exterior and interior design, to mention some of the primary aspects of naval architecture. In terms of process, the naval architects usually follow the Ship Design Spiral (Fig. 1) concept to be successful in their ship designs. The design spiral is generally an iterative process, which starts with a preliminary design, which in turn evolves to become the final design, ready for construction. Naval architects use the design spiral concept to design the exterior of the ship, to provide the basic arrangement of the compartments inside the ship, and to determine the size and shape of the hull. Relevant to the psychology of ship design, the naval architect decides on the size and position of the rooms in which the crew will live and work, commonly in the superstructure of the ship and around the engine room. They often indicate the detailed interior arrangement of such rooms; initial layouts are, however, often refined during the subsequent design processes. She or he furthermore makes preliminary estimates of speed and propulsion resistance of the hull, ship stability, seakeeping characteristics, manoeuvring properties, the weight of the ship, the cargo and consumables like fuel

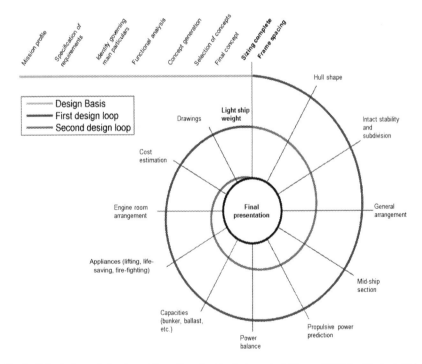

Fig. 1 Ship design spiral, adapted from Evan's ship design spiral (Evans 1959) by Linda de Vries and Per Hogström at Chalmers Technical University. Used with permission

and water on board during a voyage, and balances these properties against trading requirements and building costs for the particular ship.

It is worthwhile to note that most ship designs are bespoke, in the sense that only very few ships are built to a particular design; indeed, a design may be just for one particular ship; a series of 12 ships is considered long, and a series of 48 ships or more is seldom, if ever, seen. If a series is built, the sister ship will only very rarely be entirely identical, as refinement or even redesign takes place as the series is built, based on lessons learned with the previous ship/s.

Once the preliminary design of a new ship is in place, more detailed design activities can start, usually utilizing iterative design processes of subsystems or subassemblies, which in terms of methodology are comparable to the ship design spiral, but which involve many more specialist disciplines than naval architecture. Traditionally, a ship design—and a ship design office—is divided into the main divisions of hull, machinery and outfit. Structural engineers deal with the structural design of the hull, marine engineers usually deal with machinery, often aided by electrical engineers for the design of electrical power generation and distribution systems, while "the rest" of the ship usually is dealt with by a mixture of engineering disciplines involving hydraulics, pneumatics, electronics, ventilation and heating—indeed all the disciplines one would see in the design and construction of a middle-sized village, which is a fair comparison, when the complexity of a modern ship is understood. Furthermore, comparable to the design and construction practice of onshore facilities, each of the maritime designers involved in a particular ship design usually builds up the onboard systems from a core of readily available equipment, devices and components—there is a vast number of maritime subsuppliers, each specializing within niches; one is producing navigation equipment, one is producing pumps, one is producing remotely controlled valves. In turn, these products are also designed and developed iteratively by engineers of various disciplines; indeed, the design of a maritime radar system involves physics, mechanics, electronics and software—all engineering disciplines. For the modern ship, it is interesting to note that such subsupplies overwhelmingly are what is called COTS—commercial off-the-shelf—in other words, such subsystems are seldom made to order, but are chosen from what is available in the market matching the specification of the particular—bespoke—ship.

Consider, in this context, the example of the design of the Engine Control Room (ECR) of a new ship, the ECR being the facility from which the entire number and diversity of engine systems of a modern ship is monitored, controlled and supervised. The size and position of the ECR, as well as the overall layout of this work space, is in most cases decided upon by the naval architect when going through the first few iterations of the preliminary design phase—*en passant* noting that the space requirement for the ECR will be competing with the space needed for the machinery as well as for the cargo of the ship; maximizing the cargo space supports the profitability of the design. While preparing the plans for this part of the ship, she or he will indicate the expected size and position of the largest and most important components to be included, like the main electrical switchboard and the main ECR console, the latter which hosts the plethora of devices, computer monitors and control panels required to operate the machinery plant. The selection, however, of each of these systems is in the hands of the design engineers who are focusing on the various subsystems in the ship: the tank gauging system may well be decided upon by the engineer responsible for the bunkering and fuel oil transfer system, while the main engine control system may be decided upon by the marine engineer responsible for choosing the main engine and providing the basic design of the engine room. The power management system, which is a core component when it comes to managing and supervising the production of electrical power, could well be decided upon by the electrical engineer designing the main electrical switch-board, and the lubrication oil purifier remote control system could be part of the hardware package provided by that particular manufacturer. To compound the challenges of the psychology of ship design, all these individual control panels, which often have an interactive dimension, may end up being positioned in the main ECR console by a rather junior mechanical engineer. As will be elaborated in the following sections, such a design engineer will very likely have little or no direct experience with seagoing ships, marine engineering practice or first-hand knowledge about the operation of a large ship, for which reason the order and relevance of the individual position of the various controls in such a console may be somewhat arbitrary. Actually, under these circumstances of a limited size of the ECR, and thus the console in question, and a limited budget, the design target for the console designer could well be the one of space optimization, attempting to squeeze as much as possible into as little space as possible, function and logical interrelations aside. In any case, even if the console designer was informed by human factors, and acted upon this according to best practice, the differences in look, feel, interaction paradigms and even the alarm indication concepts of the individual devices are entirely beyond his control: such properties were decided by the design engineers working with the particular subsupplier of each component, and being the manufacturers' standard, they will not have been experientially adapted to the (bespoke) ship.

State of Knowledge

The Psychology of Ship Design

The anecdotal background provided above provides a natural starting point for a more formal discussion of the state of the knowledge of the psychology of ship design. Presently, ships appear to be designed without fully taking account of the ideas put forth by ergonomics. Lützhöft and colleagues (Lützhöft 2004) found that there is considerable room for improvement, especially with respect to the use of maritime Human Factors (HF) knowledge and Human-Centred Design (HCD) (Petersen et al. 2010; Petersen and Lützhöft 2009). In the ship design process, HF is considered to be the discipline which deals with the psychological and physical aspects of the interaction between the human and the ship systems (technical or procedural). HF can, depending on the vantage point and teleology of the beholder, equally well be identified as a scientific or an engineering discipline; irrespectively, the concern is with the analysis, research, development, design and evaluation of man/man, man/machine, and man/environment interfaces.

As outlined above, a ship is a complex human–machine system, an interwoven set of sociotechnical systems, and human interaction is a crucial factor for the safe and efficient operation of the ship. However, the gap between human and system is continually increasing due to the lack of appropriate HF consideration when introducing (new) complex technological systems, integrated computer systems and the automation of machinery, and there is a growing realization within certain parts of the maritime scientific community that consideration of HF issues is vital (Beevis et al. 2000; Grech et al. 2008; McSweeney et al. 2009). However, the uptake appears to be slow. The National Transportation Safety Board (NTSB) report on the grounding of the *Royal Majesty* (NTSB 1997) stated that "Thus, while human engineering is a known concept in the marine industry, there have not been any unifying efforts to integrate this concept into the marine engineering and manufacturing sector" (p. 40), and unfortunately the finding in the NTSB report on the *Royal Majesty* yet remains to be addressed at the time of writing (2015); indeed, no radical changes in either the mandatory rules and regulations or in the maritime design culture and practice can be clearly seen presently. On the subject of de facto inclusion of HF in marine design, only very few examples are available in the published literature (Koester 2005; Petersen et al. 2010).

It has been estimated that 60–80 % of all accidents at sea are the result of "operator error" and that this costs the maritime industry around US$541 million a year (Alert! 2003; UK P&I CLUB 2003). In terms of the psychology of ship design, the notion of "operator error" is, however, but a symptom (Dekker 2002; Grech et al. 2008), and its underlying causes are often found to be related to HF issues, including the shortcomings of training, communication, procedures and design (Alert! 2003). According to Walker (2011), the root cause of "operator errors" can often be traced back to the design and construction stages of a ship, primarily because the operator is excluded from the design process (Lützhöft et al. 2011). Insufficient integration of HF in design may translate into poorer operations, higher training costs, and an increased risk of failing at the task (Holden et al. 2013). Conversely, the application of HF knowledge can lead to better design, and facilitate the understanding of practical problems and their solutions (Norros 2014), helping to improve many dimensions, such as the habitability, maintainability, workability, controllability, manoeuvrability, survivability, safety, occupational health and emergency response, security, usability, reliability, supportability, acceptability, and affordability of the ship (Alert! 2004, 2010; Hemmen 2003; Lloyd's Register 2008). Overall, HF practice is believed to benefit the employee in terms of being a prerequisite for improved well-being and therefore for doing a better and more effective job, as well as being to the benefit of the employer in terms of improved work performance of individuals and groups in the organization (Grech et al. 2008; Ross 2009)—crew retention notwithstanding.

The Potential of Ship Psychology

Barker and Wright's theory about behaviour settings (1949), in which certain settings are posited to evoke certain behaviours, and where the environment provides cues for action, is a forerunner to the approaches that today are relevant to the psychology of ship design. Three such strands of behavioural effects are considered below: design for support of (a) democratic action, (b) emotive design to combat stress, and (c) design to increase mental well-being.

In the Hoegh experiments (mentioned in the introduction), the main outcome was "lessons learned," which were implemented in the next step, the *M/S Balao* project. The "lessons" included reorganization of work planning meetings to reduce onboard bureaucracy. At the time, the *M/S Balao* project was a completely new concept; no one at the time seemed to take into account a relationship between physical design and the social psychology of shipboard life (Lezaun 2011). During the 1970s and 1980s shipyards were in control of the design, as it was a seller's market. The only areas available for redesign in such series of ships, given these constraints, were the accommodation areas, and it was decided to focus on these areas, for socialization and private habitation. The idea was to dismantle traditional hierarchies and generate stronger social bonds across the entire crew. For this reason, the number of hallways was reduced and joint recreation spaces were included. A single mess room for all crew ranks replaced the earlier divided ones, and after dinner people would move via the joint coffee lounge to the shared dayroom. In the cabins, an effort was made to remove status symbols and other differences—leading to mostly same-sized cabins built with similar materials, furnishings and windows in all cabins. The joint mess room had been one of the largest worries of the crew, but after a few months in operation, there were only positive reactions.

However, the results of the *M/S Balao* project were mixed. On board, the democratic society did indeed flourish, with radical changes to the traditional hierarchies and ways of working, and the project is summarized as having "... been able to ... achieve job enlargement, job enrichment and ... has the properties of a completely new organization" (Johansen 1978, p. 236). The impact on other ships, ship design processes and other organizations was, however, disappointingly limited (Johansen 1978), and—discouragingly—most of the abovementioned challenges still exist today under new labels. Workload, complacency, and human error are challenges which are compounded by the smaller crews of this day and age, amplified by increased demands for communications and administrative work of today's ships, purportedly supported by technologies, more or less automated.

A more recent study comes from cross-disciplinary cooperation. Parker and colleagues identified a number of challenges in the working environment of offshore personnel, which included being away from home for extended periods, being subjected to physical motion, some MSD (Musculoskeletal Disorder) issues and high BMI (Body Mass Index, as an indicator of being overweight) issues as well as matters relating to privacy, sleep quality and fatigue (Parker et al. 1997).

Another example of how to address mental well-being issues in ship design is the RV Investigator, based in Hobart, Tasmania and owned by the Commonwealth Scientific and Industrial Research Organisation (CSIRO) on behalf of the Australian nation. RV Investigator is managed by Australia's Marine National Facility, who utilize the services of a ship management company to crew and operate the vessel. The approach has been to use an Australian initiative called "Beyond Blue"—to combat anxiety and depression. Substantial design efforts went into making spaces suited both for interaction and social life as well as quieter spaces for small meetings, reading or relaxing. Furthermore, the "media room" has space both for watching movies and playing games without disturbing each other. The benefits of the application of HF knowledge to the design of the RV Investigator are yet to be demonstrated, as she has only undertaken her first long voyages in 2015, the results of which are still to be evaluated.

The Psychology of Ship Designers

As with any other group of designers, maritime designers are likely to have their own innovative ideas, which they are interested in implementing while designing new ships and new equipment for ships. However, if these ideas do not satisfy the psychological and operational requirements of the end-users, as appears to be the case in mainstream maritime design today, such innovation may eventually end up with the tag "another poor design" (Rasmussen 2005; Squire 2014; The Nautical Institute 1998). To avoid this, we are suggesting that maritime design practice has to better include the psychology of ship design. The professional knowledge and skill of the maritime designers regarding how ships are designed to support the physiological processes, and the associated cognitive functions of its users, must be recognized to be of paramount importance, in order to get ships and equipment that are really "usable." In other words, the question that confronts all maritime design engineers should be: "How can we design a usable ship taking user requirements more completely into account?" However, this question appears to get insufficient attention; there is no evidence in the public domain to help us address it, and as we have noted above, this oversight may well be related to onboard accidents and injuries.

Improvements to the currently overlooked aspects of the psychology of ship design can only be made if the ship designers initially appreciate that there is such a problem (Petersen 2012; Schein 1996; Weick and Quinn 1999). Unfortunately, most of the design engineers involved in the ship design process seem to be unaware of the psychological and operational dimensions which ships' crew face during their sea time, in spite of an impressive, easily available literature and knowledge on maritime HF (American Bureau of Shipping 2003a, b, 2010). Many researchers have taken efforts to improve the application of ship psychology during designing, and as reported above, practical experiments have also been undertaken and reported several decades ago, but all little general to avail. Widdel and Motz (2000) sought

Table 1 Selected examples of ergonomic requirements (Widdel and Motz 2000)

Category	Ergonomic requirements (one out of each category)
1. Bridge layout	Clear route—A clear route across the wheelhouse from bridge wing to bridge wing should be provided. The width of the passageway should be at least 1.2 m
2. Work environment	Glare avoidance—Care should be taken to avoid glare and stay image reflections in the bridge environment. All prepared surfaces should be glare free
3. Workstation layout	Large charts accommodation—The chart table should have facilities to accommodate charts larger than the table depth, for example a 10 mm slit along front and back edges of the chart table surface
4. Alarms	Modes of alarms—All required alarms should be presented through both visual and auditory means
5. Input devices	Control orientation—All controls associated with ship movement should be located so that the operator faces forward

to determine ergonomic requirements for the design of ship bridges. One major finding of their work was that inappropriate ergonomic interface design, without consideration of HF, is the main reason behind many maritime accidents. They carried out task analysis, questionnaires and interviews with watchkeeping officers, and these data were used to evaluate what mariners are required to have at their disposal to achieve safe and efficient operation of ships. Further, they evaluated different bridges and devices from the mariners' point of view. To make the knowledge gained operational for ship designers, the authors developed a computer program storing all the ergonomic factors in a computer database, to serve as a ship psychology supporting tool and evaluation system for the designers (see Table 1, which contains a minimal set of examples from the five main categories of the database; all told, the database contains 652 ergonomic requirements). However, the literature lacks any reports on the utilization of this knowledge.

Another illustration of the lack of uptake of maritime HF knowledge comes from a survey on habitability, and its implications, carried out for Royal Navy ships by Strong (2000). This study provides valuable indications of personal priorities and preferences for habitability features in naval ship designs, and focuses on non-operational spaces and the living conditions and facilities at sea. The subsequent analysis highlights the requirement of adequate levels of privacy, which is facilitated for individual and social relaxation. One of the major conclusions from this study is to use concepts from social psychology and architectural design to develop criteria for ship accommodation design to reflect significant personal and social needs. However, again there is no reported impact of this knowledge in the literature regarding ship design.

Attempts have been made to disseminate and support the application of the existing psychology of ship design knowledge in the shipping world. A notable example is the Human Element Alert! initiative, driven by the Nautical Institute and sponsored by the Lloyd's Register foundation since 2003. Alert! is centred on a web page[1] and a 4-monthly newsletter, aimed to represent the views of the shipping community and increase awareness of the human element. One particular feature is the centrespread of the newsletter, separately downloadable, summarizing in info-graphic form the topic of the current issue. One of these, number 11, gives an overview of the areas in which the knowledge can be applied. These categories are presently (2015) under revision but the original ones were:

- Habitability
- Maintainability
- Workability
- Controllability
- Manoeuvrability
- Survivability
- System safety
- Occupational health and safety.

One of the benefits of this categorization is the almost self-explanatory terms—managing to combine the needs of work and life on board, physical and mental demands, as well as embracing a systemic view where humans, technology and organization can be regarded and addressed as an integrated system. Yet, also in this case there is lack of evidence of a wider uptake and the application of the psychology of ship design body of knowledge.

Holistically, the lack of awareness of psychology among ship designers is likely due to the combined effects of at least the academic nature, taxonomy and presen-tation of the present maritime HF knowledge base, the poor maritime HF education in naval architecture and engineering courses (Kuo and Houison-Craufurd 2000), and poor "post-design" contact with those who work on board the ships (The Nautical Institute 1998). Moreover, both naval architects and other designers involved in the design of ships and their equipment adhere to particular classification and International Maritime Organization (IMO) regulations[2] throughout the design process. Whether the relevant rules, regulations and recommendations help resolve the problems in designing a ship which can satisfy the psychological and operational requirements of its users is a very important issue that deserves to be systematically addressed. Rasmussen (2005) presents an overview of IMO activities relating to the role of the human element in the design, safety and operation of ships, with the emphasis on what the naval architect could and should be doing. Furthermore, he discusses whether the plethora of rules, regulations and recommendations help to solve the problems in designing and building a ship which can satisfy the

---

[1]http://www.he-alert.org/index.cfm/bulletin/Human-factors.

[2]The sheer number—in the tens of thousands—of maritime rules and regulations preclude any being specifically mentioned here. Reference is made to the home pages of the major classification societies (eagle.org, lr.org, exchange.dnv.com), to the IEC home page for electrotechnical stan-dards applicable to ships (iec.org) and to the IMO home page (imo.org), in all cases both for specific information, but also for anyone interested in getting a firmer understanding of the maritime rules regime.

requirements of its users. His conclusion is that regulations indeed help, but only to a certain extent; regulations do not replace the professional knowledge and maritime HF skill of the designers, which is a necessity to designing ships that are usable. As mentioned in the previous section, the naval architects follow the ship design spiral concept as a golden rule during the design process, but this design methodology focuses exclusively on the ship as a physical artefact, and does not have a focus on work design and human–system integration, and only implicitly assumes the physiological processes and the associated cognitive functions which essentially should be considered during the design phase. In other words, this particular design method does not explicitly consider the needs of the end-user, and thus does not employ HF concepts to their full extent (Calhoun and Stevens 2003).

In summary, maritime designers should be more aware of the particular context of use and the nature and work of the intended users of the equipment they design. Without such an understanding, they will produce designs that are less effective and efficient from the perspective of ship psychology. To those familiar with the engineering community, this should, however, not come as a surprise (Petersen 2012). The remainder of this section will elaborate on how and why design engineers are not naturally inclined towards the "softness" of the psychology of ship design. We also discuss how they are not formally taught such subjects, how engineering is thinking in terms of objects, decomposition and how the handling of uncertainty, all in combination, does not mesh well with traditional maritime HF knowledge. Indeed, the learning and subsequent application of HF knowledge present a serious challenge to the engineering profession—not out of any kind of ill will, or any lack of mental capabilities or faculties, but because humans are different—and these differences, in this case, conceivably are acting as barriers to the successful learning and usage of HF knowledge in system design (Petersen 2012).

Design Engineering Fundamentals

As a starting point, it is important to note that "engineering refers to the practice of organizing the design and construction of any artefact which transforms the physical world around us to meet some recognized need" (Rogers 1983, p. 51), which highlights that design engineering is a practical application, aimed at producing "objects" (Koen 1985, 2003; Petroski 1982; Rogers 1983; Simon 1996; Vincenti 1993). More than anything else, we suggest that appreciating this makes one appreciate that design engineering teleologically is orthogonal to science, and indeed that design engineers are not scientists (Petroski 2010). Design engineering is not a science, but

> … differ[s] from science proper in the way in which it is appropriate to ask whether their theories are true or false. One should ask of the engineering sciences only that they be adequate for the underpinning of our technologies. A theory can be of great practical use for design purposes, yet inadequate from a scientific point of view (Rogers 1983, p. 54).

As it transpires, design engineering is not primarily concerned with the production of knowledge, as is the case for science: "Unlike science, engineering does not seek to model reality, but society's perception of reality, including its myths and prejudices" (Koen 1985, p. 15). The complete focus on artefacts, which is the raison d'etre of design engineering, and their creation, which correspondingly is the raison d'etre of any design engineering organization, resonates with Vincenti's (1993) suggestion that design engineering possesses particular knowledge on two different planes; one which addresses the artefact itself, and one which addresses the design engineering method, or process—a useful division which is also adopted in the foregoing, addressing the psychology of ship design and the psychology of ship designers as separate issues.

The Natural Inclinations of Design Engineering

It is probably true that not everyone is cut out to become a design engineer; like any other discipline, design engineering requires particular skills and inclinations. We believe Gardner's descriptive intelligence is a useful tool in describing the archetypical design engineer from this perspective, starting with Gardner noting that "anyone involved with tangible products of any sort is necessarily using naturalist intelligence" (2006a, p. 38). He elaborates that the archetypical design engineer is gifted with this as well as spatial intelligence, bodily-kinaesthetic intelligence and logical-mathematical intelligence (Gardner 2006a, b).

The naturalistic intelligence, which builds on pattern recognition, gives design engineering the capability to discriminate between seemingly similar constructs, spanning functions and brands, while the spatial intelligence provides the capability to form and operate on mental images (Gardner 2006a). Indeed, "the appreciation of spatial relations may also come into play at a metaphoric level; many individuals who create ... products conceive of and work on their chosen entities in a spatial format" (Gardner 2006a, p. 34). This maps directly into one of the preferred ways of communication in design engineering: drawings, sketches, blueprints and models—the production of which is interlinked with the "technological" intelligence, which is another name for bodily-kinaesthetic intelligence: "the capacity to solve problems or to create products using your whole body, or parts of your body, like your hand ..." (Gardner 2006a, p. 35). Reflecting on the prominence of the logical-mathematical intelligence in design engineering, such thinking is inseparable from the "rigidly deterministic" (Bucciarelli 1994, p. 84), and accordingly engineering directly builds on applied mathematics and physics, including the laws that rule in these domains. Indeed, "the engineer is convinced that he can capture the essence of life in a net of numbers and logic" (Koen 2003, p. 69). This notion becomes very visible in the typical curriculum in engineering and naval architectural education programmes, which are biased towards technological and operational subjects, and which pretermit the psychological aspect of the end-user in their curriculum. In a recent survey of over 40 % of the engineering schools in the

United States (including the top universities), 51 % of the current civil engineering curriculum is found to be on "Engineering Topics," while "Maths and Science," at approximately 27 % (Kuo and Houison-Craufurd 2000; Russel and Stouffer 2005; Walker 2011), accounts for an additional quarter of the entire curriculum.

The design engineering community is not only particular in terms of the archetypical composition of intelligences, it is also exacting in terms of learning preferences—a trait, we believe, which is not limited to guiding the way of university teaching, but a characteristic which could be observed when new knowledge and information is provided to the design engineer also at later stages of her career. Felder and Silverman (1988) established a model of styles in engineering learning which defines five different dimensions, or axes: Perception, Input, Organization, Processing and Understanding, each of which has two opposite poles. Referring to Table 2, and with relevance to the transfer of ship design psychology to this target group, it is noteworthy that "many or most engineering students are visual, sensing, inductive, and active, and some of the most creative students are global" (Felder and Silverman 1988, p. 680). Thus, to address this group of students successfully, and, with great likelihood, this entire disciplinary community, one should observe that "*sensors* like facts, data and experimentation" (Felder and Silverman 1988, p. 676) and that "*visual learners* remember best when they see: pictures, diagrams, flow charts, time lines, films, demonstrations" (Felder and Silverman 1988, p. 676) (italics added for clarity). This resonates with an audience which is gifted with logical-mathematical, naturalistic and "technological" intelligences. Similarly, it seems quite unsurprising, when addressing a discipline strong on spatial intelligence (Gardner 2006a), that "films or live demonstrations of working processes should be presented whenever possible" (Felder and Silverman 1988, p. 677), and since most of the students interviewed by Felder and Silverman found themselves to be inductive, one should be mindful that

Table 2 Engineering student learning styles—Adapted from Felder and Silverman (1988)

Preferred learning styles for engineering students		
Input	Visual	Pictures, diagrams, graphs, demonstrations
	Auditory	Words, sounds
Perception	Sensory	Sights, sounds, physical sensations
	Intuitive	Possibilities, insights, hunches
Processing	Active	Engagement in physical activity or discussion
	Reflective	Introspection
Organization	Inductive	Facts and observations are given, underlying principles are inferred
	Deductive	Principles are given, consequences and applications are deduced
Understanding	Sequential	Information is provided in continual steps
	Global	Information is provided in large jumps, holistically

> ... inductive learners need motivation for learning. They do not feel comfortable with the "Trust me – this stuff will be useful to you some day" approach: like sensors, they need to see the phenomena before they can understand and appreciate the underlying theory (Felder and Silverman 1988, p. 678).

It should also be remembered that active learners do not learn much in situations which require them to be passive, like the typical lecture (Felder and Silverman 1988), and it is similarly noteworthy that active learners work well in groups, and tend to be experimentalists—something which appears to tie in with bodily-kinaesthetic intelligence and the ability to solve problems by involving your hands in the process (Gardner 2006a). Finally, the global learners, who are the "synthesizers, the multidisciplinary researchers, the systems thinkers, the ones who see the connection no else sees" (Felder and Silverman 1988, p. 679), should be encouraged by establishing "the context and relevance of the subject matter ... [and] a particularly valuable way for the instructors to serve the global learners ... is to assign creativity exercises" (Felder and Silverman 1988, p. 679).

Design Engineering Thinking

Objects and Artefacts

In the foregoing, the almost positivist nature of design engineering has become apparent, the technological focus and the natural interests are gravitating towards objects and artefacts. For those involved in the development of technology, how-ever, the interest does not stop with the object itself, but goes beyond the surface and the utility seen by the common user; engineering is captivated by what Simon (1996, p. 128) labels "the inner environment" of the object. As a design engineer, you strive to "understand the importance of seeing how things hook together" (Beyer and Holtzblatt 1998, p. 3650), and as a part of this, you do not just accept the utility of an artefact, taking the inner mechanisms for granted:

> The way in which one sees how technology works is very much a matter of the nature of the encounter ... our relations to and hence our perspectives on technology may vary, but in general, as user, traveller, player, viewer or tender, we do not have the same connection to technology that its makers have. However we appropriate technique, most of us do not see technology in terms of its formal structure, underlying form, or **inner construction** [original emphasis] (Bucciarelli 1994, p. 11).

What Bucciarelli highlights here is the pivotal status objects have to design engineering; how the engineering world essentially revolves around the objects they develop:

> ... it is the object as they see and work with it that patterns their thought and practice, not just when they must engage the physics of the device but throughout the entire design process, permeating all exchange and discourse within the subculture of the firm. This way of thinking

is so prevalent within contemporary design that I have given it a label—"object-world thinking"... [original quotation marks] (Bucciarelli 1994, p. 5).

This obviously informs the mind and actions of the design engineer. "The object serves as a kind of icon that embodies a set of attitudes and ways of thinking that are particular to engineering," Bucciarelli (1994, p. 2) notes, and furthermore argues that when it comes to the design of large, complex structures like ships, this is not a kind of thinking that is limited to the individual: the object focus is something which "pervade[s] ... beyond the realm of hardware and the modelling of physical systems to encompass the planning and management of the design process itself" (Bucciarelli 1994, p. 123)—from which another hallmark characteristic of design engineering emerges: to this discipline, objects are made of objects; any artefact is a hierarchy of other objects; any object can be, and is being, decomposed.

Decomposition

The foregoing anecdotal description of the design of an Engine Control Room (ECR) in a ship demonstrates exactly this point: the overall function of this space is being decomposed to include a set of subfunctions, which in turn are being represented by various control devices. At each level of subdivision, other specialists take over the design and management of the particular function, entirely in line with the way design engineering handles complexity: reduction and decomposition of objects and artefacts are pivotal techniques in design engineering (Bucciarelli 1994; Koen 2003; Simon 1996; Vincenti 1993), and design engineering follows the line set by "the urge to control complex affairs through a division and segmenting of process into independent components" (Bucciarelli 1994, p. 110):

> To design ... a complex structure, one powerful technique is to discover viable ways of decomposing it into semi-independent components corresponding to its many functional parts. The design of each component can then be carried out with some degree of independence of the design of others, since each will affect the others largely through its function, and independently of the details of the mechanisms that accomplish the function (Simon 1996, p. 128).

As Brooks (1995) as well as Baxter and Sommerville (2011) note, the success of decomposition as a strategy depends eventually on the robustness of the interfaces between components, to be defined at an early stage of the design, and to be kept stable as long as changes can be avoided: interface changes can and do threaten the foundation on which other components rest. For design engineering, the natural way of achieving robustness and unambiguity is to suppress potentially refractory issues by avoiding qualitative requirements, leaving design team members with only measurable, physical constructs as acceptable building blocks, preferably described in "the abstract and universal language of mathematics" (Bucciarelli 1994, p. 108).

Considering the psychology of ship design, the effects of decomposition are probably not ideal, since, conceivably, such reduction may break up workflow and human tasks utilizing more than one technological object or artefact, teamwork between departments, etc., and thus have a negative influence on the performance of humans and, indeed, the sociotechnical systems. Thinking back to the anecdotal description of an ECR design, this is likely what will happen: instruments and control devices which are to be operationally used in combination may become physically separated, and will with great likelihood have different interaction paradigms. In other words, this particular characteristic of design engineering is somewhat orthogonal to the mainstream thinking of human–systems integration (Baxter and Sommerville 2011; Kossiakoff et al. 2011), which points to one of the challenges facing future improvement in the psychology of ship design.

Uncertainty

The entire purpose of design engineering is to create something new—which unavoidably involves a certain risk of failure. Design engineers are "frequently required to make decisions of great practical consequence in the face of incomplete or uncertain knowledge," Vincenti (1993, p. 16) notes. Considering that design engineering has lived with this risk—and survived—for more than two millennia (Rogers 1983), it should not come as a surprise that this disciplinary community has learned to tackle uncertainty; actually, a core part of design engineering thinking pivots around risk management, and uncertainty appears to inform almost every stage in the design engineering development process; it seems to be second nature in engineering. In the face of uncertainty, design engineering is likely to revert to "inventing immediately from the data" (Beyer and Holtzblatt 1998, p. 3655), a potential lack of precise information notwithstanding. Since such practice potentially is unsafe, design engineering uses heuristics—robust rules of thumb—as a counterbalance (Koen 1985, 2003; Rogers 1983):

> In traditional engineering, limits have frequently been set as 'good practice' by experienced engineers, rather than on the basis of exhaustive analysis. The combination of the short time-to-market ... and the rapid changes in technologies being used, is likely to lead to continued use of engineering judgment, despite increased analysis. [original quotation marks] (Sherwood Jones 2001).

In combination, the method of decomposition, and the habit and experience in the handling of uncertainty, seems to conspire against the psychology of ship design, especially when it comes to having a distant relationship to the eventual end-users of a design, as hinted at above. For design engineering, it is not seen as a problem to "guesstimate" the context of use, user characteristics, user work methods or similar constructs (Petersen et al. 2011); such lack of information is simply "yet another" uncertainty, and not a deterrent to design engineering. On the contrary, literature demonstrates how designers often see themselves as valid representatives of the end-users (Bader and Nyce 1998; Petersen et al. 2011, 2014), which arguably results in designs which are better suited for the designers than for the intended end-users.

The Design Engineering Knowledge Base

It is important to understand how the shared knowledge base of design engineering is supplemented with new knowledge. True to form, the engineering knowledge base reflects that design engineers are practical people, who are not naturally inclined towards the ways of academia, but prefers more "hands-on" approaches, responding positively to methods and experiences demonstrated to work in practice (Bella 1987), or indeed to not having worked in practice, in the sense of having demonstrably failed (Petroski 1982); as it has been described, design engineers learn well from experiments (Felder and Silverman 1988)—no matter whether the outcome is positive or negative.

Bella (1987) introduces the term *design engineering paradigms*, which leads to the "orderly, practical and efficient accomplishment of tasks" (Bella 1987, p. 119), and provides a model of these paradigms, constituted as they are by the "integrated systems of theories, concepts, laws, procedures, examples, models and techniques" (Bella 1987, p. 119). In particular, Bella focuses on the delicate mechanism associated with the expansion of the paradigms, and how the success in this direction depends on shared professional virtues, the personal integrity of the members of the disciplinary community, on the experience of the members and on the social interplay between these professionals. According to Bella (1987), four different sets of social behaviour are involved: *innovation* and *technological actions*, which are the executive actions of engineering; the associated feedback from society at large, which Bella labels *observations*; and the intercommunitarian *discipline*, which is the community's way of policing the integrity of the paradigm (see Fig. 2).

Innovation is the driver which evolves the knowledge base. Through time, community members devise new ways of fulfilling and improving the standards set by the paradigms, and undertake *disciplined and practical observation* of the results when these are tested through technological actions (Bella 1987): "The knowledge of a community evolves as shared innovations become accepted as paradigms for technological activity" (Bella 1987, p. 122). In particular

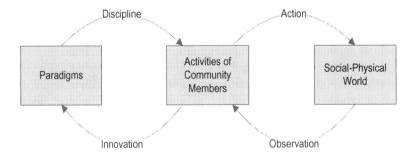

Fig. 2 The evolvement of the design engineering knowledge base (Bella 1987)

… one looks for evidence. Does it make sense? Does it work? Can you prove it? Answers to such questions, based upon discipline, observation and practical actions, provide the bases for separating valid innovations from work which is just different because of sloppiness, ineptness or fraud (Bella 1987, p. 122).

Interestingly, there seems to be consistency between Bella's description of the way the design engineer convinces himself, and his disciplinary community, and how the reflective practitioner (Schön 1983) becomes informed by practical actions and situations:

… the practitioner allows himself to experience surprise, puzzlement, or confusion in a situation which he finds uncertain or unique. He reflects on the phenomena before him, and on the prior understandings which have been implicit in his behaviour. He carries out an experiment which serves to generate both a new understanding of the phenomenon and a change in the situation. When someone reflects-in-action, he becomes a researcher in the practice context (Schön 1983, p. 68).

To conclude this discussion, we have tried to demonstrate how design engineering is practical rather than scientific in its teleology, how this disciplinary community is taught to concentrate on the design of objects, how it is naturally inclined to decompose such objects to manage complexity, how its natural inclination is to express relationships numerically, in accordance with "natural laws" of mathematics, how uncertainty is second nature in engineering process and discourse, and how, at least occasionally, these processes may be guided by heuristics rather than by deep and comprehensive analysis. Indeed, understanding the design engineer as the essential reflective practitioner, as he is described by Schön (1983), appears to provide another bit of the potential recipe for how other practices and disciplines may interact with design engineering: whatever the form—direct cooperation, or other means of knowledge transfer—the exchange has to be practical, the subject has to be observable, and the knowledge has to be immediately relevant, credible and effective, addressing an actual problem. Novel requirements, or consequences of knowledge novel to design engineering, have to be, or have to become, comparable to other design requirements, and cannot be of an ultimate nature. To make their point heard, other disciplines are best served by speaking the engineering language, and would be well advised to exploit the fact that in design engineering, "Seeing is Believing" (Petersen 2012; Petersen et al. 2014).

What is Next? Key Research Questions

Can design make safety, efficiency and satisfaction?
If ships were built by engineers with non-technical skills, would that make a difference?

We believe this chapter has answered these questions with a "yes." Now, however, the challenge is how to achieve this, taking due account of the characteristics and natural inclinations of design engineers.

Exposure to Practice

Building on Gardner (2006a; Petersen et al. 2014), a representational redescription is a potential inroad to changing minds. In the present context, one potential way of improving the uptake and application of ship psychology knowledge (also known as maritime human factors), which appears to be in harmony with the target group, could be to provide first-hand experience on the physiological processes, and the associated cognitive functions of the seafarers, rather than attempting to transfer such knowledge using more traditional teaching methods. The aim of such first-hand practice would be to address naval architects, marine engineers and other engineering disciplines who are involved in the design of ships and ship equipment, and through exposure to the real environment and the end-users, provide insight to the present inadequacy of designs (Schaffer 2004; Weick and Quinn 1999). Engineers from all disciplines could come to know that HF integration can enhance human well-being and the overall performance of the seafarers, which in turn could help to reduce the risk of shipboard errors and accidents. Exposure to practical seafaring, we suggest, could lessen their lack of awareness of maritime HF and operational problems, and moreover it could improve their communication with those who work and live aboard; previous research has proven this to be poor (Ross 2009; The Nautical Institute 1998). Looking ahead, the effectiveness of such in-practice training is, however, yet to be seen, and we see a need for a systematic, widespread effort to realize the potential of this approach.

Extension of the Design Engineering Curriculum

According to Walker (2011), an early challenge is educating designers and other stakeholders with respect to the benefits of ergonomics in design; to reiterate, the competency of design engineers who have direct influence on the design of the ship is paramount and in our view needs to be supplemented to include maritime HF. The benefit of such a successful extension of the design engineering curricula is believed to be a good long-term solution to address the subject of human element in the maritime domain. Kuo and Houison-Craufurd (2000) note that the present naval architecture education system is heavily biased towards the technological field and very few have been exposed to such topics as HF and HCD, much in line with the findings of Russel and Stouffer (2005). These authors propose a method to help naval architects to understand HF and give full attention at the design stage to include HF in order to achieve an acceptable level of safety. Their conclusion is to add a HF course to the naval architecture degree syllabus and to encourage students by demonstrating the impact of HF on each phase of a ship's life cycle.

To better match the characteristics of design engineering, problem-based learning (PBL) seems a promising approach. PBL can be identified as a student-centred pedagogy in which students learn about a subject through the experience of problem solving (Eberlein et al. 2008; Walton and Matthews 1989; Hmelo-Silver 2004); with PBL, students learn both thinking strategies and domain knowledge. PBL is an instructional learner-centred approach that empowers learners to conduct research, integrate theory and practice, and apply knowledge and skills to develop a viable solution to a defined problem, which we suggest resonates well with the fundamentals of design engineering thinking. This pedagogy seems to be able to equip students with the mindsets and methods of HCD in a fashion matching their learning preferences, making them more aware and better equipped to face and solve relevant challenges of the psychology of ship design.

There is "work-in-progress" also on this front. One example is the course on "Human Factors for Naval Architect students" (HFNA), a 5-day voluntary summer course run for 5 years at Chalmers Technical University in Sweden. It delivers basic knowledge within the field of maritime HF, human–machine interaction and how this links to ship classification and ship design. The emphasis was on using ship visits to support design tasks, and to learn how to identify design issues, e.g. recognizing "integration work." Classroom exercises and lectures supported this. The course evolved over the years, and has been used in the EU project CyClaDes, providing participants with insights into teaching interested naval architecture students, engineers and designers.

Along comparable lines, there is a HF course at University of Southampton, an optional module available to ship science students in their fourth year, and open to every student studying engineering at the university. Most of the students attending, however, come from the branches of mechanical engineering, aero and astro, acoustical engineering programmes, rather than ship science (in fact, no naval architects had attended). In terms of the HF course, the lectures cover various aspects of human capability, in terms of physical, environmental, physiological and psychological factors which enable the engineer to take account of the human element in the design of machines, displays, controls, and living and working environments. The knowledge can be applied for designing products in students' expertise/interests, including ship design (Brian Sherwood Jones, personal communication).

A third example can be found at the Faculty of Maritime Technology and Operations at Aalesund University College in Norway, which also conducts a course on "Human Factors" for students enrolled in the Master's degree in "Demanding Marine Operations". A final example (Thomas et al. 2013) describes a design project which is developed in the National Centre for Maritime Engineering and Hydrodynamics at the Australian Maritime College (AMC). This course allows final-year naval architect students to carry out a two-phase design process in multidisciplinary teams, allowing a focus on the development of teamwork skills, and uses a PBL approach together with a strong focus on practical work. Another current AMC undertaking is a research project which focuses on amalgamating maritime HF and HCD knowledge into the undergraduate naval architecture syllabus, by way of creating and injecting HCD champions (Gulliksen et al. 2003) into the design project teams, and to study the effects of this change through action research. In addition, this project aims at operationalizing maritime HF knowledge, as it includes the development of a computer-based "HF Design Support" tool.

Embryonic as the above is, as both medium-term and long-term results are yet to be seen, these courses have the potential to cement the psychology of ship design in the minds of young design engineers.

Low-key Human-Centred Design

Human-centred design (HCD), and the derivatives of this methodology, are seen as universal tools for the inclusion of user needs and characteristics in design. Thus supporting the inclusion of HF knowledge during design, HCD approaches are believed to lead to products which in turn provide a number of benefits to their users, including improved human working conditions, improved productivity, enhanced user well-being, avoidance of stress, increased accessibility and reduced risk of harm (International Organization for Standardization (ISO) 2010; Maguire 2001). HCD, and the steps described by ISO (2009) and elaborated by Maguire (2001), moreover appear to be accepted on a global scale (Quesenbery 2005). In the present context, it is entirely natural to suggest that catering for the psychology of ship design can be handled using this process, and the discussion becomes one of understanding what design engineers really do need to integrate HF, in general and in particular, into the ship design process, i.e. the ship design spiral and the present regime of rules and regulations.

The "ABCD[3] Working Group on Human Performance at Sea" (Dobbins et al. 2008), which is an international group consisting of hydrodynamicists and HF researchers, carried out notable research work on integrating HF in High Speed Craft (HSC) design. They have identified nine HF areas and detailed HF design principles to the feasibility design stage, the main design phase and the end design in order to support the integration of HF into the HSC design process (see Table 3). The authors produced an engineering design guide to support the industry and academic naval architecture and design community, by providing HF engineering guidance to enhance the specification, design, evaluation and operation of HSC. The development of this guidance was followed by consultation with stakeholders, operators and naval architects, as following the HCD cycle to develop the integrated HF naval architect concept in the design process.

McSweeney et al. (2009) similarly discuss an applied approach for human factors engineering (HFE) principles integration and implementation into ship design, throughout the conceptual, preliminary, and detailed design stages and during the construction, suggesting a comprehensive programme, including several tasks such as promotion of interaction between design personnel with end-users, review of early project design documents, the identification of HF tasks and the

---

[3]This is known as the "ABCD Group" due to the nationalities who form its membership: American, Australian, British, Canadian and Dutch researchers and defence agencies.

Table 3 HSC HF areas and HF input to design process (Dobbins et al. 2008)

HF Area	HF design principles (one out of each area)
HSC motions	The requirements of the User Requirement Document and System Requirement Document for craft ride/motion characteristics should be examined, particularly in relation to the Shock and Vibration exposure of the crew and passengers, and the subsequent requirements for Shock and Vibration mitigation
Sight	Consider the influence of the design on the coxswain and navigator's external visibility For example, to what effect will the hull design affect the coxswain's visibility of the sea close to the vessel?
Sound	Identify the major sources of noise on the HSC (e.g. engines) and estimate whether the noise levels are likely to interfere with communication in closed versus open boat designs, ensuring systems provide good coverage of all crew working areas
Environment	Design of crew and passenger work positions should take account of heating, cooling, and ventilation requirements, including the location of major components. Installation of ventilation facilities needs to consider cooling requirements (e.g. will machinery generate significant amounts of heat?) and ventilation to prevent the build-up of diesel (and other) fumes
Health and safety	Identify the main sources of potential hazard to crew and passengers. Incorporate additional space allowance in payload space and other areas where manual handling tasks are anticipated. Incorporate sufficient space allowance on deck for stowage of items. Consider crew and passenger escape and evacuation where appropriate
Man–machine interface	The designer should consider the high-level crew requirements, e.g. the coxswain will need to combine maintaining a good external view with monitoring the instrumentation panel; the navigator may need flat surfaces for conducting chartwork; the maintainer requires good access to servicing areas
Habitability	Estimate width and height requirements (to accommodate largest crew and passenger sizes) for passageways to be included within main-space estimates. Locate working areas in locations of best "ride quality," and as far as practicable away from machinery items
Maintainability	The designer should ensure that sufficient clearance is maintained around serviceable items. Additionally, serviceable items may need to be raised to provide maintained good access at a convenient working height
Design review	Designers, engineers and end-users together should review the design (CAD drawing and 3D modelling)

preparation of a HF plan, training of design personnel, design drawing review, visits to the construction yard and many more (see Table 4).

These two schemes notwithstanding, previous and ongoing research demonstrates that the application of full-scope HCD by design engineering is unlikely to be successful (Petersen 2010, 2012, 2013; Petersen et al. 2010). Duly observing the usability capability maturity level (Earthy 1998; Nielsen 2006a, b) of the maritime industry when it comes to the application of HF, it seems more promising to perform a reduced-scope set of activities, borrowed from the full application of

Table 4 Summary of McSweeney et al.'s (2009) HFE programme

Task	Description
Review/development of early project design documents	The purpose of this task is to identify any existing HFE design requirements to verify they are incorporated into the final design of the project. These documents should state the objectives for the project, how, and by whom, the project will be managed, and what technical components will be involved in the project
Identify HFE tasks and prepare the HFE plan	The HFE plan should identify the tasks to be performed, the schedule, linked to the master project schedule, to which each task will be carried out and the personnel responsible for each task. Any special studies (e.g. a link analysis of a control room) should also be laid out in the plan
Select/write the HFE design aids	HFE design aids are a collection of the most important HFE design requirements packaged to provide quick and easy access to design criteria for specific HFE design requirements (e.g. operability/maintainability envelopes or control/displays concerns) of interest to the project engineers, designers and modellers
Conduct training	This task provides introductory orientation training regarding HFE for all management, engineering and design personnel
Establish an HFE tracking database	This database allows each HFE design input to be tracked and records all HFE inputs, whether or not the input was accepted or rejected (including the rationale for rejection)
Carry out a manning assessment	Manning assessments should be conducted to determine and/or verify knowledge, skills and abilities and proposed manning levels for final designs
Conduct drawing/design reviews	Engineering drawings and design documents (including three-dimensional module drawings showing plan, section, elevation and details) should be reviewed to verify that the design and layouts comply with project HFE design requirements, providing sufficient ingress/egress throughout the design and sufficient clearance/access for the operation and maintenance of equipment
Apply HFE to vendor-supplied equipment	HFE design requirements should be incorporated into appropriate vendor-supplied hardware and software packages. Items should be selected based on the presence of HFE design requirements included in the vendor specification (e.g. consoles/panels, access clearances, etc.)
Prioritize HFE efforts for systems/equipment	It is important that the HFE personnel review the equipment/systems/subsystems lists to identify potential HFE activities and those parts of the design which should receive detailed HFE attention

(continued)

Table 4 (continued)

Task	Description
Incorporate a labelling programme	A labelling programme should cover such design issues as label colours, contrast, character sizes, content and format as well as create standards for the various types of labels, signs and job aids used throughout the facility
Prepare/review operations, maintenance, and training materials/manuals	For the manuals to benefit the operations and maintenance personnel, it is important for them to be designed in an easy-to-read and easy-to follow manner
Participate in special design studies	The HFE personnel should participate in design studies that address HFE concerns and design requirements relative to O&M, manning, training, safety, etc. The HFE personnel's primary involvement should focus on issues relating to crew member performance or safety
Visit the construction yard and vendor facilities	The objective of this HFE activity is to verify that the HFE requirements considered during the detailed design and construction phases have been implemented as per the design intention
Prepare progress reports	The report should briefly describe the HFE activities completed thus far, the general status of the HFE programme, deliverables made, number and location of visits made to the construction yard and/or vendors, and upcoming planned activities

HCD, as this is described by ISO (2009), and limit the focus to the lower key subjects of understanding the context of use, as well as understanding and being able to practise relatively simple usability testing, subjects which will be elaborated further. Such an approach is illustrated in Fig. 3, demonstrating the suggested short cut of limiting the designers' HF considerations to the first and last stages of the conventional HCD design iterations—and, at that, to use less ambitious, comprehensive and complicated processes, as is elaborated below. The axiom being that "a little bit of human factors thinking is better than none," the point here is to lower the adoption barrier to the application of the psychology of ship design to levels and complexity with which novices are likely to be more comfortable. In the figure, the dotted lines and greyed-out boxes are the parts of the full-scope HCD iterations which as such are entirely disregarded.

The first step is to "understand and specify the context of use," attaining knowledge of the end-user of the product or process being developed, as well as the circumstances under which it will be used. Such knowledge will inform the design process, aiming to make the product fit for the user and task as well. While obtaining and maintaining a correct understanding of the context of use can be time consuming and costly, and could—or, indeed, should—involve ethnographically inspired field studies and prolonged immersion in the environment, a simplified

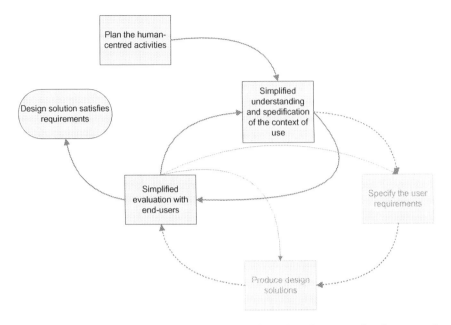

Fig. 3 The iterative HCD design activities (ISO 9241-210) adapted to a more low-key approach

method could be for ship designers to watch short video clips of the relevant work situations, to have interviews with end-users, or to visit ships in port to see with their own eyes. Be this as it may, and in slightly more detail, the following information is of importance in this step:

1. Understand primary and secondary users.
2. Skills and knowledge of the users, including experience and training.
3. Physical attributes, including any limitations.
4. Motivations, positive or negative attitudes to job, task and product.
5. Workplace design, spaces, layout, reach and postures.
6. Health and safety, hazards and protective equipment requirements.

Following the design phase, which design engineering is entirely confident and supremely competent to undertake, testing with end-users, preferably in the context of use previously defined, is a second step which will help elucidate potential product flaws—and a step which appears to be often ignored. Depending on the level of ambition and HF competence (and usability capability maturity), this step can be of low complexity; for novices, it should be kept low key. Two different approaches appear to be particularly useful under such circumstances, one being simple user testing, the other being heuristic evaluation in the earlier phases of a design.

In terms of the former, the designers could identify the perhaps 30 % most important or most frequent tasks the user will have to undertake with the artefact in question, and simply observe five to seven representative end-users perform those tasks under realistic conditions. Experience has it that not only will one find a high number of whatever usability issues the artefact may suffer from (Mack and Nielsen 1994; Nielsen 1994), the approach also seems to be capable of making the designers accept that the product—artefact—is actually flawed (Baxter and Sommerville 2011; Desurvire 1994; Eriksson et al. 2009; Schaffer 2004), and thus induce an added future focus on the psychology of ship design.

Heuristic evaluation (Mack and Nielsen 1994; Nielsen 1994; Shneiderman and Plaisant 2005; Wickens et al. 2004) pivots around the assessment of an artefact along the axes of attributes known to improve usability, such as consistency in operation, clarity of language, ease of reading, error prevention and good error handling, good error messages, intuitiveness, user control, and, importantly, a good match between the user's mental model of the system under control and the view presented by the system under scrutiny; see Petersen et al. (2014) for an overview of the various sets of well-known heuristics. This approach appears to have potential for the successful application by design engineering teams (Desurvire 1994; Karat 1994; Nielsen 1994). Considering the near future in the maritime domain, heuristic evaluation thus could be a viable approach to increased adoption —and evaluation—of the psychology of ship design; this, however, requires additional research before firm recommendations can be made.

Conclusion: Recommendations on the Psychology of Ship Design

We have produced a snapshot of the present state of the psychology of ship design in the maritime industry—including having elaborated on the systemic challenges and barriers to an increased usage of HF knowledge by design engineering; indeed these are varied and are influenced by topics as diverse as the natural inclinations of design engineers and design engineering, the culture of the maritime industry and the way ships are designed and built, to the commercial dimension which dictates what a ship designer can do, and what s/he cannot do, if the ship designed is to be a success from a business perspective.

In the final section of this chapter, we also hope we have shown a pragmatic way ahead: universities teaching naval architecture and marine engineering are advised to extend the curriculum to include maritime human factors, which will provide a basic knowledge graduates can build on in their entire career in the maritime industry. We are also calling for a universal exposure to practice; in our view, any design engineer involved in the creation of new maritime artefacts should be exposed, briefly or for longer periods, to seafaring and seafarers—it seems to us to be the perhaps simplest and most effective way of improving the usability of ships and maritime equipment. Finally, the issue of low-key user-centred design is in our view suitable for both students, new graduates and seasoned design engineers and design engineering managers; there seem to be few, if any, real barriers to the successful introduction and execution of investigating and understanding the context of use, and the performance of low-key testing of equipment with representative end-users seems simply to be a natural component in any design process striving to produce successful artefacts. We see heuristic evaluation of usability characteristics to be a powerful guide during the early design stages of an artefact; having these issues in mind is bound to reduce the risk of producing artefacts which will fail during later usability testing with end-users—but heuristic evaluation should not be seen as a replacement of testing with representative end-users. On the subject of physical ergonomics, Sanders and McCormick (1992) state that "All the anthropometric data in the world cannot substitute for a full-scale mock-up" (1992, p. 423)—we wish to extend this realization to the entire area of maritime human factors.

References

Alert! (2003). The human element: Improving the awareness of the human element in the maritime industry. *The International Maritime Human Element Bulletin, 1*.

Alert! (2004). Ergonomics: An ergonomic nightmare! Reflects a view of the bridge.. or the engineroom? *The International Maritime Human Element Bulletin, 3*.

Alert! (2010). Design, build, maintain: The ultimate aim—always keep the human element in mind. *The International Maritime Human Element Bulletin, 24*(8). Retrieved from http://www.he-alert.org/

American Bureau of Shipping. (2003a). *Guidance notes for the application of ergonomics to marine systems*. Houston, TX: American Bureau of Shipping.

American Bureau of Shipping. (2003b). *Guidance notes on ergonomic design of navigation bridges*. Houston, TX: American Bureau of Shipping.

American Bureau of Shipping. (2010). Guide for bridge design and navigational equipment/systems. Houston, TX: American Bureau of Shipping.Bader, G., & Nyce, J. M. (1998). When only the self is real: Theory and practice in the development community. Journal of Computer Documentation, 22(1), 5-10.

Bader, G., & Nyce, J. M. (1998). When only the self is real: Theory and practice in the development community. *Journal of Computer Documentation, 22*(1), 5–10.

Barker, R. G., & Wright, H. F. (1949). Psychological ecology and the problem of psychosocial development. *Child Development, 20*(3), 131–143.

Baxter, G., & Sommerville, I. (2011). Socio-technical systems: From design metods to systems engineering. *Interacting with Computers, 23*, 4–17.

Beevis, D., Davidson, P., Webb, R., & Coutu, E. (2000, September 27–29). *Software support for sharing and tracking human factors issues during ship design*. Paper presented at the Human Factors in Ship Design and Operation. London, UK: The Royal Institute of Naval Architects.

Bella, D. A. (1987). Engineering and Erosion of Trust. *Journal of Professional Issues in Engineering, 113*(2), 117–129.

Beyer, H., & Holtzblatt, K. (1998). *Contextual design—Defining customer-centered systems*. San Diego, CA: Academic Press. [Kindle ed.].

Brooks, F. P. (1995). *The Mythical Man-Month: Essays on Software Engineering*. Boston: Addison-Wesley Longman Inc. [Kindle ed.].

Bucciarelli, L. L. (1994). *Designing engineers*. Cambridge, MA: MIT Press.

Calhoun, S. R., & Stevens, S. C. (2003). Human factors in ship design. In T. Lamb (Ed.), Ship design and construction (Vol. 2, pp. 1–27). Alexandria VA: Society of Naval Architects and Marine Engineers (SNAME).

Dekker, S. (2002). *The field guide to human error investigations*. Aldershot, UK: Ashgate.

Desurvire, H. W. (1994). Faster, cheaper!! Are usability inspection methods as effective as empirical testing? In J. Nielsen & R. L. Mack (Eds.), *Usability inspection methods* (pp. 173–202). New York: Wiley.

Dobbins, T., Rowley, I., & Campbell, L. (2008). High speed craft human factors engineering design guide. Retrieved from http://www.highspeedcraft.org/HSC_HFE_Design_Guide_v1.0.pdf

Earthy, J. (1998). WP5—Deliverable D5.1.4(s)—Usability maturity model: Human centredness scale. From London: Eberlein, T., Kampmeier, J., Minderhout, V., Moog, R. S., Platt, T., Varma-Nelson, P., & White.

Eberlein, T., Kampmeier, J., Minderhout, V., Moog, R. S., Platt, T., Varma-Nelson, P., et al. (2008). Pedagogies of engagement in science. *Biochemistry and Molecular Biology Education, 36*(4), 262–273.

Eriksson, E., Cajander, Å., & Gulliksen, J. (2009, August 24–28). *Hello world!—Experiencing usability methods without usability expertise*. Paper presented at the INTERACT, Part II, Uppsala, Sweden.

Evans, J. H. (1959). Basic design concepts. *Journal of American Society of Naval Engineers*, 671–678.

Felder, R. M., & Silverman, L. K. (1988). Learning and teaching styles in engineering education. *Engineering Education, 78*(7), 674–681.

Gardner, H. (2006a). *Changing minds*. Boston, MA: Harvard Business School Publishing.

Gardner, H. (2006b). *Multiple intelligences—New horizons*. New York: Basic Books. (Kindle ed.).

Grech, M. R., Horberry, T. J., & Koester, T. (2008). *Human factors in the maritime domain* (1st ed.). Florida: CRC Press.

Gulliksen, J., Göransson, B., Boivie, I., Blomkvist, S., Persson, J., & Cajander, Å. (2003). Key principles for user-centred systems design. *Behaviour and Information Technology, 22*(6), 397–409.

Hemmen, H. F. V. (2003). *The need for additional human factors considerations in ship operations*. Paper presented at the Second International Symposium on Ship Operations. Athens, Greece: Management & Economics.

Hmelo-Silver, C. E. (2004). Problem-based learning: What and how do students learn? *Educational Psychology Review, 16*(3), 235–266.

Holden, K. L., Boyer, J. L., Ezer, N., Holubec, K., Sándor, A., & Stephens, J.-P. (2013). Human factors in space vehicle design. *Acta Astronautica, 92*(1), 110–118.

International Organization for Standardization (ISO). (2009). *Ergonomics of human-system interaction—Part 210: Human-centred design for interactive systems (ISO 9241-210)*. Geneva: ISO.

International Organization for Standardization (ISO). (2010). *Ergonomics of human-system interaction—Part 210: Human-centred design for interactive system (ISO 9241-210:2010)*. Geneva: ISO.

Johansen, R. (1978). Stress and socio-technical design: A new ship organization. In C. L. Cooper & R. Payne (Eds.), *Stress at work*. Chichester: Wiley.

Karat, C.-M. (1994). A comparison of user interface evaluation methods. In J. Nielsen & R. L. Mack (Eds.), *Usability inspection methods*. New York: Wiley.

Koen, B. V. (1985). *Definition of the engineering method*. Washington, D.C. American Society for Engineering Educations.

Koen, B. V. (2003). *Discussion of the method—Conducting the engineer's approach to problem solving*. New York: Oxford University Press.

Koester, T. (2005, February 23-24). *Human factors in the design process—A new approach to the design of maritime communication equipment*. Paper presented at the RINA, Royal Institution of Naval Architects International Conference—Human Factors in Ship Design, Safety and Operation.

Kossiakoff, A., Sweet, W. N., Seymour, S. J., & Biemer, S. M. (2011). *Systems engineering—principles and practice*. New York: Wiley.

Kuo, C., & Houison-Craufurd, S. (2000, September 27–29). *Managing human error in maritime activities*. Paper presented at the Human Factors in Ship Design and Operation. London, UK: Royal Institute of Naval Architects.

Lloyd's Register. (2008). *The human element—An introduction* (p. 24). London: Lloyd's Register Group.

Lezaun, J. (2011). Offshore democracy: launch and landfall of a socio-technical experiment. *Economy and Society, 40*(4), 553–581.

Lützhöft, M. (2004). *"The technology is great when it works": Maritime technology and human integration on the ship's bridge*. Doctor of Philosophy, University of Linköping.

Lützhöft, M., Grech, M. R., & Porathe, T. (2011). Information environment, fatigue, and culture in the maritime domain. In P. R. DeLucia (Ed.), *Reviews of human factors and ergonomics* (pp. 280–320). Thousand Oaks, CA: SAGE Publications.

Mack, R. L., & Nielsen, J. (1994). Executive summary. In J. Nielsen & R. L. Mack (Eds.), *Usability Inspection methods*. New York: Wiley.

Maguire, M. (2001). Methods to support human-centred design. *International Journal of Human-Computer Studies, 55*(4), 587–634.

McSweeney, K. P., Pray, J., & Craig, B. N. (2009, February). *Integration of human factors engineering into design—an applied approach*. Paper presented at the Human Factors in Ship Design and Operation. London, UK: Royal Institute of Naval Architects.

National Transportation Safety Board (1997). *Grounding of the Panamanian passenger ship Royal Majesty on Rose and Crown Shoal near Nantucket, Massachusetts*. Retrieved from Washington, DC.

Nielsen, J. (1994). Heuristic evaluation. In J. Nielsen & R. L. Mack (Eds.), *Usability inspection methods*. New York: Wiley.

Nielsen, J. (2006a). Corporate usability maturity: Stages 1–4. Jakob Nielsen's Alertbox. Retrieved from www.useit.com/alertbox/maturity.html

Nielsen, J. (2006b). Corporate usability maturity: Stages 5–8. Jakob Nielsen's Alertbox. Retrieved from www.useit.com/alertbox/process_maturity.html

Norros, L. (2014). Developing human factors/ergonomics as a design discipline. *Applied Ergonomics, 45*(1), 61–71.

Parker, A. W., Hubinger, L. M., Green, S., Sargent, L., & Boyd, B. (1997). *A survey of the health stress and fatigue of Australian seafarers*. Australia: Australian Maritime Safety Authority.

Petersen, E. S. (2010). *User-centered methods must also be user centered: a single voice from the field* (Lic. Eng.). Göteborg: Chalmers Technical University.

Petersen, E. S. (2012). *Engineering usability (Doctor of Technology)*. Gothenburg: Chalmers Technical University.

Petersen, E. S. (2013). *Human-centric design challenges*. Paper presented at the IMarEST MECSS 2013, Amsterdam, The Netherlands.

Petersen, E. S., Dittmann, K., & Lützhöft, M. (2010, October 7-8). *Making the phantom real: a case of applied maritime human factors*. Paper presented at the SNAME SOME 2010, Athens, Greece.

Petersen, E. S., & Lützhöft, M. (2009, February 25-26). *A human factors approach to the design of maritime software applications*. Paper presented at the Human Factors in Ship Design and Operation, London.

Petersen, E. S., Nyce, J. M., & Lützhöft, M. (2011). Ethnography reengineered: The two tribes problem. *Theoretical Issues in Ergonomics Sciences, 12*(6).

Petersen, E. S., Nyce, J. M., & Lützhöft, M. (2014). Interacting with classic design engineering. *Interacting with Computers*, 1–18.

Petroski, H. (1982). *To engineer is human—the role of failure in successful design.* New York: Vintage Books (First Vintage Books Edition)

Petroski, H. (2010). *The essential engineer—why science alone will not solve our global problems.* New York: Alfred A. Knopf.

Quesenbery, W. (2005, July 10-13). *Usability standards: Connecting practice around the world.* Paper presented at the 2005 IEEE International Professional Communication Conference Proceedings, Limerick, Ireland.

Rasmussen, J. (2005, February 23-24). *Designing usable ships.* Paper presented at the Human Factors in Ship Design, Safety and Operation. London, UK: Royal Institute of Naval Architects.

Rogers, G. F. C. (1983). *The nature of engineering—A philosophy of technology.* London: The MacMillan Press Ltd.

Ross, J. M. (2009). *Human factors for naval marine vehicle design and operation* (1st ed.). Farnham, England: Ashgate.

Russel, J. S., & Stouffer, W. B. (2005, April). Survey of the National Civil Engineering Curriculum. *Journal of Professional Issues in Engineering Education and Practice,* 118–128.

Sanders, M. S., & McCormick, E. J. (1992). *Human factors in engineering and design.* Boston: McGraw-Hill Inc.

Schaffer, E. (2004). *Institutionalization of usability—a step-by-step guide.* Boston: Addison-Wesley.

Schein, E. H. (1996). Kurt Lewin's change theory in the field and in the classroom: Notes toward a model of managed learning. *Reflections, 1*(1), 59–72.

Schön, D. A. (1983). *The Reflective practitioner—how professionals think in action.* London: Maurice Temple Smith Ltd.

Sherwood Jones, B. (2001). *Enabling and maintaining control.* Paper presented at the IEE Conference Publication.

Shneiderman, B., & Plaisant, C. (2005). *Designing the user interface.* Boston: Pearson—Addison Wesley.

Simon, H. A. (1996). *The sciences of the artificial* (3rd ed.). Cambridge, MA: The MIT Press.

Squire, D. (2014, February 26-27). *Human element competencies for the maritime industry.* Paper presented at the Human Factors in Ship Design and Operation. London, UK. Royal Institute of Naval Architects.

Strong, R. (2000, September 27-29). *RN Habitability survey: Ship design implications: Some important social and architectural issues in the design of accommodation spaces.* Paper presented at the Human Factors in Ship Design and Operation. London, UK: Royal Institute of Naval Architects.

The Nautical Institute. (1998). *Improving ship operational design.* London: The Nautical Institute.

Thomas, G., Harte, D., & Pointing, D. (2013, February 26-27). *Developing student skills through industry-aligned and team-focussed design projects.* Paper presented at the Education and Professional Development of Engineers in the Maritime Industry, Singapore.

UK P&I CLUB. (2003). Just waiting to happen: The work of the UK P&I club. *The International Maritime Human Element Bulletin, 1,* 3–4.

Vincenti, W. G. (1993). *What engineers know and how they know it—analytical studies from aeronautical history.* Baltimore: Johns Hopkins University Press.

Walker, O. (2011, November 16-17). *The human element competency required for design appraisal.* Paper presented at the Human Factors in Ship Design and Operation. London, UK: Royal Institute of Naval Architects.

Walton, H. J., & Matthews, M. B. (1989). Essentials of problem-based learning. *Medical Education, 23,* 542–559.

Weick, K. E., & Quinn, R. E. (1999). Organizational change and development. *Annual Review of Psychology, 50,* 361–386.

Wickens, C. D., Lee, J. D., Liu, Y., & Gordon Becker, S. E. (2004). *An introduction to human factors engineering* (2nd ed.). Upper Saddle River, NJ: Pearson Prentice Hall.

Widdel, H., & Motz, F. (2000, September 27-29). *Ergonomic requirements for the design of ship bridges.* Paper presented at the Human Factors in Ship Design and Operation. London UK. Royal Institute of Naval Architects.

Occupational Stress in Seafaring

Ana Slišković

'Voice' of Croatian Seafarers Employed in the International Maritime Sector

A recent study conducted on a large sample of Croatian seafarers employed on cargo ships identified a range of themes, from the seafarer's own qualitative reports, concerning their sources of job dissatisfaction (Slišković and Penezić 2015). Through answers to open questions, the study participants offered their own perspectives, experiences and insights with regard to the main sources of dissatisfaction they faced in their occupation. These themes and accompanying illustrative quotations (see Table 1) show some cultural and contextual specificities. A major concern was dissatisfaction with state laws governing seafarers' rights and obligations, clearly having a number of practical implications for the State, the Croatian Ministry of Maritime Affairs, educational institutions, agencies and labour unions.

Most of the other sources of dissatisfaction found in this study (e.g. separation from home and family, living and working conditions on board, etc.) are quite well recognized as *occupational stressors in the maritime sector* (Allen et al. 2008; Carotenuto et al. 2012; Iversen 2012; MacLachlan et al. 2012; Oldenburg et al. 2010a). This supports previous findings of negative association between job satisfaction and occupational stress, obtained both in the general working population (Faragher et al. 2005) and in seafarers (Lang 2011). However, examples of typical answers given in Table 1 offer a deeper insight into what actually makes seafarers stressed, dissatisfied or unhappy in relation to their occupation. The source of dissatisfaction labelled *changes in the maritime sector* provides insight to a seafarer's perspective on reasons for the increase of occupational stress in the maritime sector.

A. Slišković (✉)
Department of Psychology, University of Zadar, Obala kralja Petra Krešimira IV,
2, 23000 Zadar, Croatia
e-mail: aslavic@unizd.hr

© Springer International Publishing Switzerland 2017
M. MacLachlan (ed.), *Maritime Psychology*, DOI 10.1007/978-3-319-45430-6_5

Table 1 Sources of job dissatisfaction

Sources of job dissatisfaction (% of responses)[a]	Examples of responses
(1) Separation from home and family (20.9)	*"I miss being with the family, Internet helps, but does not solve the closeness with them"* *"... always missing family moments while children are growing up, which no one can replace"*
(2) Status of seafarers in the Republic of Croatia (22.8)	*"Well, generally most unhappy at the treatment of seafarers in our country, i.e. they require all sorts of things, and in return nothing ... First of all, paying taxes needs to be abolished immediately because the State does not give anything i.e. only demands, or if they want us to pay them they in turn should give something ..."* *"Neglect, from the State, of seafarers and their benefits. We can not be in the same group as others for retirement, since no one will find work in the profession to the age of 67"* *"The payment of health insurance in the Republic of Croatia during stays on board (at that time I already have health insurance through the company I work for, and my whole family)"*
(3) Status of Croatian seafarers in the international labour market (2.8)	*"Underpayment in comparison to other nations"* *"As a Croat it is hard to make progress in the offshore sector, for example. We can talk about what we want, but our passports are of no significance outside. Cheap labour will smash us"*
(4) Status of seafarers in the company and promotion opportunities (7.3)	*"Slave-holding treatment by the company of its people"* *"The fact that the work is not valued as it should be, people are being promoted by luck, because decisions about the progress of the people are made in the office of the company, not on board, where people know how one works, while the real evaluation of individual work is difficult to convey in paper reports to the people in the office"*
(5) Company and living and working conditions on board (35.8)	*"Non-respect of the contract, contract duration of 4 months on board converts to 5 months, sometimes even longer"* *"Daily work 12–14 h, after 3 months' stay I think we need a psychiatrist before coming home, because the only topic of my life is work"* *"Isolation. Today LNG ships are floating prisons"* *"The inability to use the Internet on board"* *"... in most companies food is criminally bad and poor quality, and even worse is the preparation. In addition to that, the menu is always adjusted for Asians, who are more prevalent on board, and the cook is Asian"*

(continued)

Table 1 (continued)

Sources of job dissatisfaction (% of responses)[a]	Examples of responses
(6) Interpersonal relationships on board (12.8)	*"Relationships that are sometimes negative and from which there is no escape"* *"Sometimes superiors are not correct towards the lower-ranking staff"*
(7) Changes in maritime sector (12.8)	*"The industry is moving in a direction that increases the number of tasks we perform, and which are not directly related to navigation. Autonomy of crew (especially officers) is decreasing, increasing administration..."* *"...capitalism that is relentless, and it is almost impossible to do the job by the book, i.e. to harmonize the rules imposed or required by the STCW, ISM and others"*

[a]Percentages of responses are calculated as n of responses in each category divided by n of subjects (530), but the fact that some subjects cited two or more sources of job dissatisfaction must be taken into the account
Source Slišković and Penezić (2015)

Implementing Findings of Research in the Field of Occupational Stress in Seafaring

During the conducting of recent research focused on occupational stress in Croatian seafarers, I experienced many personal reactions not only of participants, but also of those who did not want to participate. The background of their reluctance to participate was largely based on the view that the research would not help in solving their real problems. Some of the negative characteristics of their working environment are seen by them as unchangeable because it is "just so in their particular company and/or in the maritime sector". Company management is seen as primarily based on profit, while changes introduced by international regulatory bodies aimed at improvements in the maritime sector are often seen as "extra paperwork" and as "conflicting with real practices on board". Through these adverse reactions came the claim that the scientist/psychologist employed on land cannot imagine the working stressors on board. Indeed, can we imagine the depth of loneliness and worry caused by the separation from home and family? Or the level of isolation of a seafarer whose stay on board, according to the contract, is 4 or 6 months, but who, due to irregularities of shift, does not know when he is going home? Add to this picture the intense work demands, safety and health risks, overtime hours—which are often not recorded—and poor interpersonal relationships, which occur in every work team, but from which you cannot distance yourself when you are on board. The above list of adverse characteristics (stressors) is by no means exhaustive.

This chapter gives a review of previous studies focused on occupational stress in seafarers, including a detailed overview of occupational stressors in seafaring. However, before focusing on the state of knowledge in the field, let us go back to the main issue that I experienced from seafarers: "How can you help us?" Although the practical implications are commonly given at the end of a text, I believe that this question must be to the fore, and that addressing it requires collaborative work between the owners and managers of shipping companies, unions, and national and international regulatory bodies.

Occupational stress management strategies depend on perspectives or views on the stress issue, which are shaped and changed under political, cultural, social and economic influence. Generally, views on occupational stress may be divided into two broad categories. One of them is the understanding of stress at work as a "personal problem" of the employee, arising from his or her personal characteristics, while the second involves care on the part of the community, since the problems of employees result from the unfavourable characteristics of the work environment (Kenny and Cooper 2003). Therefore, stress management strategies can be targeted at the individual or at the working conditions (Michie 2007). Intervention strategies can be classified into three levels: primary, secondary and tertiary (Kendall et al. 2000; O'Driscoll and Cooper 2002). *Primary level* interventions relate to the reduction of stress in the workplace, and are typically developed following the evaluation of specific factors that induce stress in the work environment. Examples include reducing individual workloads or redesigning jobs to remove ambiguity and conflict. *Secondary level* interventions include helping individuals to cope with stress in the workplace, while *tertiary level* interventions are basically programmes of support and counselling for employees who experience the effects of occupational stress. Managers of work organizations under pressure from the public are becoming increasingly aware that they must do something, yet more often focus on the individual level than implementations of changes in organizational structure or redesigning of jobs. Programmes of support, and training in coping with stress, not only are perceived as cheaper and more convenient for implementation in relation to long-term restructuring or major organizational changes, but also divert responsibility for the excessive stress of employees from the work organizations' managers.

Regarding intervention strategies for optimizing seafarers' health and well-being, it has to be said that some countries, such as the UK and Australia, have valuable projects relating to the mental health of seafarers (Iversen 2012). However, their main activities (printed booklets and leaflets about methods of stress reduction, recognition of signs of depression, a 24/7 help hotline, etc.) are directed at the seafarers. As such, they can be regarded only as *tertiary* (dealing with stress outcomes) or in some cases *secondary* measures of intervention (help in coping with stressors). Still, since many seafarers are reluctant to seek medical and psychological help because of rigorous health requirements in the competitive job market (Iversen 2012), these measures which raise awareness and help in coping with stressors in seafarers are of great importance.

However, the main intervention strategies in reducing stress and diminishing the occupational health risk of seafaring among seafarers should focus on reducing the main occupational stressors and risks (*primary* measures). Experts in the field warn that preventive measures should be based on strong evidence, since many suggestions for stress management in seafaring are based only on questionnaire surveys conducted ashore (Oldenburg et al. 2013b). Yet people who relate in any way to the maritime sector are aware, or should be aware, of the main stressors and hazards, such as, for example extremely long separation from home and family, or long working hours. Salyga and Juozulynas (2006) showed that psycho-emotional stress was already experienced after an average of 2.7 months from the beginning of the voyage. Still, the average stay on board for non-European crew members in a study conducted by Oldenburg et al. (2009) was 9.9 months per year. Furthermore, long working hours and related fatigue (Jensen et al. 2006; Smith et al. 2006) are also prevalent in the maritime sector. Knowledge from the broader area of occupational stress can also be a starting point for stress-preventive measures in seafarers. For example, data from a representative sample of the Canadian population aged 30–59 show that the number of hours spent working is a better predictor of stress and impaired health than is the type of activity (Beaujot and Anderson 2004). Finally, although the survey method has many shortcomings, in line with the transactional view of stress it is crucial, in the measurement of stress, to cover the appraisal of stressful factors in the work environment. Therefore, on the basis of the occupational stressors reviewed in this chapter, some of the main primary interventions in seafaring should include: *reduction in long separations from families* (i.e. shorter durations of stay on board), *minimizing fatigue* (through reduction of long working hours, increased number of crew and unbroken periods of rest and sleep), and *improvements in quality of life on board* (improvements in telecommunications, nutrition and recreational opportunities, as well as the promotion of social events on board). Although communication and family life among seafarers are today very favourable compared to former times (Hagmark 2003), free and unlimited internet access on board is still just an aspiration for many seafarers.

In addition to the above suggestions, it is extremely important for managers to listen to the voices of their employees and to take them into account in making decisions. There is a large volume of evidence, in the broader area of occupational stress, that intervention on this basis—in the direction of re-designing jobs (especially those which increase control and autonomy among employees), adopting participatory management styles, developing clear role descriptions, setting effective goals and giving feedback—can reduce stress and increase the well-being of employees (O'Driscoll and Cooper 2002). These approaches include the provision of certain financial resources, as well as involvement and effort from the management, but in the long term bring benefits to the employees and the work organization (Giga et al. 2003; O'Driscoll and Cooper 2002). On the other hand, evidence of the efficacy of secondary and tertiary interventions is inconsistent and very limited (McKenna 2000; O'Driscoll and Cooper 2002). The managements of shipping organizations, as well as national and international regulatory bodies in the maritime sector, have responsibility for development activities that enhance, rather than impair, the physical and mental health of employees. A common approach in dealing with stress may result in a work environment that is productive for the shipping organizations and healthier for seafarers. Furthermore, intervention strategies should be focused not solely on the prevention of physical or psychological risk, but on practices which yield healthy organizations (Jaimez and Bretones 2011). A "healthy organization" is defined as one whose culture, management, working climate and other business practices create an environment that promotes the complete physical, mental and social well-being, effectiveness and performance of its employees (Wilson et al. 2004). According to Jaimez and Bretones (2011), there is no single solution for all types of organization, but the participation and involvement of employees is proposed as a fundamental element for creating a healthy organization. Therefore, all workers should be actively involved in the development and optimization of organizational practices which promote a healthy workplace—which, in the case of shipping companies, includes seafarers on board.

Occupational Stress in Seafaring from the Transactional Perspective

Seafaring is a demanding, high-risk and stressful occupation which cannot be compared with jobs ashore. There are a large number of stressors, risks and challenges that seafarers face, which can lead to consequences for their physical and psychological health (Allen et al. 2008; Carotenuto et al. 2012; Iversen 2012; MacLachlan et al. 2012; Oldenburg et al. 2010a). MacLachlan et al. (2012, 2013) noted that the health of seafarers has been dramatically influenced by factors such as globalization of the shipping industry, increased automation and mechanization of work on ships, improvements in navigation techniques, reduction in crew numbers, increased uncertainty and short-term contracting of seafarers in commercial fleets, multicultural crewing and ships operated under flags of convenience.

In accordance with the transactional perspective on occupational stress, in this chapter the main stressors in the field will be determined, as well as their potential effects on the health and well-being of seafarers. In addition to effects at the individual level, effects at the organizational level will also be discussed. Finally, important individual and organizational characteristics which can moderate or mediate links between occupational stressors and stress outcomes will be reviewed, some of which have been relatively neglected in the research field. However, it is important to first define the concept of occupational stress within the theoretical framework in use.

Definition of Occupational Stress

Occupational stress is a term which is often used in the scientific literature and in daily life. However, there is no general agreement on its definition, which is the result of various research approaches to *stress* in general, and also too broad a use of the term *stress* (Hart and Cooper 2001).

In scientific literature, *stress* has usually been understood in three ways: (1) stress as an external stimulus or the force exerted on the individual, i.e. *stimulus model* (2) stress as the individual psychological or physical response to an external force, i.e. *response model*, and (3) stress as the interaction of stimulus and response, i.e. *interactional* or *cognitive model* (Arnold et al. 2005; Sulsky and Smith 2005). Today, however, most researchers use the term *stressor* to identify external stimuli or events, and the terms *strain* or *distress* for the response or reaction of the individual. Thus, the term *stress* covers the general interactional process of linking stressors, coping with the stressors and the effects of stress, rather than specific elements. The key factor which determines whether the stress occurs is a personal appraisal of the situation and assessment of the risk level, unlike physical and environmental stressors, where, for example, exposure to toxic substances does not necessarily lead to appraisal, but often leads to physical reactions: "For psychosocial stressors, stress is indeed in the eye of the beholder" (Sulsky and Smith 2005, p. 12).

A great contribution to the field of stress was made by Lazarus and Folkman (1984, 1987; Lazarus 1990). They defined stress as a relationship between the individual and the environment arising from the former's estimation that the requirements of the latter exceed his capabilities to meet them. If such requirements persist over time, this can lead to chronic adverse effects. However, stress reaction is preceded by an appraisal of the stressfulness of the situation. The primary appraisal of stress depends on personal and situational factors, and it is followed by a secondary cognitive appraisal which implies the evaluation of different strategies of coping with the stressor. Lazarus and Folkman gradually formed a *transactional model* of stress and, with its formulation, theoretically moved away from the classical interactional models of stress, which assumed an additive and linear relation between environmental and individual factors in determining outcomes of stress, or a one-way causality. Under the interactional approach, stress has been studied as a static structure with fixedly divided independent and dependent variables, which does not allow reciprocal causation—for example, that the level of stress responses of an individual affects the perception of stressors. In contrast, Lazarus' transactional standpoint implies a circular nature and a feedback system. It introduces the concept of reappraisal based on new information, either from the environment or personal reaction. Because the model assumes constant change in the individual and the environment, cognitive appraisal is continuously renewing and changing (Hart and Cooper 2001). These benefits of the transactional model compared to previous models are also shortcomings from the methodological point of view, because it is difficult to determine when the stress process begins and when it ends, which creates difficulties in stress research (Lazarus 1990).

As there is no single definition of stress in general, there is no single definition of occupational stress. This ambiguity in the definition and operationalization of professional stress is one of the most important methodological problems in its research (Schonfeld et al. 1995). Kenny and McIntyre (2005) classified contemporary approaches and models of occupational stress into five categories: (1) intrapersonal approach; (2) interpersonal approach; (3) organizational and transactional occupational stress theories; (4) cybernetics and systems theory; and (5) occupational stress in the framework of the analysis of the work process.

The most comprehensive transactional perspective on occupational stress is given in the model of Cooper et al. (1988, 2001; Cooper and Baglioni 1988; O'Driscoll and Cooper 2002; Williams and Cooper 1998), as well as in that of Cox and co-workers (Cox and Mackay 1981; Cox 1987; Cox and Griffiths 1995). Considering the great influence of the transactional approach to stress in the broader area of stress, it will serve here as a broader theoretical frame to illustrate the main elements of stress in seafarers. In establishing the transactional model of occupational stress, Cooper et al. (1988) argued that the dominant models in that time period (Karasek's *demand-control model* and *person-environment fit theories*) were limited and should be incorporated into the broader multidimensional transactional model of Lazarus. In spite of differences between the different models (e.g. Cooper's vs. Cox's model), a general transactional perspective on occupational stress is focused on three elements: the sources of stress, the consequences for the individual and the organization, and individual differences in personality and behaviour. Stress transactions are the product of the individual and the environment: the individual affects the environment and at the same time responds to demands of the environment. The central place in the model is taken by appraisal or assessment, so the object of measurement of occupational stress is not work requirement or pressure, but the perception of pressure. Therefore, in examining occupational stress and stressors it is appropriate to use questionnaires. The process of stress depends on the perception of the situation or the assessment of the stressfulness of situations. Stress reaction occurs when an individual determines that the intensity of the stressors overcomes his ability to cope. Therefore, the following sections will relate to (1) sources of stress in seafarers; (2) stress reactions, i.e. effects of stress at the individual and organizational levels; and (3) individual characteristics which influence the perception of stressfulness, stress reactions and consequences.

Sources of Stress in Seafarers

Table 2 shows the different sources of stress (i.e. stressors) faced by seafarers, some of which are occupation related, while the others (work related) are typical sources of work stressors recognized in different occupations, but also found in seafarers.

One of the most frequently cited psychosocial sources of stress (i.e. stressors) in seafaring is *long-term separation* from home and family (Carotenuto et al. 2012; Iversen 2012). Although this stressor is especially evident in the cases of longer contract duration and in younger seafarers with children (Oldenburg et al. 2009, 2010a), the fact is that all seafarers are, by the nature of their work, separated from their homes. Even under the most favourable employment conditions, seafarers

Table 2 Sources of stress in seafaring

Occupation-related stressors in seafaring	Work-related stressors in seafaring
Long-term separation from home and family *Deprivation of physical and psycho-social needs on board*: sleep deprivation, limited influence on quality and quantity of food, limited opportunities for recreation, disturbed sexual life, social isolation "*Living two separate lives*" *Environmental stressors on board*: poor weather, ship motion, noise, vibration, heat *Multinational crews* *Exploitation and abuse* "*Criminalization of seafarers*"	*Demands of the job:* high workload, long working hours, shift work *Low level of control over work* *Interpersonal relationships* with supervisors, colleagues, and subordinates *Level of support received from management and colleagues* *Role in the organization* and *role conflict* *Introduction of changes and change management* *Job insecurity*

spend at least 6 months a year at sea (Alderton et al. 2004). Stress levels caused by separation from home increase significantly when family members are unwell or when contact with the family is difficult (Carotenuto et al. 2012). Being physically away from home and family can bring anxiety relating to the illness of loved ones, sexual fidelity of the partner, problematic behaviour of children, the family's general well-being and practical household matters (Alderton et al. 2004). Therefore, cyberspace communication with the partner is of great importance for peer social support and strengthening of relationships in seafaring (Tang 2012).

Alongside loneliness caused by separation from family, partner or wife and children, seafarers also report *social isolation*, caused by their characteristic way of life on board, now additionally aggravated by reduction in crew numbers, short ship-turnaround times and lack of shore leave (Iversen 2012; MacLachlan et al. 2012). Besides short ship-turnaround times, the reasons for low levels of shore leave are: working, a need for rest, difficulties in simply getting to the dockyard gate from the berthing area, lack of visa or security regulation in the country, and depression (Iversen 2012). Social isolation in seafarers is a major cause of psychological problems, such as depression, and in particular situations, and in vulnerable individuals, this can lead to suicide (Carotenuto et al. 2012; Iversen 2012).

Work-related stressors of seafaring include typical sources of work stress which are recognized in many occupational stress models, such as: the *demands of the job* (*high workload* and *long working hours*); the *level of control* seafarers have over their work; the *support* received from management and colleagues; *relationships at work*; the *seafarers' role* in the organization; *change and change management*; and *job security* (especially for non-rated seafarers who are employed on contract) (Iversen 2012). These stressors lead to typical symptoms of stress, such as insomnia, loss of concentration, anxiety, frustration, anger, headaches, heart disease and less productivity in general, but they can also lead to burnout and chronic responsibility syndrome. Chronic responsibility syndrome is defined as a kind of burnout where people become mentally and physically exhausted from high workload caused by the individual's perception that no one but them can do the work (Iversen 2012). Regarding *working hours*, the results of an international study which included 6461 seafarers from 11 countries showed that most seafarers worked every day of the week, for 67–70 h a week on average, during periods of 2.5–8.5 months at sea (Jensen et al. 2006). In addition, comparison of seafarers with non-seafarers of matched ages shows a significant difference in the *level of control* between them (Lodde et al. 2008). That is, assessments of Karasek's decision-latitude dimension were at much lower levels for seafarers than for non-seafarers. The results also showed that 17 % of seafarers (compared to 0 % of non-seafarers) were ranked in the category of heavy strain/low decision latitude, which is regarded by Karasek as a high risk of stress, and that 33 % of seafarers reached a score which indicated psychic stress according to Langner's Total Health Test. One of the work-related stressors which was highly elevated was *role conflict* (Rydstedt and Lundh 2010). Role conflict appears where conflicting requirements by other actors and interested parties in the shipping operation are directed towards the individual seafarer. It is particularly characteristic of mid-level managers "who are supposed [to] live up to their professional standards in shipping and at the same [time] operate the ship with reduced crew numbers and high speed, so as to satisfy the requirements for profitability" (Rydstedt and Lundh 2010, p. 174). The authors assumed that the rapid technological and organizational change and increased pressure for economic profitability that characterize the shipping industry have aggravated this source of stress. In the context of working stressors on board, one of the major issues is fatigue.

Fatigue in seafarers is regarded as a consequence of work stress, high job demands, insufficient crew members, long working hours, watch systems which do not allow enough rest periods (2-watch system and rotating watch system), disturbed circadian rhythms imposed by shift schedules and quick travel across multiple time zones, sleep deprivation and compromised safety standards (Allen et al. 2008; Arulanandam and Chan Chung Tsing 2009; Carotenuto et al. 2012; Hystad et al. 2013; Oldenburg et al. 2010a, 2013b; Wadsworth et al. 2006, 2008). Many maritime studies have focused on fatigue, since it is considered the most important risk factor for maritime accidents, with severe life-threatening environmental and economic consequences, as well as for the impairment of seafarers' health and well-being. Unfortunately, fatigue is more prevalent in the seafaring world than scientists are currently able or prepared to measure (Allen et al. 2008). Authors in this field warn of a concerning number of under-recorded working hours in seafarers (Smith et al. 2006). Disturbance of circadian rhythms imposed by *shift work*, especially night work, is recognized as an important factor in the development of sleep disturbance, as well as serious illnesses, such as gastrointestinal and cardiovascular diseases (Slišković 2010). Results of studies in seafarers confirm a strong independent association between longer term fatigue and physical and mental health outcome measures (Smith et al. 2006; Wadsworth et al. 2006, 2008). Data also show that measuring seafarers' fatigue on waking may be a more sensitive measure of emerging cumulative fatigue, which could relate to occupational performance, accident risk, and perhaps longer- term well-being (Wadsworth et al. 2006).

In addition to psychosocial stressors related to the seafarers' characteristic way of life (separation from home and families, isolation and loneliness) and specific work stressors and related fatigue, seafarers are continuously exposed to *environmental stressors on board*. These include *poor weather*, *ship motion*, *noise* and *vibration*, and they can significantly impact the recreational value of leisure and sleeping times (Oldenburg et al. 2010a). An additional environmental stressor for engine personnel is the *heat* in the workplace (Oldenburg et al. 2009; Rengamani and Murugan 2012). Life on board brings with it additional stressors, primarily those related to the *deprivation* of physical and psycho-social needs. During the stay on board, seafarers have *limited influence on quality and quantity of food* (Oldenburg et al. 2013a), and their nutrition issue is even more pronounced in multi-ethnic crews with different dietary habits. Recent studies showed poor food hygiene knowledge of cooking and catering staff on board (Grappasonni et al. 2013), and numerous barriers to promotion of healthy diet at sea (Hjarnoe and Leppin 2014). *Limited opportunities for recreation* are regarded as an important source of stress, since the often-observed lack of leisure-time facilities (e.g. fitness rooms or social events) impairs seafarers' physical, psychological and social well-being (Carotenuto et al. 2012; Oldenburg et al. 2010a). *Disturbed sexual life* on board is also associated with the occurrence of psycho-emotional stress in seafarers (Oldenburg et al. 2010a).

Interpersonal relationships with supervisors, colleagues, and subordinates are generally recognized as one of the major occupational stressors (Cartwright and Cooper 1996). Considering the frequent changes in working teams on board and working in the multinational and multicultural environment of the seafaring sector, interpersonal relationships may pose a specific challenge for seafarers. Regarding familiarity of working teams, Espevik and Olsen (2013) showed that unfamiliar teams use less efficient coordination strategies, which reduce efficiency and increase levels of stress in novel and critical work situations. *Multinational crews* are recognized as a specific stressor, too (Oldenburg et al. 2010a). Since crews consist not only of many different nationalities, but also of different religious and cultural backgrounds, different needs, values and expectations may lead to communication problems, conflicts, abuse, racism and isolation (Carotenuto et al. 2012; Oldenburg et al. 2010a; Iversen 2012). Adequate English language skills among crew members are prerequisite not only for work, but also for socialization on board (Sampson and Zhao 2003). Furthermore, ship owners' preferences for particular groups on the basis of skills, nationality and cost may lead to discrimination, which takes varying forms, but the most widespread is in terms of wage differentials between different nationalities (McLaughlin 2012). This could also be reflected in the crew on board in terms of poor relations between nationals and non-nationals working on vessels flying certain flags. Oldenburg et al. (2009) note that the social gradient in their study, where only 6.4 % of non-Europeans performed superior duties, likely also constitutes a source of stress on ships.

Some seafarers report *exploitation and abuse* (Iversen 2012). This is most evident in those seafarers who work in a substandard sector of merchant shipping (ships defective in structure and equipment, and those with low wages and poor working conditions). Hayashi (2001) warned that the entire maritime industry suffers from practices which disregard generally accepted standards. With regard to the evident decline in the numbers of seafarers coming from developed countries, coupled with shipping companies' desire to reduce labour unit costs (McLaughlin 2012), exploitation of the cheap workforces of the Far East and Eastern Europe is becoming a significant issue for seafarers' health and well-being.

Seafarers also report one special source of stress, known as *criminalization of seafarers*. It is a term used to describe the treatment of maritime incidents (for example, oil pollution incidents; maritime accidents beyond their control; maritime accidents where there has been some negligence, regardless of the fact that such negligence is not considered criminal in the maritime industry) as 'true crimes'. It is also used as a blanket term to describe the denial of procedural and human rights in the investigation and prosecution of those incidents (Iversen 2012).

In addition to the above stressors, the specificity shared by all seafarers is the fact that they are *living two separate lives* (Hafez 1999). The first life is the onboard ship life away from home with all specificities. The second life is the home life, where the seafarer is supposed to enjoy family life and generally relax before returning to sea. However, seafarers at home may also be exposed to different types of stress concerning their family issues. Adaptation by the seafarer and his family to differences related to the two ways of life may also be stressful. Stressfulness of their period at home may also especially be the case if they are not protected and covered by a social security system (Hafez 1999; Slišković and Penezić 2015).

Besides the stressors, it should be noted that seafaring still has many risks (Grappasonni et al. 2012; Iversen 2012; Rodríguez et al. 2011; Oldenburg et al. 2010a, b). Seafaring risks include (1) *accidents* due to harmful conditions at sea and to non-observance of safety rules; (2) *piracy,* whose incidence has been rising since the mid 1990s; (3) risk of *communicable diseases*, including those related to on-board hygiene; (4) *the limited ability to provide medical aid on board*, which is most pronounced in cases of heart failure; and (5) *exposure to hazardous substances and UV light*, which may be related to the risk of *occupational cancer*.

Effects of Stress in Seafaring at the Individual and Organizational Levels

Occupational stressors have been implicated as risk factors for many physical, psychological and behavioural problems in workers, including increased risk of heart disease, gastrointestinal problems, musculoskeletal disorders, sleep problems, headache, anxiety, depression, burnout, fatigue, accidents, substance misuse, dysfunctional behaviour, suicide, homicide, work-family conflict, and many other problems (Arnold et al. 2005; Cox and Griffiths 1995; Leka et al. 2005; Theorell and Karasek 1996). At the individual level, stressors lead to a state of being unable to perform one's duties with the usual diligence, accuracy and efficiency. The outcomes described at the individual level can also have serious consequences for employers, potentially leading to decreased performance and productivity, high turnover and absenteeism, increased unsafe working practice and accident rates, and low morale (Arnold et al. 2005; Leka et al. 2005). The financial costs of stressful work are due to a combination of two reasons: reduced productivity and increased levels of health problems associated with stress. According to Arnold et al. (2005), the UK is losing 10 % of its annual national income due to stress generated at work. The causes of these losses are manifold. In the first place are the organizational and medical costs of sick leave, since stress at work is generally the most significant cause of absenteeism. In addition, job turnover increases the costs of job training, job advertising and selection, reduces overall efficiency and disturbs other workers. Finally, the complaints of workers due to stress-related illness, and the implementation of stress management programmes in organizations, which are becoming a necessity nowadays, also contribute significantly to the aforementioned losses.

Regarding the effects of stress in seafaring at the organizational level, the main contributions are made by a Cardiff study (Smith et al. 2006) and maritime field studies (Oldenburg et al. 2013b), which showed links between working hours in reduced crewing, fatigue and performance. These results indicated that the policy of reduced crewing in the shipping industry is associated with an increase in stress and a decrease in health and safety. However, most of the research in this field focuses on outcomes at the individual level, i.e. the health and well-being of seafarers. Yet results obtained from general working populations show an association between average well-being at the organizational level and organizational performance (Daniels and Harris 2000). Furthermore, workers' attitudes, such as job satisfaction, are associated with their health and level of occupational stress (Faragher et al. 2005), and also with job performance, turnover and withdrawal behaviour (Saari and Judge 2004). Therefore, outcomes of stress at the individual and organizational levels are presumably inevitably intertwined also in the maritime sector.

Since intensive stress could be a trigger for impaired health in seafarers, further sections present the results of research relating to the mortality, health and well-being of seafarers. Potential clues about links between stressors in seafaring and health may be found in studies using biochemical parameters. For example, Lu et al. (2010) analysed blood chemistry measures in 170 Chinese seafarers before and after a 3-month voyage, and identified nine measures (monoamine oxidases, creatine kinase, lactate dehydrogenase, albumin, fructosamine, inorganic ions: calcium, phosphate, kalium and natrium) which were affected during the sailing. The authors argue that great temperature changes, poor diet structure, lack of exercise, abnormal electromagnetic radiation and stress may cause subtle changes in physiological and psychological functions in seafarers' bodies.

Mortality in Seafarers

The results of a study which involved 24,132 Danish seafarers (Hansen and Pedersen 1996) have shown that merchant seafarers have a higher mortality than the general population. (The standardized mortality ratio was 1.43 from all causes and 3.05 from accidents.) Despite a very high risk of fatal accidents in the workplace, these accidents could only explain a proportion of the observed excess mortality, while accidents ashore and diseases related to lifestyle factors made a major contribution to the observed excess mortality. The results of mortality studies in seafarers can generally be divided into three categories: (1) accident-related mortality, (2) disease- and lifestyle-related mortality, and (3) suicide mortality.

Further research on Danish seafarers (Hansen et al. 2002) focused on *occupational accidents* aboard merchant ships in international trade (time period 1993–1997). Among a total number of 1993 accidents, 209 accidents resulted in permanent disability of 5 % or more, and 27 were fatal. An analysis of traumatic work-related mortality among seafarers employed in British merchant shipping from 1976 to 2002, which was based on official mortality files, with a very large sample, has shown that the mortality rate for the 530 fatal accidents that occurred in the workplace in the observed time period was 27.8 times as high as in the general workforce in Great Britain during the same time period (Roberts and Marlow 2005). To be precise, of 835 traumatic work-related deaths, 564 were caused by accidents, 55 by suicide, 17 by homicide, and 14 by drug or alcohol poisoning. The circumstances in which the other 185 deaths occurred, including 178 seafarers who disappeared at sea or were found drowned, were undetermined. The authors conclude that, despite improvements in health and safety that have led to substantial reductions in fatal accident rates in UK merchant shipping throughout most of the last 90 years, seafaring has remained a hazardous occupation (Roberts and Marlow 2005). Actually, the data show that the relative risk of an accident in UK shipping, compared with the general British workforce, was similar in 2001 to that in 1961 (Roberts 2008). Since shipping accidents remain a major concern in the modern shipping industry, contemporary studies deal with analysis of causes of different classes of accidents and collisions (Chauvin et al. 2013), prediction of mortality count based on influencing factors, such as type and place of accident, weather and darkness conditions (Weng and Yang 2015), and differences between nationalities in the rate of accidents, such as those which were found in the Danish merchant fleet (Ádám et al. 2014). Although differences decreased over the investigated period (2010–2012), the higher accident rate of Western European than that of Eastern European, South East Asian and Indian seamen, according to the authors, may be related to national differences in reporting practice, safety behaviour and fitness to work. Further exploration of the underlying causes of nationality differences in occupational safety culture is recommended (Ádám et al. 2014).

Studies focusing on *morbidity and mortality* in seafarers are often confounded by the "healthy worker effect," i.e. better or equal health status of seafarers compared to the general population. This effect is commonly obtained in cross-sectional studies and may be explained by self-selection and adaptation. Seafarers who cannot adapt to the work on board, as well as those who are suffering from the effects of occupational stressors, leave the occupation. This effect is also known as the "survival effect," meaning that individuals capable of coping with work demands tend to remain in the workforce (Bridger et al. 2010). For example, mortality data on seafarers employed in British merchant shipping from 1939 to 2002 (Roberts 2005) show sharp reductions regarding mortality from gastrointestinal diseases and from alcoholism. These results contrast with increases among the general British population, and are largely due to the "flagging-out" of most British deep-sea ships, and consequent reductions in long voyages, as well as reductions in alcohol consumption among seafarers at work. Lower work-related mortality from cardiovascular diseases (CVD) and ischemic heart disease (IHD) among seafarers employed in British shipping than in the corresponding general population is also explained by a healthy worker effect among the seafarers (Roberts and Jaremin 2010). At the same time, mortality risk from CVD among British seafarers ashore in Britain increased, which is at least partially caused by seafarers' being discharged ashore from active service because of sickness or disability, including CVD morbidity. Results from the same study showed an increase in mortality risk from CVD among the crews of North Sea offshore ships, which may reflect particular work-related hazards in this sector. It can be concluded that cross-sectional research may underestimate health problems in seafarers, so longitudinal studies are strongly recommended. However, since an increase in morbidity and mortality occur in the function of ageing, a seafarers group followed through their work and life span (including the period after any abandonment of the occupation) should be accompanied by a control group of workers with matching characteristics.

The data on *suicides* prove that the mental health of seafarers in many cases continues to be very poor and often fatal (Iversen 2012). While the figure for suicide among total deaths in the general population ranges from 1.2 to 2 %, suicides by seafarers are much more common. Seafarers' international death statistics based on 20 reports published in the years from 1960 to 2009 show that, of a total of 17,026 seafarer deaths, 1011 (i.e. 5.9 %) were by suicide (Iversen 2012). Analysis of suicides among seafarers in UK merchant shipping (Roberts et al. 2009) show that the suicide rate among seafarers was substantially higher than the overall suicide rate in the general British population from 1919 to the 1970s, but, following reductions in suicide mortality among seafarers, it has become more comparable since. These drops are explained by reductions over time in long intercontinental voyages and changes in seafarers' lifestyles over time. The results of this study additionally show that suicide rates among seafarers in UK merchant shipping were higher for ranks below officers and for older seafarers, and higher for Asian seafarers than for British seafarers (Roberts et al. 2009). The data also indicate that suicide rates among seafarers in UK merchant shipping were typically lower than those in Asian and Scandinavian merchant fleets. The results of a mortality study among Polish seafarers and deep-sea fishermen have shown that the incidence of suicides among the observed sample during work at sea was significantly higher than suicides among the age-comparable male population of the country

(Szymanska et al. 2006). The risk is greatest for seafarers aged 30–39 years, with a period of service from 10 to 24 years, working as ratings, with known or concealed alcohol addiction and/or family problems or insufficient identification with the group.

Physical Health and Psychological Well-Being of Seafarers

According to a review of papers published in the journal *International Maritime Health* from 2000 to 2010 (MacLachlan et al. 2012), among *physical health problems* in seafarers, most papers focused on cardiovascular disease, heart attack, diabetes, and lifestyle factors which contribute to these diseases.

Although acute cardiovascular diseases are the main cause of death in industrialized countries (both at sea and on land), the results of the study show that, after taking into consideration the healthy worker effect of seafarers, cardiac risk factors are shown to occur slightly more frequently in seafarers than in the general population (Oldenburg et al. 2010b). Results of research on cardiovascular and coronary diseases in seafarers on vessels under the German flag show that, in spite of the seafarers' regular medical surveillance examination, their CHD risk was similar to that of a reference population working ashore (Oldenburg et al. 2007, 2010c).

Since seafarers may be exposed to engine exhaust, various oil products and many carcinogenic chemicals, some studies have focussed on cancer risk. The results of a study which aimed to investigate the possible work-related reasons for the increased incidence of many cancers among seafarers who worked on Finnish ships for any time during the period 1960–80 (Saarni et al. 2002) show that occupational exposure of deck crews on tankers adds to their risk of renal cancer, leukaemia and possibly lymphoma. On the other hand, engine crews have an asbestos-related risk of mesothelioma, and engine-room conditions also seem to increase the risk of lung cancer. The results of research conducted on all Danish seafarers during 1986–1999 who were followed up for cancer until the end of 2002 have shown that Danish seafarers, especially men, face an increased overall cancer risk—in particular, risk of lung cancer and other tobacco-associated cancers (Kaerlev et al. 2005).

Regarding the slightly elevated risk of cardiovascular disease in seafarers, Oldenburg (2014) allocated three potentially influential risk factors: the ship's specific stress situation (originating from specific occupational psychosocial stressors), malnutrition (unbalanced, high-fat diet) and the lack of exercise on board. Data generally show that lifestyle factors explain a large proportion of mortality and disease in seafarers. Comparison of sea captains and marine chief engineers with a group of shore-based employed men (matched with the seafarers for age, ethnic origin and level of education) has shown that certain behavioural risk factors were more dominant among the seafarers than among the control group (Carel et al. 1990). These include smoking level, alcohol consumption and lack of leisure-time physical activity. Analysis of national data for England and Wales indicates that seafarers are among the groups of occupations with the highest mortality from alcohol-related diseases and injuries (Coggon et al. 2010). The results of a stratified survey of French seafarers (Fort et al. 2009) confirmed that alcohol and nicotine consumption is a major public health issue in seafarers. Approximately 44 % of their sample was current smokers, and more than 11 % drank alcohol every day. A review study (Pougnet et al. 2014) which focused on consumption of addictive substances showed a higher prevalence of tobacco and alcohol consumption in seafarers than the general population. According to this review, which was based on international publications, 63.1 % of seafarers smoked, while 14.5 % were hazardous drinkers (according to the World Health Organization (WHO) definition). Besides smoking and alcohol consumption, one of the factors in lifestyle-related diseases that dominate among seafarers is obesity. Overweight was found, to a statistically significant extent, to be represented more highly in seafarers than a reference group ashore (Hoeyer and Hansen 2005), and this can influence seafarers' health and shipboard safety. Data also show that the best predictor of work ability in seafarers was the interaction between body mass index and age, where the adverse effect of high body mass index was greater in older seafarers (Bridger and Bennett 2011). Study results show that obesity among seafarers is favoured by compulsive eating disorder, night eating disorder and emotional eating disorder, and that eating is most frequently a reaction to stress or boredom (Jeżewska et al. 2009).

The above-mentioned review (MacLachlan et al. 2012) showed that the category *psychological functioning and health* had a relatively small, but increasing, number of papers. Papers relating to stress, fatigue, alertness levels and psychological issues such as depression and general psychological well-being featured most prominently in this category. It can be said that the area of psychological well-being and mental health has been relatively neglected in previous studies in comparison to studies which focused on physical health. For example, in a paper titled 'Mapping the knowledge base for maritime health', psychological aspects of health are also relatively unattended to (Carter 2011). Respecting the definition of health given by the WHO (1948), where health is defined as "a state of complete physical, mental and social well-being and not merely the absence of disease or infirmity", scientists and practitioners in the maritime health area need to place greater emphasis on psychological and mental aspects of health, especially regarding the numerous mental and psychosocial stressors that seafarers face.

Therefore, studies that have focused on psychological well-being (e.g. Carotenuto et al. 2013), psychological quality of life (e.g. Juozulynas et al. 2007) and burn-out syndrome (e.g. Oldenburg et al. 2012) are encouraged, especially those which aim to determine the role of working conditions in the well-being of seafarers. For example, Oldenburg et al. (2012) showed that emotional exhaustion in seafarers is associated with a subjective perception of insufficient sleep on board, lack of care provided by their superiors and/or the shipping company, with high responsibility for work organization (for senior members of crew) and with social problems due to the long periods of separation from their families.

Since job satisfaction and intent to leave are considered reliable indicators of work-related well-being, one survey study focused on these variables (Nielsen et al. 2013). The results of this study, conducted on 817 seafarers working on vessels belonging to two large Norwegian shipping companies, show that job satisfaction and intent to leave among seafarers are related to physical and psychosocial factors in the working environment, and especially safety perceptions, job demands and team cohesion. The results of a study on Danish seafarers (Haka et al. 2011) confirmed that the main motivating and demotivating factors are related to psychosocial factors rather than organizational or structural factors. The work motivators which were identified in this study include duration of home leave, level of responsibility and level of challenge, while the main demotivating factors that were identified were being away from home, the shipping company´s HRM, and regulatory requirements. However, it would be interesting to conduct similar studies on other national and cultural groups. The results of a pilot study of Croatian seafarers (Penezić et al. 2013) have shown that job satisfaction is a significant positive predictor of their life satisfaction. On the other hand, the results also showed that significant negative correlates of seafarers' life satisfaction include depression, stress and social loneliness, loneliness in love and loneliness in the family.

Individual Differences in Experience of Occupational Stressors, Health and Well-Being Among Seafarers

Regarding the various socio-demographic and working characteristics (age, cultural background and nationality, length of service, level of education, rank and type of job on board, type of employment contract and duration of onboard stay, type and size of vessel, marital status, having children, etc.), the seafaring population cannot be regarded as a whole. The results of an international study of seafarers (Jensen et al. 2006) showed that self-rated health generally declined significantly with age, and it varied by country. Obvious explanations of national differences can be found in the fact that seafarers from South-East Asian countries spent longer periods at sea, and had lower numbers of officers and older seafarers than are found among seafarers from western countries. According with that fact is the result of a study conducted by Borovnik (2011), who warned of particular health risks for seafarers from developing Pacific countries because of their long contracts on board. Oldenburg et al. (2009) noted that non-European crew members on German-flagged ships stay twice as long as Europeans: 9.9 versus 4.9 months, and sometimes exceeding 12 months.

The ageing of the workforce is particularly important within the whole of the transportation industry (Popkin et al. 2008). Regarding seafarers, the results of a study conducted by Rydstedt and Lundh (2012) suggest that rapid technological and organizational development in the shipping industry may be associated with increased mental strain for older engine-room officers. Data from a study of Lithuanian seafarers (Juozulynas et al. 2007) have confirmed age differences in the physical and psychological health-related quality of life (QOL). These results show that physical QOL is best among the youngest seafarers (20–24 years old), while psychological QOL is best among seafarers aged 20–24 and 25–34 years.

Length of service is also an important variable. Although seafarers' health declines with age (Jensen et al. 2006), the experience which is obtained with years of service could minimize the effects of work-related stressors. The results obtained by Jeżewska et al. (2006) showed that students, during their training period on merchant ships, perceive the job as highly stressful compared to the group of merchant marine officers.

The results of the abovementioned study of Lithuanian seafarers (Juozulynas et al. 2007) also show differences by profession, where health-related QOL is best among commanding group members. The physical dimension of QOL is worst among engineer ship service members, while psychological QOL is worst among ship auxiliary service seafarers. A study done by Carotenuto et al. (2013) also showed differences in some aspects of psychological well-being between seafarers of different categories. The results obtained (higher levels of anxiety and self-control among deck and engine officers than among the crew) supported the view that management responsibilities are related to higher levels of stress. A study on a sample of Danish seafarers has shown differences in the motivational profiles of officers and non-officers (Haka et al. 2011). All these results show the importance of considering the rank and job tasks on board, since they involve coping with different stressors. While non-officers stay on board for considerably longer periods than officers (8.3 months vs. 4.8 months), officers complain more frequently of time pressure and report a far higher number of working hours than non-officers (Oldenburg et al. 2009). The results of the study conducted by Oldenburg et al. (2009) also showed that low qualification of subordinate crew represents a stressor on board for superiors, and that deck and catering staff had higher stress levels due to long working days and time pressure or hectic activities, compared to engine-room personnel.

Furthermore, working conditions, occupational stressors and stress levels depend upon type of ship (cargo vs. passenger ship), type of cargo (e.g. container, tanker, etc.), size of vessel, and port frequency or average time period of voyage (short vs. long voyages) and ship route, although systematic investigation of these factors has as yet scarcely been performed (Oldenburg et al. 2009).

Regarding family situation, Oldenburg et al. (2009) noted that separation from home and family particularly affects younger seafarers with children. Peplińska et al. (2013, 2014) showed that marital satisfaction has a significant mediating role in the association between perceived stress and anxiety reactions, as well as between stress and sense of purpose of life. Marital satisfaction in seafarers thus increases their ability to cope with stressful situations at sea, reducing the likelihood of anxiety reaction, and providing a sense of purpose in life. On the other hand, low levels of marital satisfaction may intensify the poignancy of stress, increase the probability of experiencing fear and anxiety and thus negatively influence a general sense of purpose in life.

Suggestions for Further Studies

Further Research Questions

Considering the lack of systematic comprehensive investigation of the complex and multivariate process of occupational stress in seafaring, the main suggestion is implementation of an ecologically valid and theoretically rich transactional perspective into the research field. Although individual differences and subjective appraisal are seen by occupational stress authors as integral to the entire stress process, a great amount of empirical research is still based on models that focus solely on environmental stressors, neglecting individual differences (Mark and Smith 2008). Within transactional models of occupational stress an important role is given to the variables which may moderate or mediate links between sources of stress and outcomes, i.e. moderator and mediator variables. The moderator variable is a stable variable (such as gender) which affects the direction and/or strength of the relation between an independent variable (e.g. stressor) and a dependent variable (e.g. stress outcome), while the mediator variable (such as personal coping skills) is itself changing under the influence of an independent variable and in turn influences the dependent variable (Baron and Kenny 1986). A great number of individual and organizational characteristics may have a moderator or mediator role in the relationship of stressors and stress outcomes in seafaring. As noted in the previous section, while earlier studies showed the significant role of some of the socio-demographic and work-related characteristics, many important characteristics have not gained as much attention (e.g. type of cargo or ship route).

Regarding individual characteristics, along with socio-demographic and work-related characteristics, further studies in the field therefore should include personality traits, whose moderator or mediator role is shown in the broader area of occupational stress. These include anxiety as a trait, neuroticism, negative affectivity, extraversion, conscientiousness, self-esteem, work locus of control, personal hardiness, and some aspects of type-A behaviour, such as hostility, etc. (Arnold et al. 2005; Grant and Langan-Fox 2006; Hart and Cooper 2001; Kobasa 1979; Ng et al. 2006; O'Driscoll and Cooper 2002; Semmer 2003; Sulsky and Smith 2005). For example, internal locus of control in the work setting is positively related to general well-being, including psychological well-being, physical health, and job satisfaction, and also to intrinsic motivational orientation and proactive behavioural orientation of workers (Ng et al. 2006).

Further research should also incorporate coping with stress, since coping strategy may be more important for outcomes at both individual and organizational levels than frequency and intensity of stressful events (Lazarus and Folkman 1984). Therefore, further studies may investigate the use of different coping strategies (problem-focused vs. emotion-focused strategies) in dealing with different occupational stressors in seafaring. This line of research could differentiate adaptive and maladaptive coping techniques in seafarers and provide practical implications for interventions.

With regard to the important direct and/or moderator role of social support in dealing with occupational stress (Karasek and Theorell 1990; O'Driscoll and Cooper 2002), social support also deserves special attention in further studies of stress in seafarers. Thereby, different sources of social support (support from superiors, work colleagues and family), as well as different types of support (emotional vs. instrumental, actual vs. perceived) should be taken into account. Considering the relationship between social support from the supervisor and strain (Batista-Taran and Reio 2011), a special focus should be given to the identification of supportive and unsupportive behaviours of supervisors which can lead to or decrease occupational stress in seafaring.

Further, many work and organizational characteristics may moderate links between occupational stressors and strain. One of the most important is level of control in the work (Jones and Fletcher 2003; Karasek and Theorell 1990; O'Driscoll and Cooper 2002). However, links between stressors and strain depend on operationalization of control. Parkes (1989) identified three approaches to control in the working context: (1) objective characteristic of the working situation, (2) perceived control over the work, and (3) individual work locus of control. However, considering the importance of work control in both the appraisal of occupational stressors and the experience of stress reactions and long-term consequences, and the different levels of objective control present in crew members on board, it would be valuable to include work-control measurements in further studies. Since leadership behaviour and organizational culture may be related to health behaviours and practices, as well as to health problems and accidents on board (Shea 2005), organizational culture in the maritime sector should also be examined further.

Studies in the field have shown contextual and cultural implications for seafarers' health (Jensen et al. 2006; MacLachlan et al. 2012). Considering wage discrimination by nationality (McLaughlin 2012), which has implications for work motivation and mental health (MacLachlan et al. 2013), further research in the field may also include the concept of organizational justice (Greenberg 1987). Organizational justice refers to how an employee judges the behaviour of the organization and the employee's resulting attitude and behaviour. Moreover, regarding the fact that values in the workplace are influenced by culture (Hofstede 1980), some of the cultural dimensions, such as power-distance index, uncertainty avoidance, and individualism versus collectivism, appear to have relevance for the field (MacLachlan et al. 2013).

Finally, more research focusing on the families of seafarers is recommended. In spite of the fact that separation from partner and family is still one of the most important stressors for seafarers, a relatively small number of studies have focused on the effects of separation on seafarers' spouses and families (e.g. Parkes et al. 2005; Ulven et al. 2007), which is especially important in cases of longer contract duration (Thomas et al. 2003).

Methodological Considerations

Although a great number of individual and organizational variables are recommended for inclusion, design of further studies requires serious theoretical and methodological considerations. First of all, it is important to find a good balance between simplicity of models based only on objective working conditions, and complexity of models based on a transactional view of stress as a process, as it includes a great number of variables and stages, which may be hard to support empirically (Mark and Smith 2008).

Further research in this area should also seriously consider basic limitations relating to the studies of occupational stress (Sulsky and Smith 2005). In the first place, strain measures, regardless of whether they are subjective in their nature (self-reports) or objective (physiological, biochemical and behavioural), should have acceptable reliability and validity. One of the controversial issues in this area is the choice between subjective and objective strain measures. Since many studies are based on self-report conducted on land, some authors strongly recommend objective measurements, such as monitoring basic physiological parameters, to be conducted on board (Leszczynska et al. 2007; Oldenburg et al. 2013b). However, most of the maritime field studies have focused on working hours, watch systems and fatigue as univariate parameters (Oldenburg et al. 2013b). In spite of the fact that only by experimentally designed studies may causal relations between stressor and strain be tested, this approach neglects multivariate stressors present on board and numerous individual and organizational characteristics which may affect links between stressor and strain.

Taking a transactional approach, the recommendation is to use a mixture of multiple objective and subjective measures, along with careful control of the numerous confounding variables which may affect not only subjective, but also so-called objective, strain measurements. With this mixed approach, the *common method variance* characteristic of self-report studies (inflated relationships between sources and outcomes of stress) will be reduced. Studies that rely on self-report should also control negative affectivity, since some authors find that it can be a methodological nuisance in the relations between stressors and strains. Since occupational stress is a dynamic, multifaceted process, measurement of stressors and strains at one single time point do not have the capacity to capture this process. Therefore, longitudinal research is needed to examine dynamic changes in the occupational stress of seafarers over time. Such an approach, although time-consuming, would give new insight into some critical aspects of the occupation, including choice of the occupation, adaptation period, and reasons for leaving the occupation. Finally, in broadening the research field by focussing on some less-explored issues (e.g. coping with stress in seafarers, seafarers' families, cultural and contextual considerations in motivational profiles of seafarers, etc.) a qualitative approach (e.g. interviews, focus groups) is also necessary.

References

Ádám, B., Rasmussen, H. B., Pedersen, R. N. F., & Jepsen, J. R. (2014). Occupational accidents in the Danish merchant fleet and the nationality of seafarers. *Journal of Occupational Medicine and Toxicology, 9*(35), 1–8.

Alderton, T., Bloor, M., Kahveci, E., Lane, T., Sampson, H., Thomas, M., et al. (2004). *The global seafarer: Living and working conditions in a globalized industry.* Geneva: International Labour Organization.

Allen, P., Wadsworth, E., & Smith, A. (2008). Seafarers' fatigue: A review of the recent literature. *International Maritime Health, 59*(1–4), 81–92.

Arnold, J., Silvester, J., Patterson, F., Robertson, I., Cooper, C. L., & Burns, B. (2005). *Work psychology—understanding human behaviour in the workplace.* Harlow: FT Prentice Hall.

Arulanandam, S., & Chan Chung Tsing, G. (2009). Comparison of alertness levels in ship crew. An experiment on rotating versus fixed watch schedules. *International Maritime Health, 60*(1–2), 6–9.

Baron, R. M., & Kenny, D. A. (1986). The moderator-mediator variable distinction in social psychological research: Conceptual, strategic, and statistical considerations. *Journal of Personality and Social Psychology, 51*(6), 1173–1182.

Batista-Taran, L. C., & Reio, T. G. Jr. (2011). Occupational stress: Towards an integrated model. In M. S. Plakhotnik, S. M. Nielsen, & D. M. Pane (Eds.), *Proceedings of the Tenth Annual College of Education & GSN Research Conference* (pp. 9–16). Miami: Florida International University. Retrieved from http://digitalcommons.fiu.edu/cgi/viewcontent.cgi?article=1166&context=sferc. Accessed 29 May 2015.

Beaujot, R., & Anderson, R. (2004). Stress and adult health: Impact of time spent in paid and unpaid work, and its division in families. *Population Studies Centre Discussion Papers Series, 18*(8), Article 1. Retrieved from http://ir.lib.uwo.ca/pscpapers/vol18/iss8/1. Accessed 29 May 2015.

Borovnik, M. (2011). Occupational health and safety of merchant seafarers from Kiribati and Tuvalu. *Asia Pacific Viewpoint, 52*(3), 333–346.

Bridger, R. S., Brasher, K., & Dew, A. (2010). Work demands and need for recovery from work in ageing seafarers. *Ergonomics, 53*(8), 1006–1015.

Bridger, R. S., & Bennett, A. I. (2011). Age and BMI interact to determine work ability in seafarers. *Occupational Medicine, 61*(3), 157–162.

Carel, R. S., Carmil, D., & Keinan, G. (1990). Occupational stress and well-being: Do seafarers harbor more health problems than people on the shore? *Israel Journal of Medical Science, 26*(11), 619–624.

Carotenuto, A., Molino, I., Fasanaro, A. M., & Amenta, F. (2012). Psychological stress in seafarers: A review. *International Maritime Health, 63*(4), 188–194.

Carotenuto, A., Fasanaro, A. M., Molino, I., Sibilio, F., Saturnino, A., Traini, E., et al. (2013). The psychological general well-being index (PGWBI) for assessing stress of seafarers on board merchant ships. *International Maritime Health, 64*(4), 215–220.

Carter, T. (2011). Mapping the knowledge base for maritime health. *International Maritime Health, 62*(4), 209–246.

Cartwright, S., & Cooper, C. L. (1996). Coping in occupational settings. In M. Zeidner & N. S. Endler (Eds.), *Handbook of coping: Theory, research, applications* (pp. 202–220). Chichester: Wiley.

Chauvin, C., Lardjane, S., Morel, G., Clostermann, J.-P., & Langard, B. (2013). Human and organisational factors in maritime accidents: Analysis of collisions at sea using the HFACS. *Accident Analysis and Prevention, 59*, 26–37.

Coggon, D., Harris, E. C., Brown, T., Rice, S., & Palmer, K. T. (2010). Occupation and mortality related to alcohol, drugs and sexual habits. *Occupational Medicine, 60*(5), 348–353.

Cooper, C. L., & Baglioni, A. J. (1988). A structural model approach toward the development of a theory of the link between stress and mental health. *British Journal of Medical Psychology, 61* (1), 87–102.

Cooper, C. L., Sloan, S. J., & Williams, S. (1988). *Occupational stress indicator: Management guide*. Windsor: NFER-Nelson.

Cooper, C. L., Dewe, P. J., & O'Driscoll, M. P. (2001). *Organizational stress—a review and critique of theory, research and applications*. Thousand Oaks, CA: Sage Publications Inc.

Cox, T., & Mackay, C. J. (1981). A transactional approach to occupational stress. In E. N. Corlett & J. Richardson (Eds.), *Stress, work design and productivity* (pp. 91–114). Chichester: Wiley.

Cox, T. (1987). Stress, coping and problem solving. *Work & Stress, 1*(1), 5–14.

Cox, T., & Griffiths, A. (1995). The nature and measurement of work stress: Theory and practice. In J. R. Wilson & E. N. Corlett (Eds.), *Evaluation of human work: A practical ergonomics methodology*. London: Taylor & Francis.

Daniels, K., & Harris, C. (2000). Work, psychological well-being and performance. *Occupational Medicine, 50*(5), 304–309.

Espevik, R., & Olsen, O. K. (2013). A new model for understanding teamwork onboard: The shipmate model. *International Maritime Health, 64*(2), 89–94.

Faragher, E. B., Cass, M., & Cooper, C. L. (2005). The relationship between job satisfaction and health: A meta-analysis. *Occupational Environmental Medicine, 62*(2), 105–112.

Fort, E., Massardier-Pilonchery, A., & Bergeret, A. (2009). Alcohol and nicotine dependence in French seafarers. *International Maritime Health, 60*(1–2), 18–28.

Giga, S. I., Cooper, C. L., & Faragher, B. (2003). The development of a framework for a comprehensive approach to stress management interventions at work. *International Journal of Stress Management, 10*(4), 280–296.

Grant, S., & Langan-Fox, J. (2006). Occupational stress, coping and strain: The combined/ interactive effects of the Big Five traits. *Personality and Individual Differences, 41*(4), 719–732.

Grappasonni, I., Paci, P., Mazzucchi, F., De Longis, S., & Amenta, F. (2012). Awareness of health risks at the workplace and of risks of contracting communicable diseases including those related to food hygiene, among seafarers. *International Maritime Health, 63*(1), 24–31.

Grappasonni, I., Marconi, D., Mazzucchi, F., Petrelli, F., Scuri, S., & Amenta, F. (2013). Survey on food hygiene knowledge on board ships. *International Maritime Health, 64*(3), 160–167.

Greenberg, J. (1987). A taxonomy of organizational justice theories. *Academy of Management Review, 12*(1), 9–22.

Hafez, A. (1999). Seafarers' social life and its effect on maritime safety—with respect to Egyptian seafarers. Unpublished Master thesis. World Maritime University, Malmö, Sweden. Retrieved from http://dlib.wmu.se/jspui/bitstream/123456789/471/1/13208.pdf. Accessed 29 May 2015.

Hagmark, H. (2003). Women in maritime communities: A socio-historical study of continuity and change in the domestic lives of seafarers' wives in the Aland Islands, from 1930 into the New Millennium. Unpublished Ph.D. Thesis. University of Hull, UK. Retrieved from http://core.ac. uk/download/pdf/5222524.pdf. Accessed 29 May 2015.

Haka, M., Borch, D. F., Jensen, C., & Leppin, A. (2011). Should I stay or should I go? Motivational profiles of Danish seafaring officers and non-officers. *International Maritime Health, 62*(1), 20–30.

Hansen, H. L., & Pedersen, G. (1996). Influence of occupational accidents and deaths related to lifestyle on mortality among merchant seafarers. *International Journal of Epidemiology, 25*(6), 1237–1243.

Hansen, H. L., Nielsen, D., & Frydenberg, M. (2002). Occupational accidents aboard merchant ships. *Occupational and Environmental Medicine, 59*(2), 85–91.

Hart, P. M., & Cooper, C. L. (2001). Occupational stress: Toward a more integrated framework. In N. Anderson, D. S. Ones, H. K. Sinangil, & C. Viswesvaran (Eds.), *Handbook of industrial, work and organizational psychology, personnel psychology* (Vol. 2, pp. 93–114). London: Sage.

Hayashi, M. (2001). Toward the elimination of substandard shipping: The report of the International Commission on Shipping. *The International Journal of Marine and Coastal Law, 16*(3), 501–513.

Hjarnoe, L., & Leppin, A. (2014). What does it take to get a healthy diet at sea? A maritime study of the challenges of promoting a healthy lifestyle at the workplace at sea. *International Maritime Health, 65*(2), 79–86.

Hoeyer, J. L., & Hansen, H. L. (2005). Obesity among Danish seafarers. *International Maritime Health, 56*(1–4), 48–55.

Hofstede, G. (1980). *Culture's consequences: International differences in work-related values.* Beverly Hills, CA: Sage Publications.

Hystad, S. W., Saus, E. R., Sætrevik, B., & Eid, J. (2013). Fatigue in seafarers working in the offshore oil and gas re-supply industry: Effects of safety climate, psychosocial work environment and shift arrangement. *International Maritime Health, 64*(2), 72–79.

Iversen, R. T. B. (2012). The mental health of seafarers. *International Maritime Health, 63*(2), 78–89.

Jaimez, M. J., & Bretones, F. D. (2011). Towards a healthy organisation model. *Is-Guc, The Journal of Industrial Relations and Human Resource, 13*(3), 7–26.

Jensen, O. C., Sørensen, J. F. L., Thomas, M., Canals, M. L., Nikolic, N., & Hu, Y. (2006). Working conditions in international seafaring. *Occupational Medicine, 56*(6), 393–397.

Jeżewska, M., Leszczynska, I., & Jaremin, B. (2006). Work-related stress at sea: Self estimation by maritime students and officers. *International Maritime Health, 57*(1–4), 66–75.

Jeżewska, M., Babicz-Zielińska, E., Leszczyńska, I., & Grubman, M. (2009). Promotion of healthy nutrition of seafarers. *International Maritime Health, 60*(1–2), 48–50.

Jones, F., & Fletcher, B. C. (2003). Job control, physical health and psychological well-being. In M. J. Schabracq, J. A. M. Winnubst, & C. L. Cooper (Eds.), *The handbook of work and health psychology* (pp. 121–142). Chichester: Wiley.

Juozulynas, A., Sąlyga, J., Malakauskiene, R., & Lukšiene, A. (2007). Physical and psychological dimensions of health-related quality of life among Lithuanian seamen. *Acta Medica Lituanica, 14*(1), 50–53.

Kaerlev, L., Hansen, J., Hansen, H. L., & Nielsen, P. S. (2005). Cancer incidence among Danish seafarers: A population based cohort study. *Occupational and Environmental Medicine, 62*(11), 761–765.

Karasek, R., & Theorell, T. (1990). *Healthy work: Stress, productivity, and the reconstruction of working life.* New York: Basic Books.

Kendall, E., Murphy, P., O'Neill, V., & Bursnall, S. (2000). *Occupational stress: Factors that contribute to its occurrence and effective management.* Centre for Human Services, Griffith University: Work Cover Western Australia. Retrieved from http://www.mentalhealthpromotion. net/resources/occupational-stress-fractors-that-contribute-to-its-occurrence-and-effective-management.pdf. Accessed 29 May 2015.

Kenny, D. T., & McIntyre, D. (2005). Constructions of occupational stress: Nuance or novelty? In A-S. G. Antoniou & C. L. Cooper (Eds.) *Research companion to organizational health psychology* (pp. 20–58). Cheltenham, UK: Edward Elgar Publishing.

Kenny, D. T., & Cooper, C. L. (2003). Introduction: Occupational stress and its management. *International Journal of Stress Management, 10*(4), 275–279.

Kobasa, S. C. (1979). Stressful life events, personality, and health—Inquiry into hardiness. *Journal of Personality and Social Psychology, 37*(1), 1–11.

Lang, M. (2011). An investigation of organizational culture and job satisfaction on board industrial and cruise ships. Unpublished Masters thesis. The Norwegian University of Science and Technology. Retrieved from http://brage.bibsys.no/xmlui/bitstream/handle/11250/270658/ 439238_FULLTEXT01.pdf?sequence=1. Accessed 29 May 2015.

Lazarus, R. S., & Folkman, S. (1984). *Stress, appraisal and coping.* New York: Springer.

Lazarus, R. S., & Folkman, S. (1987). Transactional theory and research on emotions and coping. *European Journal of Personality, 1*(3), 141–169.

Lazarus, R. L. (1990). Theory-based stress research. *Psychological Inquiry, 1*(1), 3–13.

Leka, S., Griffiths, A., & Cox, T. (2005). Work organisation and stress: Systematic problem approaches for employers, managers and trade union representatives. *Protecting workers' health series*, 3 Geneva: World Health Organization. Retrieved from http://www.who.int/ occupational_health/publications/en/oehstress.pdf. Accessed 29 May 2015.

Leszczynska, I., Ježewska, M., & Jaremin, B. (2007). Work-related stress at sea: Possibilities of research and measures of stress. *International Maritime Health, 58*(1–4), 93–102.

Lodde, B., Jegaden, D., Lucas, D., Feraud, M., Eusen, Y., & Dewitte, J. D. (2008). Stress in seamen and non-seamen employed by the same company. *International Maritime Health, 59*(1–4), 53–60.

Lu, Y., Gao, Y., Cao, Z., Cui, J., Dong, Z., Tian, Y., et al. (2010). A study of health effects of long-distance ocean voyages on seamen using a data classification approach. *BMC Medical Informatics and Decision Making, 10*(13), 1–7.

MacLachlan, M., Kavanagh, B., & Kay, A. (2012). Maritime health: A review with suggestions for research. *International Maritime Health, 63*(1), 1–6.

MacLachlan, M., Cromie, S., Liston, P., Kavanagh, B., & Kay, A. (2013). Psychosocial and organisational aspects. In T. Carter (Ed.) *Textbook of maritime medicine*. Retrieved from http:// textbook.ncmm.no/index.php/textbook-of-maritime-medicine. Accessed 29 May 2015.

Mark, G. M., & Smith, A. P. (2008). Stress models: A review and suggested new direction. In J. Houdmont & S. Leka (Eds.), *Occupational health psychology, European perspectives on research, education and practice* (Vol. 3, pp. 111–144). Nottingham: Nottingham University Press.

McKenna, E. (2000). *Business psychology and organisational behaviour: A student's handbook*. Hove: Psychology Press.

McLaughlin, H. L. (2012). Seafarers and seafaring. In W. K. Talley (Ed.), *The Blackwell companion to maritime economics* (pp. 321–332). Oxford: Blackwell Publishing Ltd.

Michie, S. (2007). Causes and management of stress at work. *Occupational Environmental Medicine, 59*(1), 67–72.

Ng, T. W. H., Sorensen, K. L., & Eby, L. T. (2006). Locus of control at work: A meta-analysis. *Journal of Organizational Behaviour, 27*(8), 1057–1987.

Nielsen, M. B., Bergheim, K., & Eid, J. (2013). Relationships between work environment factors and workers' well-being in the maritime industry. *International Maritime Health, 64*(2), 80–88.

Oldenburg, M. (2014). Risk of cardiovascular diseases in seafarers. *International Maritime Health, 65*(2), 53–57.

O'Driscoll, M. P., & Cooper, C. L. (2002). Job-related stress and burnout. In P. Warr (Ed.), *Psychology at work* (pp. 203–229). London: Penguin Books Ltd.

Oldenburg, M., Jensen, H. J., Latza, U., & Baur, X. (2007). Coronary risks among seafarers aboard German-flagged ships. *International Archives of Occupational and Environmental Health, 81*(6), 735–741.

Oldenburg, M., Jensen, H. J., Latza, U., & Baur, X. (2009). Seafaring stressors aboard merchant and passenger ships. *International Journal of Public Health, 54*(2), 96–105.

Oldenburg, M., Baur, X., & Schlaich, C. (2010a). Occupational risks and challenges of seafaring. *Journal of Occupational Health, 52*(5), 249–256.

Oldenburg, M., Baur, X., & Schlaich, C. (2010b). Cardiovascular diseases in the modern maritime industry. *International Maritime Health, 62*(3), 101–106.

Oldenburg, M., Jensen, H. J., Latza, U., & Baur, X. (2010c). The risk of coronary heart disease of seafarers on vessels sailing under German flag. *International Maritime Health, 62*(3), 123–128.

Oldenburg, M., Jensen, H. J., & Wegner, R. (2012). Burnout syndrome in seafarers in the merchant marine service. *International Archives of Occupational and Environmental Health, 86*(4), 407–416.

Oldenburg, M., Harth, V., & Jensen, H. J. (2013a). Overview and prospect: Food and nutrition of seafarers on merchant ships. *International Maritime Health, 64*(4), 191–194.

Oldenburg, M., Hogan, B., & Jensen, H. J. (2013b). Systematic review of maritime field studies about stress and strain in seafaring. *International Archives of Occupational and Environmental Health, 86*(1), 1–15.

Parkes, K. R. (1989). Personal control in an occupational context. In A. Steptoe & A. Appels (Eds.), *Stress, personal control and health* (pp. 21–47). Chichester: Wiley.

Parkes, K. R., Carnell, S. C., & Farmer, E. L. (2005). Living two lives. *Community, Work and Family, 8*(4), 413–437.

Penezić, Z., Slišković, A., & Kevrić, D. (2013). Some correlates of life satisfaction in seamen [Neki korelati zadovoljstva životom kod pomoraca]. *Contemporary Psychology [Suvremena psihologija], 16*(1), 83–92.

Peplińska, A., Jeżewska, M., Leszczyńska, I., & Połomski, P. (2013). Stress and the level of perceived anxiety among mariners: The mediating role of marital satisfaction. *International Maritime Health, 64*(4), 221–225.

Peplińska, A., Jeżewska, M., Leszczyńska, I., & Połomski, P. (2014). Purpose in life and work-related stress in mariners. Mediating role of quality of marriage bonds and perceived anxiety. *International Maritime Health, 65*(2), 87–92.

Popkin, S. M., Morrow, S. L., Di Domenico, T. E., & Howarth, H. D. (2008). Age is more than just a number: Implications for an aging workforce in the US transportation sector. *Applied Ergonomics, 39*(5), 542–549.

Pougnet, R., Pougnet, L., Loddé, B., Canals, L., Bell, S., Lucas, D., et al. (2014). Consumption of addictive substances in mariners. *International Maritime Health, 65*(4), 199–204.

Rengamani, J., & Murugan, M. S. (2012). A study on the factors influencing the seafarers' stress. *AMET International Journal of Management, 4*, 44–51.

Roberts, S. E. (2005). Work-related mortality from gastrointestinal diseases and alcohol among seafarers employed in British merchant shipping from 1939 to 2002. *International Maritime Health, 56*(1–4), 29–47.

Roberts, S. E., & Marlow, P. B. (2005). Traumatic work-related mortality among seafarers employed in British merchant shipping, 1976–2002. *Occupational and Environmental Medicine, 62*(3), 172–180.

Roberts, S. E. (2008). Fatal work-related accidents in UK merchant shipping from 1919 to 2005. *Occupational Medicine, 58*(2), 129–137.

Roberts, S. E., Jaremin, B., Chalasani, P., & Rodgers, S. E. (2009). Suicides among seafarers in UK merchant shipping, 1919–2005. *Occupational Medicine, 60*(1), 54–61.

Roberts, S. E., & Jaremin, B. (2010). Cardiovascular disease mortality in British merchant shipping and among British seafarers ashore in Britain. *International Maritime Health, 62*(3), 107–116.

Rodríguez, J. L., Portela, R. M., & Carrera, P. V. (2011). Legal gaps relating to labour safety and health in the maritime transport sector in Spain. *International Maritime Health, 62*(2), 91–97.

Rydstedt, L. W., & Lundh, M. (2010). An ocean of stress? The relationship between psychosocial workload and mental strain among engine officers in the Swedish merchant fleet. *International Maritime Health, 62*(3), 168–175.

Rydstedt, L. F., & Lundh, M. (2012). Work demands are related to mental health problems for older engine room officers. *International Maritime Health, 63*(4), 176–180.

Saari, L. M., & Judge, T. A. (2004). Employee attitudes and job satisfaction. *Human Resource Management, 43*(4), 395–407.

Saarni, H., Pentti, J., & Pukkala, E. (2002). Cancer at sea: A case-control study among male Finnish seafarers. *Occupational and Environmental Medicine, 59*(9), 613–619.

Salyga, J., & Juozulynas, A. (2006). Association between environment and psycho-emotional stress experienced at sea by Lithuanian and Latvian seamen. *Medicina (Kaunas), 42*(9), 759–769.

Sampson, H., & Zhao, M. (2003). Multilingual crews: Communication and the operation of ships. *World Englishes, 22*(1), 31–43.

Schonfeld, I. S., Rhee, J., & Xia, F. (1995). Methodological issues in occupational-stress research: Research in one occupational group and wider applications. In S. L. Sauter & L. R. Murphy

(Eds.), *Organizational risk factors for job stress* (pp. 323–339). Washington DC: American Psychological Association.

Semmer, N. K. (2003). Individual differences, work stress and health. In M. J. Schabracq, J. A. M. Winnubst, & C. L. Cooper (Eds.), *The handbook of work and health psychology* (pp. 83–120). Chichester: Wiley.

Shea, I. P. (2005). The organisational culture of a ship: A description and some possible effects it has on accidents and lessons for seafaring leadership. Unpublished Ph.D. thesis. University of Tasmania. Retrieved from http://eprints.utas.edu.au/1023/1/01Front.pdf. Accessed 29 May 2015.

Slišković, A. (2010). Adverse effects of shiftwork—a review [Problemi rada u smjenama]. *Archives of Industrial Hygiene and Toxicology, 61*(4), 465–477.

Slišković, A., & Penezić, Z. (2015). Descriptive study of job satisfaction and job dissatisfaction in a sample of Croatian seafarers. *International Maritime Health, 66*(2), 97–105.

Smith, A., Allen, P. H., & Wadsworth, E. (2006). *Seafarer fatigue: The Cardiff research programme*. MCA Research Report, 464. Cardiff: Centre for Occupational and Health Psychology, Cardiff University. Retrieved from http://orca.cf.ac.uk/48167/1/research_report_464.pdf. Accessed 29 May 2015.

Sulsky, L., & Smith, C. A. (2005). *Work stress*. Belmont, CA: Thomson Wadsworth.

Szymanska, K., Jaremin, B., & Rosik, E. (2006). Suicides among Polish seamen and fishermen during work at sea. *International Maritime Health, 57*(1–4), 36–45.

Tang, L. (2012). Waiting together: Seafarer-partners in cyberspace. *Time & Society, 21*(2), 223–240.

Theorell, T., & Karasek, R. A. (1996). Current issues relating to psychosocial job strain and cardiovascular disease research. *Journal of Occupational Health Psychology, 1*(1), 9–26.

Thomas, M., Sampson, H., & Zhao, M. (2003). Finding a balance: Companies, seafarers and family life. *Maritime Policy & Management, 30*(1), 59–76.

Ulven, A. J., Omdal, K. A., Herløv-Nielsen, H., Irgens, A., & Dahl, E. (2007). Seafarers' wives and intermittent husbands—social and psychological impact of a subgroup of Norwegian seafarers' work schedule on their families. *International Maritime Health, 58*(1–4), 115–128.

Wadsworth, E. J. K., Allen, P. H., Wellens, B. T., McNamara, R. L., & Smith, A. P. (2006). Patterns of fatigue among seafarers during a tour of duty. *American Journal of Industrial Medicine, 49*(10), 836–844.

Wadsworth, E. J. K., Allen, P. H., McNamara, R. L., & Smith, A. P. (2008). Fatigue and health in a seafaring population. *Occupational Medicine, 58*(3), 198–204.

Weng, J., & Yang, D. (2015). Investigation of shipping accident injury severity and mortality. *Accident Analysis and Prevention, 76*, 92–101.

World Health Organization (1948) *WHO health definition*. World Health Organization. Retrieved from: http://www.who.int/about/definition/en/print.html

Williams, S., & Cooper, C. L. (1998). Measuring occupational stress: Development of the pressure management indicator. *Journal of Occupational Health Psychology, 3*(4), 306–321.

Wilson, M. G., Dejoy, D. M., Vandenberg, R. J., Richardson, H. A., & McGrath, A. L. (2004). Work characteristics and employee health and well-being: Test of a model of healthy work organization. *Journal of Occupational and Organizational Psychology, 77*(4), 565–588.

Risk Factors for Fatigue in Shipping, the Consequences for Seafarers' Health and Options for Preventive Intervention

Jørgen Riis Jepsen, Zhiwei Zhao, Claire Pekcan, Mike Barnett and Wessel M.A. van Leeuwen

Background

Although there are several recent marine casualties in European waters which have been caused by watchkeepers falling asleep while on watch, for example, the grounding of the *Danio* in 2013 (Marine Accident Investigation Board 2014), one of the most influential accidents is the grounding of the *Shen Neng 1* on the Great Barrier Reef off the coast of Australia (Australian Transport Safety Bureau 2011). At 17:05 on 3 April 2010, the Chinese-registered bulk carrier *Shen Neng 1* grounded

J.R. Jepsen (✉) · Z. Zhao
Centre of Maritime Health and Society, University of Southern Denmark,
Niels Bohrs Vej 9-10, 6700 Esbjerg, Denmark
e-mail: jriis@cmss.sdu.dk; jorgen.riis.jepsen@rsyd.dk

Z. Zhao
e-mail: zhaozhiwei2006@hotmail.com; zhao@sdu.dk

J.R. Jepsen
Department of Occupational Medicine, Hospital of South-Western Jutland,
Østergade 81-83, 6700 Esbjerg, Denmark

Z. Zhao
Seafarers Development Research Centre, Dalian Maritime University, 1 Linghai Rd.,
Ganjingzi District, 116026 Dalian City, China

C. Pekcan · M. Barnett
Warsash Maritime Academy, Southampton Solent University, Newton Rd., Warsash,
Southampton SO31 9ZL, UK
e-mail: claire.pekcan@solent.ac.uk

M. Barnett
e-mail: mike.barnett@solent.ac.uk

W.M.A. van Leeuwen
Stress Research Institute, Stockholm University, 106 91 Stockholm, Sweden
e-mail: wessel.vleeuwen@su.se

© Springer International Publishing Switzerland 2017   127
M. MacLachlan (ed.), *Maritime Psychology*, DOI 10.1007/978-3-319-45430-6_6

on Douglas Shoal, about 50 miles north of the entrance to the port of Gladstone, Queensland. The ship's hull was seriously damaged by the grounding, with the engine room, ballast and fuel oil tanks being breached, resulting in pollution in a highly environmentally sensitive area. The subsequent investigation found that the grounding occurred because the chief mate did not alter the ship's course at the designated course alteration position. His monitoring of the ship's position was ineffective and his actions were affected by fatigue. The loading of cargo in Gladstone prior to this grounding was the chief mate's first loading operation on the ship, and he was concerned that the ship may suffer delays if de-ballasting could not keep pace with the loading. Consequently, he stayed awake for most of the time in port, and so when he relieved the second mate on the ship's bridge after departure, the chief mate had slept for only $2\frac{1}{2}$ h in the previous $38\frac{1}{2}$. One of the findings of the investigation was that there was no effective fatigue management system in place, and despite recommendations to the company, the investigators remained concerned that there was no proper guidance provided to the master or crew with regard to how fatigue levels should be managed on board and when someone should make the fact known that they might not be fit to undertake a navigational watch.

Fatigue in a health sense represents a state of physical and/or mental duress that can affect any person, regardless of occupation or cultural background. Fatigue is also a symptom accompanying numerous diseases and one of the most frequent reasons for seeking medical attention (Kaltsas et al. 2010). At the same time, however, fatigue is also linked to specific circumstances of work.

Fatigue and sleepiness are often used as synonyms but differ because sleepiness will always end with an amount of sleep, while this is not necessarily the case for fatigue, which has also serious physical aspects. Physical fatigue follows prolonged periods of physical activities and causes weakness and reduced endurance. Mental fatigue is mainly the consequence of mental stress and emotional exhaustion, or high workload such as long working hours. In particular, disruption of the sleep–wake cycle and circadian rhythm, which occurs in jet lag and shift work, causes irregularity of work and of sleep, reducing both the amount and quality of sleep between work cycles. Mental fatigue occurs gradually and insidiously, and may appear as cognitive impairment, reduced performance, mental symptoms such as a sense of weariness, and reduced alertness. Three characteristic patterns of fatigue have been described. One pattern predominated by drowsiness and dullness was frequent among people who reported many as well as few symptoms and was not characteristic of any particular type of work. A second pattern, in which an inability to concentrate was prominent, was more frequent among those who reported many symptoms and characteristic of mental workers, especially after night work. A third pattern characterized by an awareness of physical discomfort was found mainly among those who reported few symptoms and were engaged in physical work (Yoshitake 1978). The International Maritime Organization (IMO) defines fatigue as "a reduction in physical and/or mental capability as the result of physical, mental or emotional exertion, which may impair nearly all physical abilities including: strength; speed; reaction time; decision-making; or balance" (IMO 2002, p. 22).

We suggest a feasible definition of fatigue as "a progressive loss of mental and physical alertness possibly ending in sleep".

Work-related fatigue is particularly an issue in safety-sensitive occupational sectors, such as transportation (both on land, at sea and in the air). The consequences of work-related fatigue have been widely studied in occupational settings. Many experiences from land-based trades such as road and rail transport, as well as from air transport, can be extrapolated to the maritime context (Smith et al. 2007).

The shipping industry is characterized by the necessity of seafarers to work in shifts to keep the vessel going continuously. Various forms of shifts have been applied, but common to most of them is that shifts permit less sleep because they break up the day in portions that leave insufficient time for rest and restitution. Sleeping may take place under unfavourable circumstances due to continuous exposures such as noise, vibration, movements of the ship and other disturbing factors at sea. Consequently, quantity and quality of sleep is prone to be disadvantageous, which is even worse if being forced to sleep at unfavourable times of the day when working outside the regular daytime hours (Ohayon et al. 2010).

The work patterns and life on board vary enormously according to factors such as cargo, type of trade, the crew nationality and flag state and so does the extent of fatigue. Working in the short sea sector appears to cause more fatigue due to more port calls and the associated increase of workload (Smith et al. 2003). Compared to shore-based workers, seafarers report higher levels of lethargy and poor quality sleep (Smith et al. 2001). It is, however, impossible to globally estimate the extent and impact of fatigue on seafarers. Previous studies suffer from low response rates and consequently it is difficult to compare with the fatigue rate of the general population. However, patterns of day-to-day changes in fatigue have been shown to be measurable and vary considerably among particular subgroups of seafarers and between the start and end of voyages (Wadsworth et al. 2006). There is evidence of under-recording of seafarers' working hours, and that this may be related to cultural and commercial pressures (Allen et al. 2006, 2008).

Measuring fatigue is complicated because fatigue represents an integration of subjective perceptions, performance and physiological functioning. The lack of a universal tool to measure fatigue challenges research that aims to relate fatigue to health and safety outcomes. However, subjective rating of sleepiness by the Karolinska Sleepiness Scale (KSS) is a simple approach for which there is evidence of good validity in comparison with electroencephalographic and behavioural variables (Kaida et al. 2006; van den Berg et al. 2005). KSS may therefore represent a feasible proxy for fatigue, and has been used in several studies on fatigue (van den Berg et al. 2005; Åkerstedt et al. 2004, 2008; Bonnefond et al. 2006; Harma et al. 2008; Eriksen et al. 2006; Lutzhoft et al. 2010; van Leeuwen et al. 2013). It is, however, emphasized that subjective rating of sleepiness differs from the subjective rating of performance (Kaida et al. 2007). Sleepiness has been shown to be context dependent (National Transportation Safety Board 1999), meaning that sleepiness can be regarded as the lack of ability to maintain a wakeful state of attention without the aid of situational factors. Consequently, the context of sleepiness may influence the KSS rating (Åkerstedt et al. 2008). Sleep diaries can serve as a proxy for the amount of sleep, while actigraph monitoring, which is applicable at sea, or elec-troencephalographic recordings, represent more objective measures of rest and sleep but cannot provide information as to what extent the person is suffering from fatigue.

A variety of specific fatigue measuring instruments exist as reviewed by Dittner and colleagues (Dittner et al. 2004). The majority of these currently available tools have the problem that they are aimed at measuring fatigue in very specific medical circumstances, such as in people suffering, for instance, from specific medical conditions whose symptoms include fatigue. This makes the majority of these instruments unsuitable for measuring fatigue in a potentially healthy population such as seafarers. In our opinion, one of the more suitable available scales to measure fatigue is the multidimensional fatigue inventory (MFI-20) developed in 1995 by Smets and colleagues (Smets et al. 1995) for measuring fatigue in cancer patients; however this instrument has also been validated in healthy volunteers (Lin et al. 2009). The scale consists of 20 items, rated on a 1–7 scale, divided over five dimensions of fatigue; namely, (1) general fatigue, (2) physical fatigue, (3) mental fatigue, (4) reduced motivation and (5) reduced activity.

This chapter aims to describe the causes of work-related fatigue in seafarers and the associated acute and chronic consequences of fatigue and risk factors for fatigue. The issue is complex. A simple illustration of the major relationships is provided in Fig. 1. In addition, ways of mitigating the risk of fatigue will be discussed.

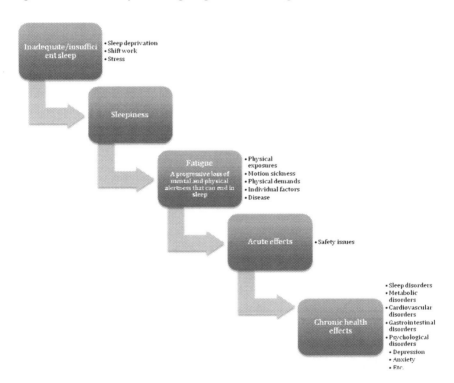

Fig. 1 Diagram illustrating the main determinants and outcomes of fatigue

Risk Factors for Fatigue

Studies of risk factors for seafarer fatigue may be related to either of the acknowledged maritime risk factors or their combination, or to occupational risk factors for fatigue that have been demonstrated among workers other than seafarers.

In a major questionnaire study of seafarers, symptoms of fatigue were found related to a range of occupational and environmental risk factors at sea (sleep quality, work hours and shifts, tour length, job demands, work stress, sleep disturbances, time zone crossings, etc.). The rate of fatigue correlated with the number of risk factors as well as with poorer cognitive and health outcomes, with fatigue as the most important risk factor for the latter (Wadsworth et al. 2008). Other recent studies confirmed that these factors in combination must be considered, in order to understand fatigue at sea, and emphasized that working more than 2×6 h per 24 h should be avoided since this leads to significantly high levels of sleepiness (Smith et al. 2006). In a study of a representative Swedish sample of 58,115 individuals interviewed at regular intervals over a period of 20 years on issues related to work and health, Åkerstedt et al. found that significant predictors for fatigue were female gender, age below 49 years, high socio-economic status, present illness, hectic work, overtime work and physically strenuous work (Åkerstedt et al. 2002a).

Seafarers in the merchant fleet are the most studied among maritime workers. However, there is evidence that, at times, fishermen may be even more prone to fatigue. A review of fatigue in fishermen resulted in five studies that all confirmed fatigue to represent a serious risk in the trade (Hovdanum et al. 2014). One study of fishermen showed that 23 % of days at sea permitted less than 4 h sleep, and, understandably, the fishermen's perceived fatigue rating remained high after sleep (Gander et al. 2008). In another study, 60 % of fishermen believed that their personal safety had been at risk due to fatigue at work, and 16 % had been involved in a fatigue-related accident. 44 % said that they had worked to the point of exhaustion or collapse (Allen et al. 2010).

Work stress, shift work and physical workload are among the most important risk factors that are related to fatigue (Åkerstedt et al. 2002a, b). Sleep deprivation, rather than perceived sleep quality, correlates best with observed biological and metabolic changes. Most studies on the association between sleep and health are based on sleep length (Cappuccio et al. 2011; Xi et al. 2014; Wang et al. 2012) but there are an increasing number of epidemiological studies on the association between sleep quality and health (Ferrie et al. 2011). A causal relation is indicated by experimental demonstration of adverse health effects following a significant reduction of the sleep duration (Tobaldini et al. 2014; van Leeuwen et al. 2010).

Stress

When it comes to the effect on sleep and fatigue of psychosocial work characteristics, the picture is complex. Unfavourable psychosocial work characteristics have only minor effects. While high job strain is found to be associated with difficulties initiating sleep and reduced psychomotor vigilance during night shifts, the average sleep duration and efficiency was not affected (Harma 2013). A literature review on psychological stress in seafarers concluded that seafaring is associated with mental, psychological and physical stressors, with the most important stressors being separation from family, loneliness on board, fatigue, multinationality, limited recreation activity and sleep deprivation. The stressors differed in between ranks and departments on board. The associated mental health risks are suggested to be addressed by helping seafarers to lower their stress level and to develop strategies for coping with "inevitable" stress conditions (Carotenuto et al. 2012). The social situation and stress at work are strongly linked to disturbed sleep and impaired awakening. Gender and age may modify these relations and the inability to stop worrying about work during free time seems to be an important link between stress and sleep (Åkerstedt et al. 2002b). Increased stress/worry at bedtime about work, for instance, is associated with impaired sleep (Åkerstedt et al. 2007) and work stress is typically associated with increased sleep latency due to work rumination (Åkerstedt 2006).

A recent review found only a small to moderate effect of work demands and job control on sleep quality (van Laethem et al. 2013). A longitudinal study of the relationship between job demands and job control demonstrated that a transition from a non-high-strain towards a high-strain job was associated with significantly reduced sleep quality and increased fatigue, while the opposite transition improved sleep-related problems (de Lange et al. 2009). This conclusion is in line with the outcome of a study of the influence of work-time control and variability of working time on recovery from fatigue, sleep quality, and work–life balance, and on the occurrence of self-reported "near misses" at work. High work-time control and variability had favourable influences on health and work–life balance (Kubo et al. 2013a, b).

One study has shown that objective sleep efficiency based on actigraphy recordings was unrelated to variations in both psychosocial work characteristics and negative affective responses, while self-recorded poor sleep was more prevalent among those overcommitted to work or with lower social support at work (Jackowska et al. 2011). Another study showed that a working week with a high workload and much stress increases sleepiness and impairs sleep, and affects the pattern of diurnal cortisol secretion with a more flattened pattern probably due to increased evening levels during the stress week (Dahlgren et al. 2005). Day-to-day variations in self-reported fatigue by sleep diaries are related to poor sleep quality, reduced sleep duration the previous night (measured by actigraphy recordings), higher stress level and to the occurrence of a cold or fever during the same day (Åkerstedt et al. 2014).

Irregular Work and Sleep Quantity

While most adults need between 7 and 9 h of sleep per day, preferably during a single major sleep period at night, this may be difficult to obtain at sea—in particular with work in shifts. Fatigue related to shift work has been studied in seafarers and clear differences between daytime workers and shift workers, and between various watch systems, have been observed (Lutzhoft et al. 2010; Project HORIZON 2012). In a case-control study of rotating shift workers and daytime workers, the sleep profile was similar in the two groups, but insomnia was found to be closely related to sleep time, anxiety, depression, fatigue and impaired quality of life (Vallieres et al. 2014). Alertness was found to be lower in rotating watch systems than in a steady watch system (Arulanandam and Tsing 2009).

Shift work causes difficulties getting to sleep, shortened sleep, and sleepiness during working days that continues into successive days off. This can only be partly improved by manipulating shift patterns. There is no clear indication that chronic sleep problems result from long-term shift work (Åkerstedt 2003), although this is suggested by retrospective studies (Dumont et al. 1997).

Shift work and long working hours contribute to sleep debt (Bayon et al. 2014). When shift work includes night work, it has pronounced negative effects on sleep, subjective and physiological sleepiness, performance, and accident risk, as well as on secondary health outcomes such as cardiovascular diseases. The reason for that is the conflict between the day-oriented circadian physiology and the requirement for work and sleep at the "wrong" biological time of day. Other factors that negatively impact work shift sleepiness and the associated accident risk include long-duration work shifts in excess of 12 h and individual vulnerability for phase intolerance, which may lead to a shift work-related disorder in workers with the greatest impairment of sleepiness and performance during the biological night and insomnia during the biological day (Åkerstedt and Wright 2009).

Shift work-related insomnia differs between various work schemes, with evening shift insomnia more prevalent in 2-shift rotation than 3-shift rotation schedules (29.8 and 19.8 %, respectively). Night-shift insomnia was higher among 3-shift rotation workers compared with permanent night workers (67.7 and 41.7 %, respectively). Rest-day insomnia was more prevalent among permanent night workers compared with 2- and 3-shift rotations (11.4 % compared with 4.2 and 3.6 %, respectively) (Flo et al. 2013).

Changing from a forward rotating to a backward rotating shift system is likely to increase sleep difficulties between successive afternoon shifts but to decrease social disruption (Barton et al. 1994). Fatigue is more pronounced in 2-watch systems (e.g. 6 on/6 off) than in 3-watch systems (e.g. 4 on/8 off) and most obvious between 04:00 and 06:00 h when the biological pressure to sleep is at its highest (Harma et al. 2008).

Eriksen and colleagues have demonstrated that, within a 6 on/6 off system, the levels of sleepiness are highest during 00–06 h shifts and rise towards the end of the shift (Eriksen et al. 2006). The 6/6-watch system (12 daily work hours) is related to higher risk of severe sleepiness for marine officers during the early morning hours compared to the 4/8 (8 daily work hours). The officers reported shorter sleep duration, more frequent nodding off on duty and excessive sleepiness. 17.6 % had fallen asleep at least once while on duty during their career (Harma et al. 2008).

These findings were confirmed in the HORIZON project, in which maritime simulators were linked to create a sustainable and realistic voyage experience. Bridge and engine crew were studied on a 4 on/8 off and 6 on/6 off watch system for a simulated voyage of 7 days in coastal and congested waters. Sleep and sleepiness were objectively assessed by polysomnographic recordings (van Leeuwen et al. 2013; Maurier et al. 2011; Barnett et al. 2012a, b). There was a high frequency of severe sleepiness, indicated by several officers actually falling asleep whilst on watch. The 6 on/6 off watch regime appeared to be more sleepiness inducing than the 4 on/8 off, with more incidents of seafarers falling asleep. The onset of sleepiness on 6 on/6 off was apparent over a shorter time frame than predicted from previous research. Watchkeepers were shown to be most sleepy during night watches and showed signs of sleepiness in the afternoon. Sleepiness increased gradually during the work periods as the week progressed. This study has also demonstrated a profound impact of sleep disturbances during rest periods, and that the actual amount of sleep obtained by watchkeepers when off watch was less than anticipated. The total amount of sleep that watchkeepers managed to obtain on 6 on/6 off was less than normally required for full rest. Watchkeepers averaged 6.5 h in total, split up into two sessions: the main one during the "night" time, followed by a "nap" during the other rest period (Project HORIZON 2012). The subjective as well as objective peaks of sleepiness during night and early morning watches coincided with the time frame in which most maritime accidents occur (Marine Accident Investigation Branch (MAIB) 2004). Overtime work was shown to have a strong impact on sleepiness. A striking number of participants fell asleep during work after a short period of mild overtime work (van Leeuwen et al. 2013).

Similar findings were reported in a study by Lützhöft and colleagues, who also found shorter sleep periods within a 6/6 system, where sleep was more often split into two episodes (Lutzhoft et al. 2010). The level of sleepiness was higher on the 00:00–06:00 and 06:00–12:00 watch, with increasing sleepiness towards the end of the watch. The sleep duration differed in between the various watches, with longer sleep during the 06:00–12:00 and 18:00–24:00 off-duty period (Eriksen et al. 2006).

Whether sleep was fragmented into 2/3 episodes on an oceanographic vessel or 5/6 episodes on a fishing vessel, the 24-h circadian alertness rhythm, assessed by Visual Analogue Scales (VAS) and actigraphs, was preserved in both instances, with seafarers having a circadian alertness dip during night time and a pronounced afternoon dip. The sleep fragmentation should be viewed not only as an occupational phenomenon but also with social factors such as meal times playing a role (Tirilly 2004).

Sleep Quality

Not all sleep is of the same quality and contains the same recuperative benefits. The highest sleep quality is obtained at night, while sleeping at other times is prone to be more disrupted and shorter, and therefore of lower quality. Good recuperation requires about 6 h of uninterrupted sleep for a person who normally sleeps 8 h.

Objective measures of sleep continuity are closely related to perceived sleep quality in the sense that sleep quality is essentially comparable to sleep continuity (Åkerstedt et al. 1994). Disturbed sleep seems to be a stronger predictor for fatigue than other well-established risk factors for fatigue (Åkerstedt et al. 2004). This is in accordance with the observation that subjective calmness of sleep and ease of falling asleep improves sleep quality and that the duration of wakefulness prior to sleep and the timing of sleep determines the subjective experience of sleep quality (Åkerstedt et al. 1997). Difficulty awakening after sleep is shown to be related more to high work demands, low social support, being male, being younger and smoking (Allen et al. 2010). Disturbed sleep is related more to female gender, age above 49 years, present illness, hectic work, physically strenuous work, and shift work (Åkerstedt et al. 2002a).

Physical Risk Factors

Exposure to a ship's engine noise at 65 dB(A) can have an adverse effect on sleep (Tamura et al. 1997), but this seems to be more a subjective effect, e.g. relating to sleep quality, which was not apparent with actigraphy (Tamura et al. 2002). Sleep tended to be often interrupted through noise and ships' movement in several studies (Wadsworth et al. 2006; Smith et al. 2006). Related to a moving environment, motion sickness—experienced by many seafarers—is a major cause of fatigue (Wertheim 1998). There is, however, little evidence about the severity of ships' motions that degrade physical and mental performance (Pisula et al. 2012). It has, however, been demonstrated that crews experience more constraints in terms of motion sickness and fatigue on days when vessel motions increased, with certain activities (balancing, moving, carrying) and responses (sleep problems, cognitive aspects of task performance, stomach awareness, dizziness) being particularly influenced by vessel motions (Haward et al. 2009).

Individual Risk Factors

Large individual differences in the effects of shift duty scheduling were shown in a study of naval day workers and night workers, so that the strategies addressing fatigue need to take into account that different individuals may be more suited to different shifts (Goh 2000). Out of several individual factors with a detrimental effect on circadian rhythms, age is an issue because there is a tendency towards an ageing workforce in the maritime industry. Ageing decreases the speed of circadian adaptation to night work and has a major impact on sleep quality and chronic disease risk factors (Ramin et al. 2015). Sleep disorders are also more prevalent in older workers. Practical countermeasures to improve the conditions of older workers should aim to fit work demands flexibly to ageing workers with different levels of work ability, health and social needs (Harma and Ilmarinen 1999). In a study of naval seafarers, older personnel did not suffer from more work-related fatigue than younger personnel, but work-related fatigue was found to accumulate over time with continuous exposure to work demands on board (Bridger et al. 2010).

While older shift workers tend to report more subjective sleepiness that decreases their work performance during morning and night shifts (Bonnefond et al. 2006), a systematic review of tolerance to shift work for older people reached conflicting results and concluded that there is only limited evidence for older people to be less tolerant. Nevertheless, it is argued that age-specific aspects should be considered in shift work planning (Blok and de Looze 2011). However, subjective sleep quality becomes worse and difficulties awakening and feelings of not being well rested after sleep increase with age (Åkerstedt et al. 2002a, b). In contrast, fatigue appears to be more prominent for younger subjects below the age of 49 years (Åkerstedt et al. 2002a, b).

Acute Responses

Acute Safety Effects

Within occupational medicine and traffic medicine, the concerns relating to safety issues are the main focus for the interest in fatigue.

Transport workers are prone to become sleepy and eventually to fall asleep during work (Harma et al. 2008; Project HORIZON 2012). In the driving sector, sleepy drivers have been estimated to be involved in at least 15–20 % of accidents (Horne and Reyner 1996). It is not easy to clearly relate sleepiness to maritime accidents retrospectively, but in a study of 279 maritime incidents, the US Coast Guard estimated that fatigue contributed to 16 % of the critical vessel casualties and 33 % of the personal injuries (National Transportation Safety Board 1999). In a study of 1647 collisions, groundings, contacts and near collisions, the British Marine Investigation Branch estimated that a third of all groundings involved a fatigued officer alone at the bridge at night, that two-thirds of vessels involved in collisions were not keeping a proper lookout, and that a third of all accidents that occurred at night involved a sole watchkeeper on the bridge. The main concerns from this study were fatigue, lookout, safe manning and the role of the master (MAIB 2004).

While reduced sleep and sleepiness in itself is an explanatory factor of accidents, the context of reduced sleep is also important since suboptimal work schedules and lifestyle, and sleep pathology are equally important factors (Åkerstedt et al. 2011). A review of 20 studies of safety in shipping across fatigue, stress, health, situation awareness, teamwork, decision-making, communication, automation, and safety culture concluded that modifications of human factor issues should be a focus for interventions (Hetherington et al. 2006). The risk of accidents is higher at night (and to a lesser degree afternoon) compared to the morning. It increases over a series of shifts and as shifts exceed 8 h (Folkard et al. 2005).

Acute Health-Related Effects

Disturbed sleep is the most common acute health-related effect of shift work, in particular with regard to difficulty getting to sleep, shortened sleep and sleepiness during working hours that continues into successive days off (Åkerstedt 2003). Falling asleep during wake time is another consequence of fatigue (Harma et al. 2008; van Leeuwen et al. 2013; Åkerstedt et al. 2002b). Since shift work and the associated fatigue impair cognition it can potentially lead to misjudgements and accidents (Marquie et al. 2015).

Chronic Responses

Chronic fatigue may follow repeated exposures to acute fatigue or represent a persistent failure of sufficient rest and recuperation to overcome fatigue. The pathways from fatigue to chronic disease are complex and not fully understood but involved mechanisms include metabolic, autonomous, and immunological pathways.

Chronic sleep debt leads to chronic circadian disruption of the immune response (van Mark et al. 2010) and increases the risk of developing cardiovascular diseases (van Leeuwen et al. 2009). Autonomic changes relating to a reduced parasympathetic modulation may result from lifetime shift work (Bernardes Souza et al. 2015; Kubo et al. 2013a, b). Disruption of the circadian regulation of the human transcriptome is another implicated mechanism behind fatigue that is related to mistimed sleep. Delaying sleep by 4 h for 3 consecutive days has been found to lead to a sixfold reduction in human blood transcriptome, while the centrally mediated circadian rhythm of melatonin remains unaffected (Archer et al. 2014). Fatigue from night and shift work alters the hormonal and sleepiness cycles and the lipid and glucose metabolism (Garbarino et al. 2002). Despite signs indicating these possible disease mechanisms, compelling evidence is still lacking (Puttonen et al. 2010).

Chronic Psychosocial Effects and Sleep Disorders

Experimental studies have demonstrated that chronic sleep loss cumulatively increases the rate of deterioration in performance across wakefulness, in particular during the circadian "night" (Cohen et al. 2010). Fatigue favours sleeping disorders such as insomnia, and delayed or advanced sleep-phase disorders and interferes with behaviour and social life (Harma and Ilmarinen 1999; Garbarino et al. 2002).

Insomnia, the inability to fall asleep and/or to stay asleep as long as desired, is the most common sleep disorder related to irregular work hours such as shift work. Sleep apnoea/hypopnoea is a common sleep disorder among overweight men who snore. The affected subject may not be aware of the condition, which causes sleepiness and fatigue when awake. While this condition is not caused by fatigue per se, it is related to fatigue in the sense that fatigue related to sleep deprivation contributes to a preference for high-caloric food that may result in overweight and metabolic changes. Delayed or advanced sleep-phase symptoms occur when the circadian rhythm is out of phase with the environment. Delayed sleep-phase syndrome causes difficulties in sleeping at night and mainly affects younger persons, while advanced sleep-phase syndrome causes problems staying awake in the evening and waking up early in the morning (Zhu and Zee 2012).

Chronic Somatic Health Effects

In addition to impaired cognition (Marquie et al. 2015), chronic exposure to shift work has been demonstrated to cause a number of other significant health implications (van Mark et al. 2006). Fatigue from night and shift work may affect the gastrointestinal and cardiovascular functions through altered hormonal and sleepiness cycles (Knutsson 2003).

Peptic ulcers and symptoms related to irritable bowel syndrome are increased in shift workers and there is no doubt that shift work is a significant risk factor for coronary heart disease (Harma and Ilmarinen 1999). The autonomous consequences of lifetime shift work lead to increased blood pressure (Bernardes Souza et al. 2015; Kubo et al. 2013a, b). The intake by shift workers of more proinflammatory diets compared to day workers (Wirth et al. 2014) contributes to their cardiovascular risk, which may also be increased through additional interrelated factors, for example, psychosocial (difficulties in controlling work hours, decreased work–life balance, poor recovery following work), behavioural (weight gain and smoking) and physiological mechanisms (activation of the autonomic nervous system, inflammation, altered lipid and glucose metabolism with related changes in risks for atherosclerosis, metabolic syndrome and type II diabetes). Again, in spite of signs indicating these possible disease mechanisms, compelling evidence remains to be elucidated (Puttonen et al. 2010). However, it has been demonstrated that incomplete recovery from work is an aspect of the overall risk profile of cardiovascular disease mortality among employees, and workers who seldom recovered from work during free weekends were particularly at risk (Kivimaki et al. 2006). This aspect may be highly relevant for seafarers subjected to extended periods (months) at sea.

Many studies have linked short sleep duration to obesity through pathways of increased high-caloric food intake and reduced energy expenditure during daytime, which is related to sedentary behaviour. Fatigue, adverse sleep patterns and shift work are known risk factors for obesity, and lead to high levels of triglycerides and low HDL cholesterol. These metabolic changes indicate an increased risk of metabolic syndrome (Kaltsas et al. 2010; Karlsson et al. 2001; Anonymous 2011), which is more prevalent among former shift workers than in workers who have never worked in shifts (Puttonen et al. 2012) and among seafarers than in the general population (Moller Pedersen and Jepsen 2013). Short sleep duration is correlated to an increased risk of adult overweight/obesity and some studies claim this to be related to a reduced circulating leptin level relative to what is predicted by fat mass (Chaput et al. 2007), whereas others have found increased circulating leptin levels after a period of short sleep (van Leeuwen et al. 2010). It should be noted, however, that experimental studies are far from consistent where it concerns the metabolic consequences of short sleep duration (Wright et al. 2015; van Cauter et al. 2008; Horne 2010). Shift work has been found to be associated with unfavourable dietary habits and consequently to overweight and related chronic diseases such as coronary heart disease, metabolic syndrome and type 2 diabetes (Hemio et al. 2015). Night-shift work, in particular for workers of older ages, increases obesity (Kubo et al. 2011a, b), calorie intake, and smoking, and causes shorter sleep duration (Ramin et al. 2015). A meta-analysis has recently demonstrated that shift work is associated to an increased risk of diabetes mellitus, in particular among men with rotating shifts (Gan et al. 2015).

Shift work has also been shown to be associated with a higher risk of common infections such as the common cold, flu-like illness, and gastroenteritis (Mohren et al. 2002). This may be explained by impaired immune function consequent to sleep deprivation (Toth 1995).

The joint additional effect of adverse lifestyle factors such as smoking, sedentary lifestyle, and obesity, which is also prevalent among seafarers, is regarded as multiplicative (Harma and Ilmarinen 1999). Individuals whose working hours exceed standard recommendations are more likely to increase their alcohol use to levels that pose a health risk (Virtanen et al. 2015).

The International Agency for Research on Cancer has classified shift work as a probable human carcinogen but research on this issue is complex (Stevens et al. 2011). For males, prostate carcinoma has been particularly implicated (Kubo et al. 2011a, b). Along with other psychosocial stressors, fatigue is regarded as associated with mental health risks (Carotenuto et al. 2012). Psychiatric conditions such as major depression are increased among shift workers and their prevalence increases with the length of exposure and age (Harma and Ilmarinen 1999).

Fatigue Mitigation

Countermeasures for fatigue in transportation, including seafaring, have been recently reviewed in a comprehensive Swedish report (Anund et al. 2015). Reducing seafarers' fatigue requires external and company regulation and control as well as individual preventive intervention and human resilience. Fatigue-mitigating factors include alertness management strategies, of which proper work–rest scheduling and adequate sleep hygiene are of primary importance (Caldwell et al. 2008). Whereas countermeasures (scheduling, education, naps, caffeine etc.)—preferably in combination—may ameliorate the negative impact of shift work on night time sleepiness and day time insomnia, there seems at present to be no way of eliminating most negative effects of shift work on human physiology and cognition (Åkerstedt and Wright 2009). Recent advice on best practices has been published by Seahealth—the occupational health service for the Danish merchant fleet (Seahealth 2010).

International Regulation

The ILO Convention 180 on Seafarers' Hours of Work and Manning of Ships, which came into force in 2002, dictates a maximum amount of work of 14 h in any 24-h period and up to 72 h in any 7-day period. The minimum hours of rest should be not less than 10 h in any 24-h period and 77 h in any 7-day period. The hours of rest may be divided into no more than two periods, one of which must be at least 6 h in length and the interval between consecutive periods must not exceed 14 h.

Other ILO Conventions 92, 133, 140, 141 and 147 introduce additional minimal habitability requirements on board ships such as noise control and air conditioning. IMO instruments concerning hours of rest and work include the International Convention on Standards of Training, Certification and Watchkeeping for Seafarers (STCW) Code, which requires alertness to factors that can contribute to fatigue including excessive or unreasonable overall working hours and to the frequency and length of leave periods as material factors in preventing fatigue from building up over a period of time. The limits of hours at work and hours at rest contained in the Maritime Labour Convention (MLC) 2006 are similar to those in ILO 180 and the revised STCW Code of 2010.

IMO also produced the "Guidelines on Fatigue Mitigation and Management" in 2001 (IMO 2001), which contains useful information on the causes and consequences of fatigue. In 2015, IMO took the decision to review these guidelines and the new guidelines will be produced by 2017, and will contain sections on managing fatigue, as well as a section on FRMS.

The International Safety Management (ISM) Code states that if fatigue, excessive hours of work, or lack of adequate rest are or should be apparent, the master and the company management should intervene to immediately remedy the problem.

The Code reiterates the important position held by the master of a ship but also states that the company will not absolve itself from responsibility by delegating the responsibility for managing safety on board to the master. The company is also responsible for ensuring their masters' monitoring and managing of their own hours of work/rest so that they do not suffer from fatigue. The company must ensure that master, officers and crew are properly qualified, experienced, trained and familiarized and sufficient in number. The safe manning certificate determines the required manning of a particular ship safely at a particular time. The Code requires the company to prepare plans and instructions, including checklists for "key shipboard operations," which will depend on the type of ship and its operational requirements (navigation and bridge management, cargo operations and management, etc.). The management of personnel and their hours of work and rest should ensure that the various tasks can be performed safely and that fatigue is prevented. Seafarers who are too tired to act safely should not perform operational tasks, and procedures should prevent this from happening.

While the ISM Code cannot achieve immediate perfection it should initiate a cycle of continuous improvement and proactive steps. It also allows a reactive approach by learning from experienced system failures, including previous corrective actions. Any situation on board where a seafarer is not achieving the minimum hours of rest or works excessive hours and is possibly suffering from fatigue must be recorded and reported.

Collective Fatigue Mitigation Management

Fatigue should be regarded as a serious health and safety issue and therefore securing sufficient quality sleep is the first and most important method of fatigue mitigation. This will promote recovery, while insufficient rest and suboptimal sleep will exacerbate fatigue, which may eventually accumulate over time (van Mark et al. 2010). Keeping fixed watch schedules for mitigating fatigue has been proposed (Arulanandam and Tsing 2009), but the feasibility in a broader context remains to be shown.

Houtman et al. emphasized proper implementation of the ISM Code as essential to reduce fatigue (Houtman et al. 2005) and consequently a focus upon company-based strategic solutions. This requires a more robust and realistic approach to regulation and manning. While vessels may already operate with more crew than demanded by their flag state, the operational mode must also be taken into account (Allen et al. 2007). The crew size may be adequate for open sailing but insufficient for maintenance, recovery, port turnarounds, or with specific security requirements. A level of redundancy requires manning specifications to be universal for all vessels to prevent economic advantage accruing to companies who operate with bare minimums. A comparison between a ship with a 24-man crew and a ship with an 18-man crew demonstrated that the latter had longer working hours, a higher level of catecholamine excretion and higher stress levels (Wegner et al. 2008).

To cope with fatigue, learning experiences should be drawn from different sectors in the maritime sector as well as from other transport sectors that are prone to fatigue, notably the aviation industry, which has dealt significantly with this issue (Hartzler 2014). Learning from best practices requires the collaborate efforts of all stakeholders such as the workforce, regulators and academics.

Under-recording of working hours to comply with the legislation is contra-active in relation to fatigue mitigation. It has been shown that seafarers who underreported (at least occasionally) their working hours were significantly more fatigued and less healthy than non-under-recording seafarers (Allen et al. 2006, 2008). To promote good quality sleep, the cabins should be quiet, dark and cool, i.e. protected from noise and vibration to the extent possible, with an option for shielding off daylight, and with efficient air conditioning facilities. Single cabins should be offered for undisturbed sleep.

Individual Fatigue Mitigation Management

Taking into account that legislation and compliance cannot solve all issues relating to fatigue, and that certain circumstances on board cannot be changed, e.g. the weather, and the sea state, and that naval architects, at best, are only likely to modify/reduce the ship's motion, collective mitigation cannot stand alone. The seafarer's own behaviour is also important.

The seafarer would benefit from taking actions such as calming down and avoiding caffeine and alcohol prior to sleep. It is important to spend as much time as possible in daylight, and to be active (physically and mentally) during the day, but not too close to bedtime. The seafarer should attempt to follow his own circadian rhythm by sleeping and waking early if a morning person and sleeping and waking late if an evening person.

The cabin should be prepared for sleep by shielding out light and by securing coolness (below 20 °C). Phone and doorbell should be switched off. Relaxing, reading or listening to soothing music before sleeping can help getting ready for sleep. Nicotine and alcohol should be avoided 2 h before sleep, and caffeine 6 h before sleep. Heavy exercise should also be avoided 2 h before going to bed. If hungry, only light food is recommended.

There are several additional countermeasures to ameliorate the negative impact of irregular work on night time sleepiness while working and daytime insomnia when there is a need of sleeping during the day. Even when these measures are applied (probably best in combination), however, there seems at present to be no way to eliminate most of the negative effects of shift work on human physiology and cognition (Åkerstedt and Wright 2009).

Blue light exposure (Taillard et al. 2012), caffeine (Philip et al. 2006; Sagaspe et al. 2007) and naps (Philip et al. 2006; Sagaspe et al. 2007; Ferguson et al. 2008) have all been demonstrated to mitigate fatigue. Naps should be kept short (15–40 min) to avoid waking up from deep sleep. A nap should be scheduled for the last

2 h before a night shift and end 1 h before starting work. Lifestyle issues such as regular exercise and healthy diet habits promote the general health, and at the same time affect positively sleep and reduce fatigue. Worksite healthy sleep programmes have shown the effectiveness of tailored interventions (Steffen et al. 2015).

A recent Cochrane review concluded that melatonin had only a limited effect on sleep duration during daytime after night shifts but no effect on sleep quality. There is insufficient knowledge for an effect of hypnotics on sleep length (Liira et al. 2014). In spite of melatonin and hypnotics being available over the counter in many countries, medications addressing sleep problems are not recommended by the authors. Their side effects may well be worse than the problem that one tries to solve by taking them.

Fatigue Prediction

Various models for fatigue prediction have been recently reviewed (CASA 2014) and the current generation of such models is regarded as an appropriate element in an FRMS to be applied in field settings by organizations and regulators. It is, however, emphasized that individual and task variables are not included in the current models (Dawson et al. 2011) and the user interphase has limited user friendliness. One of the outcomes of the EU-funded Project HORIZON (2012) was the production of a prototype fatigue prediction model for use in shipping opera- tions. This prototype is based on a theoretical model of fatigue, and uses the results of many years of research effort from other industries to produce algorithms which predict the levels of sleepiness of watchkeepers (Barnett et al. 2012a, b).

Such models may be used within an FRMS, and the authors are now involved in a follow-up project called MARTHA, one of the aims of which is to evaluate these systems in practice at sea. FRMS are new to aviation, but are virtually unknown in shipping, so this represents the first known trial of FRMS at sea. Guidance and support through self-help manuals and incident reporting are also measures being introduced in the trial by the consortium, and these will be evaluated using specific fatigue-related key performance measures. The particular challenge in this type of research is to find ways to change the culture of a diverse and multinational workforce, where fatigue is accepted as the norm, and there is resistance to acknowledging and reporting fatigue. This is exacerbated by the fact that ships work literally "over the horizon", are prone to sudden changes in voyage plan, and are therefore difficult places to monitor and to collect meaningful data.

The MARTHA project, which commenced in 2013 and lasts for 3 years, is also exploring the longer term psychosocial issues affecting crews at sea. In addition to a questionnaire given to 1000 seafaring employees, volunteer crew members have been rating their fatigue and stress levels in a weekly diary for 3–4 months, which is then sent directly to the research team by email. Some crew members are also wearing Actiwatches at the beginning and end of the study period to record their physical activity levels. In addition to this personal data, information is also being collected on the voyages, including the times of their port calls, weather conditions and any other situations which are likely to affect the quality of sleep. When all the data is collected, it will comprise a large database of the sleep experiences of about 1000 seafarers of all ranks. The authors hope that the database will provide more knowledge on the complex issues surrounding seafarer fatigue.

While there is much knowledge about the risk factors for seafarer fatigue and the many and serious consequences of fatigue in terms of health and safety effects, there is still insufficient knowledge about individual differences with respect to the impact of fatigue, the effectiveness of different mitigating interventions and the relative impact of legislation and cultural change management in relation to company policies on fatigue risk management. Future research into sleepiness and the longer term fatigue problems of seafarers is likely to focus on the following areas of interest:

- The link between individual levels of fatigue and performance on tasks associated with shipboard roles
- The recovery mechanisms for long-term fatigue and effective interventions to improve the psychological well-being of seafarers
- The effectiveness of different FRMS
- The way in which the organizational practices and cultural differences in interpretation of regulatory frameworks can affect fatigue mitigation.

References

Åkerstedt, T. (2003). Shift work and disturbed sleep/wakefulness. *Occupational Medicine (Lond), 53*(2), 89–94.

Åkerstedt, T. (2006). Psychosocial stress and impaired sleep. *Scandinavian Journal of Work, Environment & Health, 32*(6), 493–501.

Åkerstedt, T., Axelsson, J., Lekander, M., Orsini, N., & Kecklund, G. (2014). Do sleep, stress, and illness explain daily variations in fatigue? A prospective study. *Journal of Psychosomatic Research, 76*(4), 280–285.

Åkerstedt, T., Fredlund, P., Gillberg, M., & Jansson, B. (2002a). Work load and work hours in relation to disturbed sleep and fatigue in a large representative sample. *Journal of Psychosomatic Research, 53*(1), 585–588.

Åkerstedt, T., Hume, K., Minors, D., & Waterhouse, J. (1994). The meaning of good sleep: A longitudinal study of polysomnography and subjective sleep quality. *Journal of Sleep Research, 3*(3), 152–158.

Åkerstedt, T., Hume, K., Minors, D., & Waterhouse, J. (1997). Good sleep—Its timing and physiological sleep characteristics. *Journal of Sleep Research, 6*(4), 221–229.

Åkerstedt, T., Kecklund, G., & Axelsson, J. (2007). Impaired sleep after bedtime stress and worries. *Biological Psychology, 76*(3), 170–173.

Åkerstedt, T., Kecklund, G., & Axelsson, J. (2008). Effects of context on sleepiness self-ratings during repeated partial sleep deprivation. *Chronobiology International, 25*(2), 271–278.

Åkerstedt, T., Knutsson, A., Westerholm, P., Theorell, T., Alfredsson, L., & Kecklund, G. (2002b). Sleep disturbances, work stress and work hours: A cross-sectional study. *Journal of Psychosomatic Research, 53*(3), 741–748.

Åkerstedt, T., Knutsson, A., Westerholm, P., Theorell, T., Alfredsson, L., & Kecklund, G. (2004). Mental fatigue, work and sleep. *Journal of Psychosomatic Research, 57*(5), 427–433.

Åkerstedt, T., Philip, P., Capelli, A., & Kecklund, G. (2011). Sleep loss and accidents—Work hours, life style, and sleep pathology. *Progress in Brain Research, 190*, 169–188.

Åkerstedt, T., & Wright, K. P., Jr. (2009). Sleep loss and fatigue in shift work and shift work disorder. *Sleep Medicine Clinics, 4*(2), 257–271.

Allen, P., Wadsworth, E., & Smith, A. (2006). The relationship between recorded hours of work and fatigue in seafarers. *Contemporary ergonomics*. London: Taylor and Francis.

Allen, P., Wadsworth, E., & Smith, A. (2007). The prevention and management of seafarers' fatigue: A review. *International Maritime Health, 58*(1–4), 167–177.

Allen, P., Wadsworth, E., & Smith, A. (2008). Seafarers' fatigue: A review of the recent literature. *International Maritime Health, 59*(1–4), 81–92.

Allen, P., Wellens, B. T., & Smith, A. (2010). Fatigue in British fishermen. *International Maritime Health, 61*(3), 154.

Anonymous. (2011). Shift work and sleep: Optimizing health, safety, and performance. *Journal of Occupational and Environmental Medicine, 53*(5 Suppl), S1–10; quiz S11-2.

Anund, A., Fors, C., Kecklund, G., van Leeuwen, W., & Akerstedt, A. (2015). *Countermeasures for fatigue in transportation—A review of existing methods for drivers on road, rail, sea and in aviation*. Stockholm: VTI Rapport.

Archer, S. N., Laing, E. E., Moller-Levet, C. S., van der Veen, D. R., Bucca, G., Lazar, A. S., et al. (2014). Mistimed sleep disrupts circadian regulation of the human transcriptome. *Proceedings of the National Academy of Science USA, 111*(6), E682–E691.

Arulanandam, S., & Tsing, C. G. (2009). Comparison of alertness levels in ship crew. An experiment on rotating versus fixed watch schedules. *International Maritime Health, 60*(1–2), 6–9.

Australian Transport Safety Bureau. (2011). *Independent investigation into the grounding of the Chinese registered bulk carrier Shen Neng 1 on Douglas Shoal, Queensland 3 April 2010, in ATSB Transport Safety Report Marine Occurrence Investigation*. Report no. 274/2011, ATSB.

Barnett, M., Lützhöft, M., & Åkerstedt, T., (2012). *HORIZON. Fatigue Management Toolkit*, Doc Ref: hzn047v5. Luxemburg: EU Commission. http://www.warsashacademy.co.uk/about/resources/horizon-fatigue-management-toolkit.pdf

Barnett, M., Pekcan, C., & Gatfield, D. (2012, April 23–27). The use of linked simulators in project "HORIZON": Research into seafarer fatigue. In *MARSIM, 2012*, Singapore.

Barton, J., Folkard, S., Smith, L., & Poole, C. J. (1994). Effects on health of a change from a delaying to an advancing shift system. *Occupational and Environmental Medicine, 51*(11), 749–755.

Bayon, V., Leger, D., Gomez-Merino, D., Vecchierini, M. F., & Chennaoui, M. (2014). Sleep debt and obesity. *Annals of Medicine, 46*(5), 264–272.

Bernardes Souza, B., Mussi Monteze, N., Pereira de Oliveira, F. L., de Oliveira, J. M., Nascimento de Freitas, S., Marques do Nascimento Neto, R., et al. (2015). Lifetime shift work exposure: Association with anthropometry, body composition, blood pressure, glucose and heart rate variability. *Occupational and Environmental Medicine, 72*(3), 208–215.

Blok, M. M., & de Looze, M. P. (2011). What is the evidence for less shift work tolerance in older workers? *Ergonomics, 54*(3), 221–232.

Bonnefond, A., Harma, M., Hakola, T., Sallinen, M., Kandolin, I., & Virkkala, J. (2006). Interaction of age with shift-related sleep-wakefulness, sleepiness, performance, and social life. *Experimental Aging Research, 32*(2), 185–208.

Bridger, R. S., Brasher, K., & Dew, A. (2010). Work demands and need for recovery from work in ageing seafarers. *Ergonomics, 53*(8), 1006–1015.

Caldwell, J. A., Caldwell, J. L., & Schmidt, R. M. (2008). Alertness management strategies for operational contexts. *Sleep Medicine Reviews, 12*(4), 257–273.

Cappuccio, F. P., Cooper, D., D'Elia, L., Strazzullo, P., & Miller, M. A. (2011). Sleep duration predicts cardiovascular outcomes: A systematic review and meta-analysis of prospective studies. *European Heart Journal, 32*(12), 1484–1492.

Carotenuto, A., Molino, I., Fasanaro, A. M., & Amenta, F. (2012). Psychological stress in seafarers: A review. *International Maritime Health, 63*(4), 188–194.

Chaput, J.-P., Despres, J.-P., Bouchard, C., & Tremblay, A. (2007). Short sleep duration is associated with reduced leptin levels and increased adiposity: Results from the Québec family study. *Obesity, 15*(1), 253–261.

Civil Aviation Safety Authority. (2014). *Biomathematical fatigue models—Guidance document,* CASA (Ed.) Albert Park, Australia: Dédale Asia Pacific.

Cohen, D. A., Wang, W., Wyatt, J. K., Kronauer, R. E., Dijk, D. J., Czeisler, C. A., et al. (2010). Uncovering residual effects of chronic sleep loss on human performance. *Science Translational Medicine, 2*(14), 14ra3.

Dahlgren, A., Kecklund, G., & Akerstedt, T. (2005). Different levels of work-related stress and the effects on sleep, fatigue and cortisol. *Scandinavian Journal of Work, Environment & Health, 31*(4), 277–285.

Dawson, D., Ian Noy, Y., Harma, M., Akerstedt, T., & Belenky, G. (2011). Modelling fatigue and the use of fatigue models in work settings. *Accident Analyses and Prevention, 43*(2), 549–564.

de Lange, A. H., Kompier, M. A., Taris, T. W., Geurts, S. A., Beckers, D. G., Houtman, I. L., et al. (2009). A hard day's night: A longitudinal study on the relationships among job demands and job control, sleep quality and fatigue. *Journal of Sleep Research, 18*(3), 374–383.

Dittner, A. J., Wessely, S. C., & Brown, R. G. (2004). The assessment of fatigue: A practical guide for clinicians and researchers. *Journal of Psychosomatic Research, 56*(2), 157–170.

Dumont, M., Montplaisir, J., & Infante-Rivard, C. (1997). Sleep quality of former night-shift workers. *International Journal of Occupational and Environmental Health, 3*(Supplement 2), S10–S14.

Eriksen, C. A., Gillberg, M., & Vestergren, P. (2006). Sleepiness and sleep in a simulated "six hours on/six hours off" sea watch system. *Chronobiology International, 23*(6), 1193–1202.

Ferguson, S. A., Lamond, N., Kandelaars, K., Jay, S. M., & Dawson, D. (2008). The impact of short, irregular sleep opportunities at sea on the alertness of marine pilots working extended hours. *Chronobiology International, 25*(2), 399–411.

Ferrie, J. E., Kumari, M., Salo, P., Singh-Manoux, A., & Kivimaki, M. (2011). Sleep epidemiology—A rapidly growing field. *International Journal of Epidemiology, 40*(6), 1431–1437.

Flo, E., Pallesen, S., Akerstedt, T., Mageroy, N., Moen, B. E., Gronli, J., et al. (2013). Shift-related sleep problems vary according to work schedule. *Occupational and Environmental Medicine, 70*(4), 238–245.

Folkard, S., Lombardi, D. A., & Tucker, P. T. (2005). Shiftwork: Safety, sleepiness and sleep. *Industrial Health, 43*, 20–23.

Gan, Y., Yang, C., Tong, X., Sun, H., Cong, Y., Yin, X., et al. (2015). Shift work and diabetes mellitus: A meta-analysis of observational studies. *Occupational and Environmental Medicine, 72*(1), 72–78.

Gander, P., van den Berg, M., & Signal, L. (2008). Sleep and sleepiness of fishermen on rotating schedules. *Chronobiology International, 25*(2), 389–398.

Garbarino, S., Beelke, M., Costa, G., Violani, C., Lucidi, F., Ferrillo, F., et al. (2002). Brain function and effects of shift work: Implications for clinical neuropharmacology. *Neuropsychobiology, 45*(1), 50–56.

Goh, V. H. (2000). Circadian disturbances after night-shift work onboard a naval ship. *Military Medicine, 165*(2), 101–105.

Harma, M. (2013). Psychosocial work characteristics and sleep—A well-known but poorly understood association. *Scandinavian Journal of Work, Environment & Health, 39*(6), 531–533.

Harma, M. I., & Ilmarinen, J. E. (1999). Towards the 24-hour society—New approaches for aging shift workers? *Scandinavian Journal of Work, Environment & Health, 25*(6), 610–615.

Harma, M., Partinen, M., Repo, R., Sorsa, M., & Siivonen, P. (2008). Effects of 6/6 and 4/8 watch systems on sleepiness among bridge officers. *Chronobiology International, 25*(2), 413–423.

Hartzler, B. M. (2014). Fatigue on the flight deck: The consequences of sleep loss and the benefits of napping. *Accident Analyses and Prevention, 62*, 309–318.

Haward, B. M., Lewis, C. H., & Griffin, M. J. (2009). Motions and crew responses on an offshore oil production and storage vessel. *Applied Ergonomics, 40*(5), 904–914.

Hemio, K., Puttonen, S., Viitasalo, K., Harma, M., Peltonen, M., & Lindstrom, J. (2015). Food and nutrient intake among workers with different shift systems. *Occupational and Environmental Medicine, 72*(7), 513–520.

Hetherington, C., Flin, R., & Mearns, K. (2006). Safety in shipping: The human element. *Journal of Safety Research, 37*(4), 401–411.

Horne, J. (2010). Habitual 'short sleep': Six hours is 'safe'. *Journal of Sleep Research, 19*(1 Pt 1), 119–120.

Horne, J. A., & Reyner, L. A. (1996). Counteracting driver sleepiness: Effects of napping, caffeine, and placebo. *Psychophysiology, 33*(3), 306–309.

Hovdanum, A. S., Jensen, O. C., Petursdottir, G., & Holmen, I. M. (2014). A review of fatigue in fishermen: A complicated and underprioritised area of research. *International Maritime Health, 65*(3), 166–172.

Houtman, I., Miedema, M., Jettinghoff, K., Starren, A., Heinrich, J., Gort, J., et al. (2005). *Fatigue in the shipping industry*. The Hague: TNO.

International Maritime Organization. (2001). *Guidance on fatigue mitigation and management*. London: IMO.

International Maritime Organization. (2002). *Guidelines on fatigue*. London: IMO.

Jackowska, M., Dockray, S., Hendrickx, H., & Steptoe, A. (2011). Psychosocial factors and sleep efficiency: Discrepancies between subjective and objective evaluations of sleep. *Psychosomatic Medicine, 73*(9), 810–816.

Kaida, K., Åkerstedt, T., Kecklund, G., Nilsson, J. P., & Axelsson, J. (2007). The effects of asking for verbal ratings of sleepiness on sleepiness and its masking effects on performance. *Clinical Neurophysiology, 118*(6), 1324–1331.

Kaida, K., Takahashi, M., Akerstedt, T., Nakata, A., Otsuka, Y., Haratani, T., et al. (2006). Validation of the Karolinska sleepiness scale against performance and EEG variables. *Clinical Neurophysiology, 117*(7), 1574–1581.

Kaltsas, G., Vgontzas, A., & Chrousos, G. (2010). Fatigue, endocrinopathies, and metabolic disorders. *Physical Medicine and Rehabilitation, 2*(5), 393–398.

Karlsson, B., Knutsson, A., & Lindahl, B. (2001). Is there an association between shift work and having a metabolic syndrome? Results from a population based study of 27,485 people. *Occupational and Environmental Medicine, 58*(11), 747–752.

Kivimaki, M., Leino-Arjas, P., Kaila-Kangas, L., Luukkonen, R., Vahtera, J., Elovainio, M., et al. (2006). Is incomplete recovery from work a risk marker of cardiovascular death? Prospective evidence from industrial employees. *Psychosomatic Medicine, 68*(3), 402–407.

Knutsson, A. (2003). Health disorders of shift workers. *Occupational Medicine (Lond), 53*(2), 103–108.

Kubo, T., Fujino, Y., Nakamura, T., Kunimoto, M., Tabata, H., Tsuchiya, T., et al. (2013a). An industry-based cohort study of the association between weight gain and hypertension risk among rotating shift workers. *Journal of Occupational and Environmental Medicine, 55*(9), 1041–1045.

Kubo, T., Oyama, I., Nakamura, T., Kunimoto, M., Kadowaki, K., Otomo, H., et al. (2011a). Industry-based retrospective cohort study of the risk of prostate cancer among rotating-shift workers. *International Journal of Urology, 18*(3), 206–211.

Kubo, T., Oyama, I., Nakamura, T., Shirane, K., Otsuka, H., Kunimoto, M., et al. (2011b). Retrospective cohort study of the risk of obesity among shift workers: Findings from the Industry-based Shift Workers' Health study. *Japan. Occupational and Environmental Medicine, 68*(5), 327–331.

Kubo, T., Takahashi, M., Togo, F., Liu, X., Shimazu, A., Tanaka, K., et al. (2013b). Effects on employees of controlling working hours and working schedules. *Occupational Medicine (Lond), 63*(2), 148–151.

Liira, J., Verbeek, J. H., Costa, G., Driscoll, T. R., Sallinen, M., Isotalo, L. K., et al. (2014). Pharmacological interventions for sleepiness and sleep disturbances caused by shift work. *Cochrane Database Systematic Reviews, 8*, CD009776.

Lin, J. M., Brimmer, D. J., Maloney, E. M., Nyarko, E., Belue, R., & Reeves, W. C. (2009). Further validation of the multidimensional fatigue inventory in a US adult population sample. *Population Health Metrics, 7*, 18.

Lutzhoft, M., Dahlgren, A., Kircher, A., Thorslund, B., & Gillberg, M. (2010). Fatigue at sea in Swedish shipping—A field study. *American Journal of Industrial Medicine, 53*(7), 733–740.

Marine Accident Investigation Board. (2014). *Report on the investigation of the grounding of Danio off Longstone, Farne Islands, England, 16 March 2013*. Report no. 8/2014, MAIB.

Marine Accident Investigation Branch. (2004). *Bridge watchkeeping safety study*. Southampton: MAIB.

Marquie, J. C., Tucker, P., Folkard, S., Gentil, C., & Ansiau, D. (2015). Chronic effects of shift work on cognition: Findings from the VISAT longitudinal study. *Occupational and Environmental Medicine, 72*(4), 258–264.

Maurier, P., Barnett, M., Pekcan, C., Gatfield, D., Corrignan, P., & Clarke, G. (2011, November 16–17). Fatigue and performance in bridge and engine control room watchkeeping on a 6on/6off watch regime. In *International Conference on Human Factors in Ship Design*. London.

Mohren, D. C., Jansen, N. W., Kant, I. J., Galama, J., van den Brandt, P. A., & Swaen, G. M. (2002). Prevalence of common infections among employees in different work schedules. *Journal of Occupational and Environmental Medicine, 44*(1), 1003–1011.

Moller Pedersen, S. F., & Jepsen, J. R. (2013). The metabolic syndrome among Danish seafarers. *International Maritime Health, 64*(4), 183–190.

National Transportation Safety Board. (1999). Evaluation of US Department of Transportation. Efforts in the 1990s to address operator fatigue. In: *Safety Report NTSB/SR-99-01*. Washington DC: National Transportation Safety Board.

Ohayon, M. M., Smolensky, M. H., & Roth, T. (2010). Consequences of shiftworking on sleep duration, sleepiness, and sleep attacks. *Chronobiology International, 27*(3), 575–589.

Philip, P., Taillard, J., Moore, N., Delord, S., Valtat, C., Sagaspe, P., et al. (2006). The effects of coffee and napping on nighttime highway driving: A randomized trial. *Annals of Internal Medicine, 144*(11), 785–791.

Pisula, P. J., Lewis, C. H., & Bridger, R. S. (2012). Vessel motion thresholds for maintaining physical and cognitive performance: A study of naval personnel at sea. *Ergonomics, 55*(6), 636–649.

Project HORIZON—Final Report Findings. (2012). Retrieved from: http://www.warsashacademy. co.uk/about/resources/final-horizon-report-final-as-printed.pdf. Accessed March 3, 2015.

Puttonen, S., Harma, M., & Hublin, C. (2010). Shift work and cardiovascular disease—Pathways from circadian stress to morbidity. *Scandinavian Journal of Work, Environment & Health, 36* (2), 96–108.

Puttonen, S., Viitasalo, K., & Harma, M. (2012). The relationship between current and former shift work and the metabolic syndrome. *Scandinavian Journal of Work, Environment & Health, 38* (4), 343–348.

Ramin, C., Devore, E. E., Wang, W., Pierre-Paul, J., Wegrzyn, L. R., & Schernhammer, E. S. (2015). Night shift work at specific age ranges and chronic disease risk factors. *Occupational and Environmental Medicine, 72*(2), 100–107.

Sagaspe, P., Taillard, J., Chaumet, G., Moore, N., Bioulac, B., & Philip, P. (2007). Aging and nocturnal driving: better with coffee or a nap? *A randomized study. Sleep, 30*(12), 1808–1813.

Seahealth. (2010). *Shipping and rest: How can we do better?*. Copenhagen: Seahealth.

Smets, E. M., Garssen, B., Bonke, B., & De Haes, J. C. (1995). The Multidimensional Fatigue Inventory (MFI) psychometric qualities of an instrument to assess fatigue. *Journal of Psychosomatic Research, 39*(3), 315–325.

Smith, A., Allen, P., & Wadsworth, E. (2006). *Seafarers fatigue: The Cardiff Research Programme*. Cardiff: Centre for Occupational and Health Psychology.

Smith, A. P., Allen, P. H., & Wadsworth, E. M. (2007). *A comparative approach to seafarers' fatigue.* Proceedings of the International Symposium on Maritime Safety, Science and Environmental Protection, Athens.

Smith, A. P., Lane, T., & Bloor, M. (2001). *Fatigue offshore: A comparison of offshore oil support shipping and the offshore oil industry.* Cardiff: Seafarers International Research Centre/Centre for Occupational and Health Psychology, Cardiff University.

Smith, A. P., Lane, T., Bloor, M., Allen, P., Burke, A., & Ellis, N. (2003). *Fatigue offshore: Phase 2. The short sea and coastal shipping industry.* Cardiff: Seafarers International Research Centre/Centre for Occupational and Health Psychology, Cardiff University.

Steffen, M. W., Hazelton, A. C., Moore, W. R., Jenkins, S. M., Clark, M. M., & Hagen, P. T. (2015). Improving sleep: Outcomes from a worksite healthy sleep program. *Journal of Occupational and Environmental Medicine, 57*(1), 1–5.

Stevens, R. G., Hansen, J., Costa, G., Haus, E., Kauppinen, T., Aronson, K. J., et al. (2011). Considerations of circadian impact for defining 'shift work' in cancer studies: IARC Working Group Report. *Occupational and Environmental Medicine, 68*(2), 154–162.

Taillard, J., Capelli, A., Sagaspe, P., Anund, A., Akerstedt, T., & Philip, P. (2012). In-car nocturnal blue light exposure improves motorway driving: A randomized controlled trial. *PLoS ONE, 7*(10), e46750.

Tamura, Y., Horiyasu, T., Sano, Y., Chonan, K., et al. (2002). Habituation of sleep to a ship's noise as determined by actigraphy and a sleep questionnaire. *Journal of Sound and Vibration, 250*(1), 107–113.

Tamura, Y., Kawada, T., & Sasazawa, Y. (1997). Effect of ship's noise on sleep. *Journal of Sound and Vibration, 205*(4), 417–425.

Tirilly, G. (2004). The impact of fragmented sleep at sea on sleep, alertness and safety of seafarers. *Medicina Maritima, 4*(1), 96–105.

Tobaldini, E., Pecis, M., & Montano, N. (2014). Effects of acute and chronic sleep deprivation on cardiovascular regulation. *Archives Italiennes de Biologie, 152*(2–3), 103–110.

Toth, L. A. (1995). Sleep, sleep deprivation and infectious disease: Studies in animals. *Advances in Neuroimmunology, 5*(1), 79–92.

Vallieres, A., Azaiez, A., Moreau, V., LeBlanc, M., & Morin, C. M. (2014). Insomnia in shift work. *Sleep Medicine, 15*(12), 1440–1448.

van Cauter, E., Spiegel, K., Tasali, E., & Leproult, R. (2008). Metabolic consequences of sleep and sleep loss. *Sleep Medicine, 9*(Suppl 1), S23–S28.

van den Berg, J., Neely, G., Nilsson, L., Knutsson, A., & Landstrom, U. (2005). Electroencephalography and subjective ratings of sleep deprivation. *Sleep Medicine, 6*(3), 231–240.

van Laethem, M., Beckers, D. G., Kompier, M. A., Dijksterhuis, A., & Geurts, S. A. (2013). Psychosocial work characteristics and sleep quality: A systematic review of longitudinal and intervention research. *Scandinavian Journal of Work, Environment & Health, 39*(6), 535–549.

van Leeuwen, W. M., Hublin, C., Sallinen, M., Harma, M., Hirvonen, A., & Porkka-Heiskanen, T. (2010). Prolonged sleep restriction affects glucose metabolism in healthy young men. *International Journal of Endocrinology, 2010*, 108641.

van Leeuwen, W. M., Kircher, A., Dahlgren, A., Lutzhoft, M., Barnett, M., Kecklund, G., et al. (2013). Sleep, sleepiness, and neurobehavioral performance while on watch in a simulated 4 hours on/8 hours off maritime watch system. *Chronobiology International, 30*(9), 1108–1115.

van Leeuwen, W. M., Lehto, M., Karisola, P., Lindholm, H., Luukkonen, R., Sallinen, M., et al. (2009). Sleep restriction increases the risk of developing cardiovascular diseases by augmenting proinflammatory responses through IL-17 and CRP. *PLoS ONE, 4*(2), e4589.

van Mark, A., Spallek, M., Kessel, R., & Brinkmann, E. (2006). Shift work and pathological conditions. *Journal of Occupational Medicine and Toxicology, 1*, 25.

van Mark, A., Weiler, S. W., Schroder, M., Otto, A., Jauch-Chara, K., Groneberg, D. A., et al. (2010). The impact of shift work induced chronic circadian disruption on IL-6 and TNF-alpha immune responses. *Journal of Occupational Medicine and Toxicology, 5*, 18.

Virtanen, M., Jokela, M., Nyberg, S. T., Madsen, I. E., Lallukka, T., Ahola, K., et al. (2015). Long working hours and alcohol use: Systematic review and meta-analysis of published studies and unpublished individual participant data. *British Medical Journal, 350*, g7772.

Wadsworth, E. J., Allen, P. H., McNamara, R. L., & Smith, A. P. (2008). Fatigue and health in a seafaring population. *Occupational Medicine (Lond), 58*(3), 198–204.

Wadsworth, E. J., Allen, P. H., Wellens, B. T., McNamara, R. L., & Smith, A. P. (2006). Patterns of fatigue among seafarers during a tour of duty. *American Journal of Industrial Medicine, 49*(10), 836–844.

Wang, Q., Xi, B., Liu, M., Zhang, Y., & Fu, M. (2012). Short sleep duration is associated with hypertension risk among adults: A systematic review and meta-analysis. *Hypertension Research, 35*(10), 1012–1018.

Wegner, R., Felixberger, F. X., Nern, E., et al. (2008) Projekt 18-Mann-Schiff. In X. Baur (Ed.), *Ergebnisse arbeitsmedizinischer Untersuchungen bei Seeleuten auf Shiffen verschiedener besatzungsstärken im Tansatlantikverkehr 1979–1981*. Hamburg: Graciela Madrigal.

Wertheim, A. H. (1998). Working in a moving environment. *Ergonomics, 41*(12), 1845–1858.

Wirth, M. D., Burch, J., Shivappa, N., Violanti, J. M., Burchfiel, C. M., Fekedulegn, D., et al. (2014). Association of a dietary inflammatory index with inflammatory indices and metabolic syndrome among police officers. *Journal of Occupational and Environmental Medicine, 56*(9), 986–989.

Wright, K. P., Jr., Drake, A. L., Frey, D. J., Fleshner, M., Desouza, C. A., Gronfier, C., et al. (2015). Influence of sleep deprivation and circadian misalignment on cortisol, inflammatory markers, and cytokine balance. *Brain, Behavior, and Immunity, 47*, 24–34.

Xi, B., He, D., Zhang, M., Xue, J., & Zhou, D. (2014). Short sleep duration predicts risk of metabolic syndrome: A systematic review and meta-analysis. *Sleep Medicine Reviews, 18*(4), 293–297.

Yoshitake, H. (1978). Three characteristic patterns of subjective fatigue symptoms. *Ergonomics, 21*(3), 231–233.

Zhu, L., & Zee, P. C. (2012). Circadian rhythm sleep disorders. *Neurologic Clinics, 30*(4), 1167–1191.

Motion Sickness Susceptibility and Management at Sea

John F. Golding

Case Study

Rob was a young healthy man who was a volunteer lifeboatman from a coastal town in England. Unfortunately he suffered from seasickness. He found difficulty in adapting (habituating) to motion and he found that anti-motion sickness tablets were not effective. But he was highly motivated and did not want to give up lifeboat crewing, which would have been the obvious solution to his problem. He sought help and advice. He was estimated to be in the extremely motion susceptible portion of the population, scoring above the 80th percentile on a validated Motion Sickness Susceptibility Questionnaire (MSSQ-short: see in this chapter the section on 'Susceptibility'). He was tested on a laboratory motion simulator capable of eliciting motion sickness in almost all the population. The usual metric on such simulators is the time tolerated before onset of various stages of motion sickness; for example, differences between drug and placebo in tolerance times to sickness are used to assess the effectiveness of anti-motion sickness medications. This objective test confirmed his extreme sensitivity by comparison with normative data. He was then given an hour of training on the controlled breathing technique, which also involves an attentional component (see section on 'Non-Pharmacological Countermeasures'). He was then instructed to practise this technique further that same day but on his own in a quiet room. Later that day the same motion simulator test was repeated while he employed controlled breathing. He still became sick, but almost doubled his tolerance time on the motion simulator. While not an ideal design to estimate the effect of the countermeasure (better to have retested several days later to have washed out any 'carry-over' effects from the initial simulator exposure), Rob saw that controlled breathing could benefit him. It also enabled him

J.F. Golding (✉)
Department of Psychology, Faculty of Science and Technology,
University of Westminster, 115 New Cavendish Street, London W1W 6UW, UK
e-mail: goldinj@westminster.ac.uk

© Springer International Publishing Switzerland 2017
M. MacLachlan (ed.), *Maritime Psychology*, DOI 10.1007/978-3-319-45430-6_7

to feel some 'control' over his situation; this aspect has also been shown to be important in motion sickness. Rob was advised to become well practiced in the breathing technique in his own time in the absence of motion, and then to use it when at sea. He was also advised that if he took anti-motion sickness tablets, these should be well before the start of any sea trip. It is often not realized that motion sickness initiates gastric stasis (a protective reflex), which occurs well before the onset of subjective motion sickness symptoms. Gastric stasis prevents any further progression of stomach contents, prevents absorption of the anti-motion sickness drug and thus renders the tablet completely ineffective (see section 'Pharmacological Countermeasures').

So far research has produced no 'magic bullets' or complete cures for motion sickness but the outcome in this case appears to have been a partial success

> … I have been out on our lifeboat this morning, and on an exercise that would normally leave me feeling at the very least nauseous. So with the breathing exercises, and NO help from tablets, instead of going to stage 3, or probably stage 4, I barely got to stage 2 ….

(Extract from subsequent email from 'Rob the Lifeboatman' to the author. The 'stages' he refers to are from the Sickness Rating scale he was trained on, where 1 = OK, 2 = Initial symptoms, 3 = Mild nausea, 4 = Moderate nausea, 5 = Severe nausea &/or retching, 6 = Vomiting; see section 'Signs, symptoms and effects on performance').

Signs, Symptoms and Effects on Performance

Over 2000 years ago the Greek physician Hippocrates wrote, '… *sailing on the sea proves that motion disorders the body* …'. Indeed the word 'nausea' derives from the Greek root word 'naus', hence 'nautical' meaning relating to ship, sailing or sailors. However, motion sickness can also be provoked by a wide variety of transport environments, including land, sea, air and space. The general term 'motion sickness' embraces sickness provoked by a wide variety of environments and often denominated by the class of provocative environment, sea sickness, car sickness, air sickness, space sickness, cinerama sickness, simulator sickness, etc. Irrespective of environment, the primary signs and symptoms of motion sickness are nausea and vomiting (Reason and Brand 1975). Other related symptoms include stomach awareness, sweating and facial pallor (sometimes called 'cold sweating'), increased salivation, sensations of bodily warmth, dizziness, drowsiness (also denoted as the 'sopite syndrome'), sometimes headache, and, unsurprisingly, loss of appetite and increased sensitivity to odours. The importance and negative impact on performance of 'sopite' (drowsiness) is often underestimated (Lackner 2014). Yawning has been shown to be a behavioural marker for the sopite syndrome and consequent reduced task performance (Matsangas and McCauley 2014). A typical motion sickness questionnaire is shown in Table 1, which lists the more frequent symptoms, excluding vomiting and facial pallor. This is an adaptation of the simulator sickness

Table 1 Symptom self-report questionnaire for motion sickness

Do you have any of the following symptoms right now? (tick boxes)				
	0	1	2	3
	None	Slight	Moderate	Severe
General discomfort				
Fatigue				
Headache				
Eye strain				
Difficulty focusing				
Increased salivation				
Sweating				
Nausea				
Difficulty concentrating				
Fullness of head				
Blurred vision				
Dizziness (eyes open)*				
Dizziness (eyes closed)*				
Vertigo				
Stomach awareness				
Burping				

*illusory feelings of motion
Note excludes facial pallor and vomiting

questionnaire (Kennedy and Fowlkes 1992). Oculomotor symptoms are relatively more frequent in situations where visual mismatches may be the provoking stimulus, such as in simulators and virtual reality systems, as opposed to motion sickness due to whole-body accelerative stimuli such as during ship motion. Similarly, headache is provoked more by visual than by real motion, even when the real motion is twice as provocative as visual motion in terms of nauseogenicity (Bijveld et al. 2008). For a more rapid assessment, the following global sickness rating scale has proved reliable and useful: 1 = no symptoms; 2 = initial symptoms of motion sickness but no nausea; 3 = mild nausea; 4 = moderate nausea; 5 = severe nausea and/or retching; 6 = vomiting (Golding et al. 2003).

Physiological responses associated with motion sickness may vary between individuals. These include autonomic changes such as sweating and vasoconstriction of the skin causing pallor (less commonly, skin vasodilation and flushing in some individuals), with the simultaneous opposite effect of vasodilation and increased blood flow of deeper blood vessels, changes in heart rate which are often an initial increase followed by a rebound decrease, and inconsistent changes in blood pressure (Benson 2002). Gastric stasis occurs for the stomach and increased frequency and reduced amplitude of the normal electro gastric rhythm (Stern et al. 1985; Koch 2014). The drop in stomach fundus and sphincter pressure correlates with the nausea of motion sickness (Schaub et al. 2014). A host of hormones are released, mimicking a generalized stress response amongst which vasopressin is thought to be most closely associated with the time course of motion sickness (Eversmann et al. 1978). The occurrence of cold sweating suggests that motion sickness may disrupt aspects of temperature regulation (Golding 1992). This notion is also consistent with the observation that motion sickness reduces deep-core body temperature during cold water immersion, accelerating onset of hypothermia (Cheung et al. 2011).

Although motion sickness is unpleasant in its own right, under some circumstances it may have adverse consequences for performance and even for survival. Approximately 80 % of personnel have difficulty working while seasick (Pethybridge 1982). Motion sickness preferentially causes decrements in performance of tasks which are complex, require sustained performance and offer the opportunity to the person to control the pace of their effort (Hettinger et al. 1990). Simple tasks and overlearned tasks are less susceptible to performance decrements caused by motion sickness, whereas novel tasks and cognitive tasks involving spatial orientation processing are particularly vulnerable (Gresty and Golding 2009). Although tiredness and drowsiness have been ascribed in the past to exertion caused by extra physical effort in a motion environment, it is now realized that it reflects a symptom of motion sickness, not simply tiredness due to physical exertion. This is often termed the 'sopite syndrome' and is especially important during long-term chronic exposure to motion. The classic situation would be a long-duration sea voyage, as opposed to a short-duration acute exposure to provocative motion in aerobatic flight. Apart from possible loss of alertness during watch-keeping, less immediately critical effects include neglect of routine tasks such as maintenance tasks, cleaning routines, etc., which are important in the longer term. For pilots and air crew, acute motion sickness can slow training in the air and in simulators and even cause a minority to fail training (Benson 2002). The majority of novice astronauts suffer some degree of space sickness in the first day of weightlessness of space. Although vomiting in space is doubtless unpleasant, the possibility of vomiting while in a spacesuit in weightlessness is potentially life threatening, consequently precluding extravehicular activity for at least the first 24 h of spaceflight (Heer and Paloski 2006). For survival at sea, such as in liferafts, seasickness can reduce survival chances by a variety of mechanisms, including reduced morale and the 'will to live', failure to consistently perform routine survival tasks, and dehydration due to loss of fluids through vomiting (Benson 2002). An additional hazard to survival at sea may be the increased risk of hypothermia, since motion sickness can reduce deep-core body temperature (Cheung et al. 2011).

Provocative Circumstances and Incidence of Motion Sickness

There is a potential for motion sickness to be caused in a wide range of situations—at sea, in cars, tilting trains, funfair rides, aircraft, weightlessness in outer space, virtual reality and simulators (Table 2).

Table 2 Stimuli capable of provoking motion sickness

Context	Examples of provocative stimuli
Sea	Boats, ferries, survival rafts, divers' lines under sea
Land	Cars, coaches, tilting trains, ski, camels, elephants, funfair rides
Air	Transport planes, small aircraft, hovercraft, helicopters, parabolic flight
Space	Shuttle, spacelab
Optokinetic	Widescreen cinemas, virtual reality, head mounted displays (HMD), microfiche-readers, 'Haunted Swing', simulators, rotating visual drums or spheres, pseudo-coriolis, reversing prism spectacles
Laboratory	Cross-coupled (Coriolis), low frequency translational oscillation (vertical or horizontal), Off Vertical Axis Rotation (OVAR), counter-rotation, g-excess in human centrifuges, Auditory vection (a very weak stimulus)
Associated stimuli	Emetic toxins, chemotherapy, Post-Operative Nausea and Vomiting (PONV), extreme arousal (fear increases/fight decreases)

Estimates for incidence rates of motion sickness vary widely, partly due to individual differences in susceptibility and also because superficially similar transport environments can vary dramatically in terms of their motions and consequent nauseogenicity. For example, air travel in small aircraft which can encounter low altitude air turbulence can provoke motion sickness incidence of around 25 %, but flights in large airliners which have less motion show incidence rates of less than 1 % (Murdin et al. 2011). In zero-G parabolic flights which mimic the weightlessness of space for repeated brief periods of time, 33 % of fliers experience nausea and 12 % vomit despite being pre-medicated with anti-motion sickness drugs (Golding et al. 2015). In the more challenging environment of space, up to 70 % of novice astronauts may suffer some degree of space sickness in the first 24 h of flight (Heer and Paloski 2006). In an extensive survey of a cruise ship, motion sickness was the most common reason for physicians' consultations; the incidence of 4.2 per 1000 person/days being higher than for infections or injuries (Schutz et al. 2014). Incidences can be much higher in small boats and rough seas. In liferafts incidence rates of over 50 % vomiting have been observed after 1 h of moderate sea motion (Benson 1999). Seasickness affects approximately 25 % of military personnel adversely in moderate seas and 70 % in rough seas (Pethybridge 1982). Long-distance coach journeys can cause some symptoms of motion sickness in over a third of passengers (Turner and Griffin 1999b). In the more challenging motion environment of rally car racing, a quarter of co-drivers may become motion sick (Perrin et al. 2013). Cinerama sickness has been noted since the birth of the moving picture cinema, but this is usually mild and affects only a small percentage of the population, usually sitting at the front near the screen, with less than 6 % experiencing minor symptoms (Golding 2006a). But the widespread introduction of newer visual technologies may pose more of a problem. Whole-field visual motion triggers some degree of motion sickness in roughly 30 % of naval simulator trainees and 60 % of virtual environment users (Lawson et al. 2002). Such technologies as virtual reality and 3D stereoscopic video films may provoke more motion sickness than 2D films. The majority of studies suggest that 3D visual technologies are more provocative of motion sickness and pose a problem for some users (Naqvi et al. 2013; Solimini 2013; Bos et al. 2013).

How Do the Mechanisms for Motion Sickness Work?

In the past it was thought that the mechanism of motion sickness was the great severity of motions acting on the vestibular apparatus of the inner ear and on the gut, such as experienced by a sailor in rough seas. These were called the 'vestibular overstimulation' or 'gut stimulation' hypotheses. Such ideas have been discarded because they cannot account for evidence which contradicts their predictions. Thus it has been shown that motion sickness can be induced by purely visual stimuli in the complete absence of any real physical motion. Equally, some very violent types of physical motion such as riding a horse at full gallop are incapable of causing motion sickness.

The generally accepted explanation of the 'how' of motion sickness, i.e. the mechanism, is based on some form of sensory conflict or sensory mismatch between actual versus expected invariant patterns of vestibular, visual, and kinaesthetic inputs as predicted by an 'internal model' (Golding 2006b). The key observation leading to the understanding of this concept is that the physical intensity of the stimulus is not necessarily related to the degree of nauseogenicity. To take one example, with optokinetic stimuli the motion is implied but not real. A susceptible person sitting at the front in a widescreen cinema experiences motion and 'cinerama-sickness' but there is no physical motion of the body in the real world. In this situation, the vestibular and somatosensory systems are signalling that the person is sitting still, but the visual system is signalling illusory movement of the self, usually termed 'vection'. Consequently the generally accepted explanation of the 'how' of motion sickness is based on some form of sensory conflict or sensory mismatch. Sensory conflict or sensory mismatch is between actual versus expected invariant patterns of vestibular, visual and kinaesthetic inputs (Claremont 1931; Reason and Brand 1975). There may be many possible sensory conflicts, perhaps the most important classes being visual–vestibular conflicts and intravestibular conflicts. The latter class of conflict is between rotational accelerations sensed by the semi-circular canals of the vestibular apparatus and linear-translational accelerations (including gravitational) sensed by the otoliths of the vestibular apparatus.

A variety of detailed hypotheses have been developed to explain the exact nature of sensory conflict, sometimes called sensory or neural mismatch (e.g. Oman 1990; Benson 1999). Benson (2002) categorized conflicts into two main types: (i) conflict between visual and vestibular inputs, and (ii) conflict between the canals and the otoliths. In addition, moving sound sources (under laboratory conditions) can provide conflicting cues for spatial orientation, and a type of auditory vection which may provoke sensory conflict and mild motion sickness in a minority of people (Keshavarz et al. 2014). However, this is of little practical significance outside of the laboratory. A simplified conflict model was proposed by Bos and Bles (1998). They postulated that there is only one conflict: between the subjective expected vertical and the sensed vertical. Despite this simplification their underlying model is necessarily complex and finds difficulty in accounting for the observation that motion sickness can be induced by types of optokinetic stimuli which pose no conflict concerning the Earth vertical (Bubka et al. 2006). Most good models of motion sickness also incorporate integrator and decay systems in which the rate of accumulation of 'sensory conflict' is processed by leaky integrators with different time constants (Oman 1990). This process can be below conscious experience, the person feeling quite OK, until a threshold is reached, triggering the onset of overt symptoms and the awareness of the beginning of motion sickness (Golding and Stott 1997a).

The 'rule of thumb' model originally advanced by Stott (1986) is not the most elegant in theoretical terms but arguably is still the most practical. This model proposes a set of simple rules, which if broken will lead to motion sickness

Rule 1. Visual–Vestibular: motion of the head in one direction must result in motion of the external visual scene in the opposite direction.
Rule 2. Canal–Otolith: rotation of the head, other than in the horizontal plane, must be accompanied by appropriate angular change in the direction of the gravity vector.
Rule 3. Utricle-Saccule (i.e. the two types of otolith organs): any sustained linear acceleration is due to gravity, has an intensity of 1 g and defines 'downwards'.

In other words, the visual world should remain space stable, and the sustained force vector is gravity, which should always point down and average over a few seconds to 1 g.

In some environments there may be only one provocative stimulus. At sea it is the low frequency 'heave' motion of the vessel that provokes seasickness. However, in many environments multiple stimuli and conflicts may be involved. For example, airsickness in a pilot produced by the flight of an agile military aircraft may be due to up to five sources (Golding 2006b). Flying through air turbulence produces low-frequency translational oscillation of the aircraft, which may cause airsickness. In addition, during aircraft turns there may be provocation from the four following sources: visual–vestibular mismatches as the pilot senses 'down' to remain through the axis of the body but the external visual world to be tilted; sustained changes in the scalar magnitude of gravito-inertial force (GIF) due to centripetal acceleration; cross-coupling (Coriolis) due to head movements during rotation of the aircraft if the turn is tight enough, and also the g-excess illusion if the pilot tilts the head during increased GIF.

In virtual reality systems, head-mounted displays or simulators, important provocative stimuli are vection, retinal slip and poor eye collimation. But phase (time) lag between real motion and the corresponding update of the visual display may be equally or more important. Vestibular ocular reflexes (VORs) automatically control eye muscle adjustments of eyeball orientation despite disruptions caused by

head movements, enabling the retinal image to be motion stabilized and consequently the visual world to remain stable despite walking, jogging or rapidly
moving the head. These compensatory VORs to head movements are as fast as
10 ms or so, consequently visual update time lag disparities not much longer than
this may be easily detectable by subjects. If visual display update lags are much
longer than this then they may provoke sickness, since it has been shown that
virtual reality sickness has been induced with update lags as short as 48 ms
(Golding 2006b).

Low-frequency translational motion is a major source of motion sickness in land
vehicles, ships, and aircraft and has been sufficiently well described to provide
engineering design parameters (exposure time, acceleration, frequency) for standards regulated by the International Standards Organisation (ISO 2631, 1997) (see
Fig. 1). The frequency weighting function is of theoretical as well as applied
interest. Laboratory experiments (O'Hanlon and McCauley 1974; Golding et al.
2001) and ship motion surveys (Lawther and Griffin 1988) have shown that nauseogenicity increases as a function of exposure time and acceleration intensity as
might be expected, but more unusually that nauseogenicity peaks at the
low-frequency motion of around 0.2 Hz. Such low frequency motions are present in
transportation in ships, coaches, aircraft flying through air turbulence, and on
camels and elephants, all of which can provoke motion sickness. Low frequency
sway can also cause motion sickness at the top of very tall buildings during high
winds (Lamb et al. 2014). This frequency relationship also explains why some
forms of transport or motion environments are not provocative, for example people
do not experience 'horse-sickness'. During horse riding, walking, running, riding
off-road trail bikes, the motion frequencies are higher than 1 Hz. Consequently,
although these motions can be quite severe (capable of bruising the person), they
are not nauseogenic (Golding 2006b). Hypotheses for the frequency dependence of
nauseogenicity of translational oscillation are a phase error in signalling motion
between canal–otolith and somatosensory systems (Von Gierke and Parker 1994;
Benson 1999), or a frequency-dependent phase error between the sensed vertical
and the subjective or expected vertical (Bos and Bles 1998). It has also been
proposed that a zone of perceptuo-motor ambiguity around 0.2 Hz triggers sickness, since at higher frequencies imposed accelerations are usually interpreted as
translation of self through space, whereas at lower frequencies imposed accelerations are usually interpreted as a shift in the main force vector, i.e. tilt of self with
respect to the assumed gravity vertical (Golding et al. 2003; Golding and Gresty
2005). The region of 0.2 Hz would be a crossover between these two interpretations
and, thus, a frequency region of maximal uncertainty concerning the correct frame
of reference for spatial orientation. More recently, Golding and Gresty (2016)
proposed a related biodynamic explanation, that this frequency tuning of motion
sickness is related to mechanical limitations on human body motion. This proposes
that a cause of motion sickness may be difficulty in selecting appropriate tactics to
maintain body stability at vehicle motion circa 0.2 Hz, between whole-body GIF
alignment seen at lower frequencies versus lateropulsion seen at higher frequencies
(Golding and Gresty 2016).

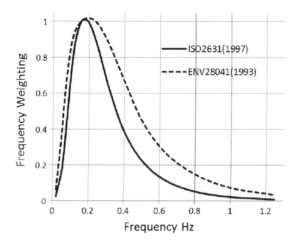

Fig. 1 Frequency weightings are shown for the potential to cause motion sickness (nauseogenicity) by oscillatory vertical motion. The lines are predictions from the International Standardisation Organisation (ISO). Similar relationships between motion frequency and nauseogenicity occur for horizontal motion. Nauseogenicity peaks at around 0.2 Hz. At lower or at higher frequencies motion has less potential to cause motion sickness. Ship motion is often around 0.2 Hz and consequently causes seasickness. Similarly, braking, accelerating and cornering in vehicles can produce horizontal motions also around 0.2 Hz which cause coach or car sickness. By contrast the frequencies of motions involved in walking, jogging, horse riding etc. are above 1 Hz and thus do not cause motion sickness

Although the physiological mechanisms are still not fully known, understanding of the brain mechanisms which underpin sensory conflict and motion sickness has progressed greatly. In a series of elegant experiments Oman and Cullen (2014) have identified brainstem and cerebellar neurons whose activity corresponds to what might be expected of putative 'sensory conflict' neurons. The concept of a discrete brainstem area postrema 'vomiting centre' has been superseded by the picture of a network of nuclei, including the nucleus tractus solitarius (NTS) and the medullary reticular formation. It seems that the same brainstem areas mediate vomiting and nausea irrespective of the triggering mechanism, whether motion or toxins. These brainstem areas not only include the NTS, but also the dorsolateral reticular formation of the caudal medulla (lateral tegmental field, LTF), and the parabrachial nucleus (PB), which act together to integrate signals that lead to nausea and vomiting (Yates et al. 2014). The NTS is the terminus of many visceral afferents and it also receives efferent projections from the area postrema and the NTS is now known to relay signals to the emesis pattern generator. In addition, neurons in the vestibular cerebellum, including the fastigial nucleus, are also influenced by visceral afferents. Galvanic vestibular stimulation in the cat has been shown to produce patterns of neural activation revealed by c-fos labelling, some of which correlate with overt signs of motion sickness, others of which show no such relationship but may relate to covert affective aspects such as nausea (Balaban et al. 2014). In humans, visually induced nausea has been studied using fMRI (Napadow et al. 2013a). Increased activity was observed in a variety of brain regions, but activity in a network including insular, anterior cingulate, orbitofrontal, somatosensory and prefrontal cortices appeared to be most specific to nausea (Napadow et al. 2013a).

Why Should Motion Sickness Exist at All?

In contrast with the 'how' of motion sickness (i.e. the mechanisms), for which there is consensus concerning sensory conflict, there are widely differing opinions concerning the 'why' of motion sickness. These hypotheses can be classified broadly into: poison detector; vestibular–cardiovascular-autonomic reflex; disorientation/motor warning; and non-functional 'Bad Luck' evolutionary maladaptation.

The poison or toxin detector hypothesis states that the vestibular system can act as a toxin detector. The evolutionary purpose of what we call 'motion sickness' is postulated to be the same as for any emetic response, which is to protect the organism from the toxic effects of potentially harmful substances that it may have ingested (Treisman 1977). The toxin detector hypothesis proposes that the brain has evolved to recognize any derangement of expected patterns of vestibular, visual, and kinaesthetic information as evidence of central nervous system malfunction and to initiate vomiting as a defence against a possible ingested neurotoxin. It provides a 'backup' to the main toxin detector system of chemoreceptors of the afferent vagal nerves and the chemoreceptor trigger zone of the brainstem. Motion sickness in pedestrian man or other animals is simply the inadvertent activation of this ancient defence reflex by the sensory conflicts induced by the novel altered visual and force environments of sea, air, land transport, space, virtual reality (Golding 2006b). This is consistent with the observation that motion sickness is evolutionarily well preserved, from man down to the level of the fish (ironically, fish can become seasick during aquarium transport) (Reason and Brand 1975). It is also consistent with the observation that people who are more susceptible to motion sickness are also more susceptible to toxins, chemotherapy, and post-operative nausea and vomiting (PONV) (Morrow 1985; Golding 1998). Further attempts to test the toxin detector hypothesis examined whether bitter taste sensitivity and aversion, which reflects activity of one part of the 'primary' toxin detector system, correlates with motion sickness susceptibility. However, unlike the well-proven associations of motion sickness susceptibility with chemotherapy sickness or PONV, these bitter taste studies have provided contradictory results, with positive (Sharma et al. 2008), negative (Benson et al. 2012), or no significant correlations (Golding and Tayyaba 2014) reported. More recently it has been proposed that reductions in core temperature observed with motion sickness (see earlier section 'Signs, symptoms and effects on performance') may be part of a coordinated defence system to cope with toxins, since, in animals at least, it has been shown that reductions in core temperature improve survival chances during toxin poisoning (Nalivaiko et al. 2014). Finally, perhaps the most convincing evidence is that the toxin detector hypothesis has been experimentally tested in animals. This demonstrated that emetic responses to a variety of emetogenic toxins were significantly reduced after bilateral vestibular ablation, which also abolished motion sickness to motion stimuli (Money and Cheung 1983).

The vestibular–cardiovascular/autonomic reflex hypothesis is based on the observation that tilt stimulation of the otoliths, which transduce linear accelerations, provoke a pressor response (increased blood pressure and cardiac output) mediated via vestibular–cardiovascular projections (Yates et al. 1998). It has been proposed that motion sickness is caused by the inappropriate activation of such vestibular–cardiovascular reflexes. The vestibular and visual systems influence autonomic control for the purpose of maintaining homeostasis during movement and changes in posture. Thus motion sickness arises from an aberrant activation of neural pathways that serve to maintain a stable internal environment (Yates et al. 1998). A somewhat similar, but non-functional, explanation has been proposed by Balaban (1999). The vestibular–cardiovascular reflex hypothesis has a good historical pedigree in the ninenteenth century concept of 'cerebral anaemia' as the cause of motion sickness (Nunn 1881). Some support is provided by the observation that cerebral hypoperfusion preceded nausea during gravito-inertial force (GIF) variation induced by centrifugation (Serrador et al. 2005), but the situation is unclear since there is considerable overlap between sick and non-sick individuals' pressor responses to motion sickness induced by the GIF variation of parabolic flight (Schelgel et al. 2001). The importance of the vestibular–cardiovascular reflexes in maintaining blood pressure may be limited, at least in humans. Bilateral labyrinthectomized patients' pressor responses to rapid tilts are only minimally slower than normal (<500 ms) (Radtke et al. 2003). Moreover, although not a formal disproof, this hypothesis does not predict the relative nauseogenicity of the various gravity-referenced and body-referenced directions of motions which would be expected to alter blood pressure (Golding et al. 1995, 2003).

The disorientation/motor warning hypothesis postulates that motion sickness is a punishment system which has evolved to discourage development of perceptual-motor programmes that are inefficient or cause spatial disorientation (Guedry et al. 1998). In other words, this system has evolved to discourage self-exposure to circumstances causing disorientation or motor instability. An extension of this hypothesis is that prostration caused by motion sickness reduces the likelihood of injury or vulnerability to predators (Bowins 2010) and other variants of the last idea have been proposed (Thornton and Bonato 2013; Knox 2014). However, an unanswered difficulty with all disorientation/motor warning hypotheses is why would evolution select such a slow warning system as nausea and vomiting, rather than the rapid warning systems of fear and pain?

The most reductionist approach is the 'Bad Luck' evolutionary maladaptation hypothesis (Oman 2012). Evolution is not perfect: an example of evolutionary maladaptation is the co-location of the entries to the respiratory airways and the oesophagus in many land animals which makes them susceptible to death by choking. From the perspective of the evolutionary maladaptation hypothesis, motion sickness is just an unfortunate consequence of the physical proximity of the motion detector (vestibular) and vomiting circuitry in the brainstem. It is just bad luck. Oman (2012) has stated that adaptive hypotheses for motion sickness such as the toxin detector hypothesis are '… naïve 'just-so' stories …' (Oman 2012, p. 125), the reference being to the children's stories by the author Rudyard Kipling providing amusing and fanciful explanations for differing animal characteristics, for example as to how the elephant got its trunk, the leopard its spots, etc.

To summarize, all of the above hypotheses remain in contention to provide explanations for the 'why' of motion sickness. If motion sickness is just a random and complicated evolutionary maladaptation, then it has been remarkably well preserved across species from fish to man and by implication over many millions of years. At present, the balance of evidence would seem to favour either the functional explanation of the toxin detector hypothesis or the 'Bad Luck' evolutionary maladaptation hypothesis.

Predictors of Motion Sickness Susceptibility

Concept of Motion Sickness Susceptibility

Determinants of motion sickness susceptibility are doubtless multifactorial. At least three general processes are thought to be at work: initial sensitivity to motion, rate of adaptation, and the retention of adaptation in the longer term (Reason and Brand 1975). In addition there can be differential sensitivity in individuals to different types of motion (Lentz 1984). Self-report questionnaires suggest the existence of independent latent susceptibilities to different types of provocative environments, usually forming factors that might be termed transportation by land, air, sea, or funfair rides (Golding 1998). This might seem to contradict the notion of a general motion susceptibility dimension. Nevertheless, these apparently contradictory views can be argued to both be true, i.e. a general motion susceptibility factor and specific factors exist. Other limitations are imposed by the test–retest reliability of response to the same motion challenge, which may be estimated from repeated exposures in the laboratory to be around $r = 0.8$–0.9 (Golding 2006b).

Motion Sickness Susceptibility Questionnaires (MSSQ) (sometimes called Motion History Questionnaires) enable a rapid estimate to be made of an individual's susceptibility. A typical questionnaire is shown in Table 3, which has been validated to predict motion sickness to motion stimuli in the laboratory and in transport environments (Golding 2006a). An overall indicator of susceptibility may be calculated as the MSSQ score = (total sickness score) $\times$ (18)/(18 $-$ number of types not experienced), this formula corrects for differing extent of exposure to different motion stimuli in individuals. For the normal young adult population, the median MSSQ score is 11.3, where higher scores indicate greater susceptibility and vice versa. More details are given in the original reference (Golding 2006a).

Table 3 Motion Sickness Susceptibility Questionnaire Short-form (MSSQ-Short) (adapted from Golding 2006a)

This questionnaire is designed to find out how susceptible to motion sickness you are, and what sorts of motion are most effective in causing that sickness. Sickness here means feeling queasy or nauseated or actually vomiting

Your CHILDHOOD Experience Only (before 12 years of age), for each of the following types of transport or entertainment please indicate:

1. As a CHILD (before age 12), how often you **Felt Sick or Nauseated** (tick boxes):

	Not Applicable–Never Travelled	Never felt Sick	Rarely felt sick	Sometimes felt sick	Frequently felt sick
Cars					
Buses or coaches					
Trains					
Aircraft					
Small boats					
Ships, e.g. channel ferries					
Swings in playgrounds					
Roundabouts in playgrounds					
Big dippers, funfair rides					
	t	0	1	2	3

Your Experience over the LAST 10 YEARS (approximately), for each of the following types of transport or entertainment please indicate:

2. Over the LAST 10 YEARS, how often you **Felt Sick or Nauseated** (tick boxes):

	Not applicable– Never travelled	Never felt sick	Rarely felt sick	Sometimes felt sick	Frequently felt sick
Cars					
Buses or coaches					
Trains					
Aircraft					
Small boats					
Ships, e.g. channel ferries					
Swings in playgrounds					
Roundabouts in playgrounds					
Big dippers, funfair rides					
	t	0	1	2	3

Genetics

Monozygotic and dizygotic twin studies suggest that the heritability of motion sickness is high at around 70 % in childhood and declines through puberty and the early adult years to around 55 % (Reavley et al. 2006). This decline of heritability with age may be due to differing experiences between each individual of a pair of twins to provocative environments as they grow older and to their consequent differential habituation. Selective breeding for high versus low motion sickness susceptibility strains of shrews has shown the importance of genetic determinants for motion sickness and that this extends to anaesthesia-induced emesis, indicating some common mechanisms under genetic control (Horn et al. 2014). There is evidence for Chinese hypersusceptibility to motion sickness, and this may provide some indirect evidence for a genetic contribution to such differences (Stern et al. 1993; Klosterhalfen et al. 2005). The nature of the genes involved is not yet clear. One example is that a single-nucleotide polymorphism of the alpha2-adrenergic receptor increases autonomic responses to stress in humans and also contributes to individual differences in autonomic responsiveness to provocative motion (Finley et al. 2004). This may be a marker for motion sickness susceptibility or simply a general marker for autonomic reactivity. A recent large-scale genome study has isolated 35 single-nucleotide polymorphisms (SNPs) associated with motion sickness susceptibility (Hromatka et al. 2015), demonstrating that multiple genes are involved.

General Predictors

Infants and very young children are immune to motion sickness but have no difficulty vomiting for other reasons. Susceptibility motion sickness appears to onset from 6 to 7 years of age (Reason and Brand 1975) and peaks around 9 years (Turner and Griffin 1999a; Henriques et al. 2014). The reasons for this are uncertain. Puberty begins later (around 10–12 years) than the 6–7 years age for onset of motion sickness susceptibility, indicating that puberty is not the critical reason. Another possibility is that the perceptuo-motor map is still highly plastic and not fully formed until around 7 years of age. Most theories of motion sickness propose that this perceptuo-motor map provides the 'expected' invariant patterns for detecting possible sensory mismatches in the relationships between vestibular, visual and kinaesthetic inputs, i.e. the 'internal model' (see section above 'Mechanisms of Motion Sickness'). Following this peak susceptibility, there is a subsequent decline of susceptibility during the teenage years toward adulthood around 20 years. This doubtless reflects habituation. It is often observed that this decline in susceptibility continues in a more gradual fashion throughout life toward old age (Paillard et al. 2013). However, the interpretation maybe limited because older people may avoid motion environments if they know that they are susceptible.

Indeed, longitudinal evidence from individuals who have been studied objectively in the laboratory suggests that toward older age, susceptibility may increase in a minority of individuals.

Surveys of transportation by sea, land and air indicate that women are more susceptible to motion sickness than men, although it must be emphasized that this sex difference is an overall trend, with considerable overlap. Women show higher incidences of vomiting and report a higher incidence of symptoms such as nausea (Kennedy et al. 1995). Surveys of passengers at sea indicate a 5 to 3 female to male risk ratio for vomiting (Lawther and Griffin 1988). This difference in vomiting suggests that the increased susceptibility in women is likely to be objective and not due to differential subjective reporting of symptoms. The elevated susceptibility in women does not seem related to extra habituation to greater ranges of motion environments experienced by risk-taking males (Dobie et al. 2001), nor to gender-biased differential self-selection between males and females, e.g. when volunteering for laboratory motion sickness experiments (Flanagan et al. 2005). Moreover, this sex difference is not exclusive to humans because in animals, such as the shrew Suncus murinus, females show significantly more emetic episodes and shorter latencies to emesis in experimental exposures to motion (Javid and Naylor 1999). The cause of greater motion sickness susceptibility in women has been suggested to involve the female hormonal cycle. Susceptibility varies over the menstrual cycle, peaking around menstruation. But this cannot fully account for the greater susceptibility in females because the magnitude of fluctuation in suscepti-bility across the menstrual cycle is only around one-third of the overall difference between male and female susceptibility (Golding et al. 2005). The elevated sus-ceptibility of females to sickness extends to post-operative nausea and vomiting as well as chemotherapy-induced nausea and vomiting (Morrow 1985; Golding 1998). This may reflect an evolutionary function. Thus greater susceptibility to sickness in females may serve to prevent exposure of the foetus to harmful toxins during pregnancy, or subsequently through milk. Elevated susceptibility in females may be 'hard-wired' but capable of upregulation, albeit variably, by hormonal influences during the menstrual cycle and even further during pregnancy (pregnancy sickness).

Relatively few other predictors of susceptibility have been found. Individuals with high levels of aerobic fitness appear to be more susceptible to motion sickness, and longitudinal experiments show aerobic fitness training increases motion sickness susceptibility (e.g. Cheung et al. 1990). A more reactive autonomic nervous system (including hypothalamic–pituitary–adrenal axis) in aerobically fit individuals may sensitize them. Psychological variables such as mood may modify susceptibility in contradictory directions: 'state' variables such as extreme fear or anxiety conditioned to motion may contribute indirectly to motion sickness susceptibility; by contrast extreme arousal 'fight-flight' such as observed in warfare may suppress motion sickness (Reason and Brand 1975). Personality trait variables such as extraversion or neuroticism do not strongly predict motion sickness susceptibility. Only weak cor-relations occur between extraversion or similar personality traits with reduced susceptibility (Reason and Brand 1975; Gordon et al. 1994) and higher levels of trait anxiety associated with increased susceptibility (Paillard et al. 2013).

Reliable physiological markers for predicting individual motion sickness susceptibility have proved elusive. The otoliths in the vestibular apparatus (labyrinths) sense linear accelerations including gravity, whereas the semi-circular canals sense rotational or angular accelerations. Individual variation in sensory thresholds to angular or translational accelerations does not seem to relate to susceptibility in any obvious fashion. Otolith asymmetry may occur naturally between left and right labyrinths in some individuals but is compensated for by neurological adaptations under the usual background acceleration of one gravity on Earth. However, such asymmetries become suddenly revealed again when measured during zero-G parabolic flight, and this has been proposed as an indicator of individual susceptibility for space sickness under weightlessness (Diamond and Markham 1991). However, this mechanism has not been definitely proven. Although motion sickness produces profound autonomic changes, baseline autonomic characteristics are unlikely to provide useful predictors for motion sickness susceptibility (Farmer et al. 2014). Similarly, although motion sickness can cause postural instability, the evidence that individual differences in postural stability or perceptual style (e.g. Riccio and Stoffregen 1991) are major predictors of motion sickness susceptibility seems limited (Golding and Gresty 2005; Diels and Howarth 2013; Lackner 2014). Indeed, postural sway evoked by visual motion has been demonstrated to be dissociable from the visually induced motion sickness (Lubeck et al. 2015). Shorter time constants of the central vestibular velocity store have been suggested to correlate with reduced motion sickness susceptibility (Lackner 2014; Dai et al. 2011), but others have found no evidence of such a relationship (Golding and Gresty 2005; Furman et al. 2011). It has been proposed that it may not be the absolute duration of the time constant per se, but the ability to modify readily the time constant that may be a candidate marker for success in motion sickness habituation (Golding and Gresty 2005). Similarly, observations on cervical Vestibular Evoked Myogenic Potentials (cVEMP) suggest that individuals with a broader dynamic range of vestibular reflexes can respond and adapt to a wider array of stimulus amplitude, predicting better future habituation to seasickness (Tal et al. 2013). Finally, individual differences in brain white matter structure revealed by fMRI may relate to nausea susceptibility, although this remains to be confirmed as a reliable predictor (Napadow et al. 2013b).

Special Groups: Blind, Migraine and Vestibular Disorders

Blind or blindfolded normally sighted individuals can be made motion sick using real physical motion, although obviously optokinetic stimuli (Table 1) will be ineffective. Blind individuals, ranging from congenital to late acquired blindness, are as susceptible to motion sickness as sighted individuals with eyes closed and their range of susceptibility tends to be comparable to normal-sighted people when exposed to provocative cross-coupled motion (Graybiel 1970).

Migraineurs tend to have elevated motion sickness susceptibility. However, the reason is not known. There may be a genetic link caused by defective calcium ion channels shared by the brain and inner ear, leading to reversible hair cell depolarization, producing vestibular symptoms and that the headache might just be a secondary phenomenon (Baloh 1998). Alternatively it may be due to altered serotonergic system functioning in migraineurs (Drummond 2005; Brey 2005). Support for this possibility was provided by the observation that the serotonin 1B/1D agonist rizatriptan provided some anti-motion sickness effects in migraineurs (Furman et al. 2011). It is possible that there are several mechanisms for this link, including pain pathways and autonomic reactivity (Cuomo-Granston and Drummond 2010). The complexity of any association between migraine and motion sickness is illustrated by Bosser et al. (2006), who surveyed the general population. This survey demonstrated the expected association between elevated motion sickness susceptibility and migraine. However, when these data were reanalyzed using multivariate techniques, the existence of any independent association of motion sickness with migraine disappeared and was replaced by other more important predictors such as syncope (faintness) and autonomic reactivity (Bosser et al. 2006).

Certain groups of patients with vestibular pathologies have reduced or elevated risk for motion sickness. Individuals who have complete bilateral loss of labyrinthine (vestibular apparatus) function appear to be largely immune to motion sickness provoked by physical motion (Murdin et al. 2015) but may have some slight susceptibility to visually induced motion sickness (Johnson et al. 1999). Patients with Vestibular Neuritis (VN) or benign paroxysmal positional vertigo (BPPV) show no overall difference in susceptibility compared to controls. But within this broad picture many individuals up- or downregulate their sensitivity to motion in response to their vestibular disease. Patients with Vestibular Migraine (VM) have greatly elevated susceptibility (Boldingh et al. 2011; Paillard et al. 2013; Murdin et al. 2015), as do those suffering from Meniere's Disease (Sharon and Hullar 2014).

Mal-de-debarquement

When a sailor returns to land after a time at sea, he or she often experiences the sensation of unsteadiness and tilting of the ground. This is termed Mal-de-debarquement. A similar effect is observed in astronauts returning to 1 g on Earth after extended time in weightlessness in space. Whittle (1689) provided an early description of Mal-de-debarquement, after the landing and during the advance of the troops of William of Orange in Torbay in 1688: '*As we marched here upon good Ground, the Souldiers would stumble and sometimes fall because of a dissiness in their Heads after they had been so long toss'd at Sea, the very Ground seem'd to rowl up and down for some days, according to the manner of the Waves*'.

Mal-de-debarquement can lead to motion sickness but symptoms usually resolve within a few hours as individuals readapt to the normal land environment. Individuals susceptible to Mal-de-debarquement may have reduced reliance on vestibular and visual inputs and increased dependence on the somatosensory system for the maintenance of balance (Nachum et al. 2004). It has long been known that the view of a stable horizon reference can increase resistance to motion sickness (see next section) but provision of an artificial horizon failed to have any effect on Mal-de-debarquement (Tal et al. 2014).

In a very small minority of individuals symptoms persist for months and years and are troublesome. Patients with persistent Mal-de-debarquement syndrome exhibit impaired postural stability but do not exhibit differences in cortical excitability compared to controls (Clark et al. 2013). Customized vestibular exercises have been proposed as a treatment (Murdin et al. 2011). Some temporary relief can be obtained by re-exposure to motion but this is not a viable treatment. It has been suggested that repetitive transcranial magnetic stimulation can reduce symptoms for persistent Mal-de-debarquement syndrome (Cha et al. 2013). Standard anti-motion sickness drugs appear ineffective but benzodiazepines appear to offer some relief (Cha 2009).

Non-pharmacological Countermeasures Against Motion Sickness

Behavioural countermeasures to motion sickness may be broadly classified into habituation versus more immediate short-term behavioural modifications such as changes in body posture or visual attention. The most useful ones are summarized in Table 4.

Habituation offers the surest countermeasure to motion sickness but by definition is a long-term approach. Habituation is superior to anti-motion sickness drugs, and it is free of side effects (Cowings and Toscano 2000). The most extensive habituation programmes, often denoted 'motion sickness desensitization', are run by the military, where anti-motion sickness medication is contra-indicated for pilots because of side effects including drowsiness and blurred vision. These programmes have success rates exceeding 85 % (Benson 1999; Lucertini et al. 2013) but can be extremely time consuming, lasting many weeks. Critical features include: (a) the massing of stimuli (exposures at intervals greater than a week almost prevents habituation), (b) use of graded stimuli to enable faster recoveries and more sessions to be scheduled, which may help avoid the opposite process of sensitization, and (c) maintenance of a positive psychological attitude to therapy (Yen-Pik-Sang et al. 2005). Whether or not anti-motion sickness drugs are of any practical use in this context is debatable. For example, although some studies appear to show that anti-motion sickness drugs can improve the rate of adaptation (Lackner and Graybiel 1994; Cohen et al. 2008), other studies in both the laboratory (Wood et al. 1986) and

Table 4 Behavioural countermeasures against motion sickness

Countermeasure	Comments	Possible Limitations
Habituation (desensitization)	The most effective of any countermeasure. Fully acquired habituation is more effective than any current anti-motion sickness drugs and also free of side effects	Can be slow to acquire, often stimulus specific. It may need periodic re-exposure to motion to maintain adaptive protection
Obtaining visual horizon reference	Shown to provide some protection in ships, ship simulators, coaches and cars	Often not possible, e.g. if below decks at sea or passenger in rear inside seat in land transport
Avoiding reading or visual scanning	Shown to reduce motion sickness in a variety of transport or simulator environments	Not compatible with performance of visual tasks such as map reading, monitoring displays, etc.
Avoid head movements	Reduces motion sickness in a variety of transport environments	Often not compatible with effective performance of tasks
Laying supine	May be acting by reducing head movements rather than posture per se	Likely to be incompatible with effective performance of most tasks
Aligning Body with Gravito-Inertial Force vector (GIF), sometimes called 'Wave-riding'	Shown to be effective both in the laboratory and outside: at sea align the standing posture (cf. 'sea-legs'); as a car passenger lean into the bends when cornering	Requires experience and some degree of accurate anticipation of motion
Avoiding locations of maximum motion	For example, avoid locations such as the bows of a ship	Sometimes passenger or crew work location cannot be chosen.
Being in control	For example being the driver or the pilot. Also evidence that perception of 'controllability' is important	Often not possible as a passenger
Systematic controlled breathing	Laboratory trials show it to be around half as effective as anti-motion sickness drugs and reliable. Also free of side effects	Requires some degree of training. Also requires some degree of attention, which may interfere with very complex tasks

Note that apart from Habituation, other behavioural countermeasures are only partially effective

at sea (Van Marion et al. 1985) have shown that although anti-motion sickness medications may speed habituation compared to placebo in the short term, in the longer term it is disadvantageous. This is because when the anti-motion sickness medication is discontinued, the medicated group relapses and is worse off than those who were habituated under placebo.

Habituation, itself, is often stimulus specific, producing the problem of lack of generalization and transfer of habituation from one type of motion to another. For example, tolerance acquired to car travel may confer no protection to seasickness (Murdin et al. 2011). Thus to foster generalization, it is useful to use as wide a variety of provocative motions as possible (see Table 2: 'Stimuli'). The specificity of habituation to different types of motion has been shown in animals to be reflected in different anatomical patterns of neuronal functional changes (presumably reflecting learning) in the vestibular–cerebellar network to different classes of provocative stimuli (Kaufman 2005). Other neural structures such as the amygdala and such areas as the nucleus tractus solitarius are thought to be important in habituation to motion sickness (Nakagawa et al. 2003; Pompeiano et al. 2004). The scope of applications of habituation training are diverse, e.g. ranging from habit-uating pilots suffering airsickness, to reducing motion sickness produced by short-arm rotors intended to provide artificial gravity in future space flight (Young et al. 2003). Research continues to optimize habituation approaches (Cheung and Hofer 2005; Stroud et al. 2005). On a positive note, although stimulus specificity of motion habituation may be a problem for some people, some generalization of habituation acquired from one type of stimulus to another can be demonstrated. Exposing subjects to visual–vestibular interaction in the laboratory reduces their sensitivity to motion sickness during travel in buses for example (Dai et al. 2011). Similarly, a controlled trial demonstrated that optokinetic habituation training generalized, giving subsequent reductions of seasickness in 71 % of those treated versus 12 % of controls (Ressiot et al. 2013).

Immediate behavioural countermeasures include reducing head movements, aligning the head and body with GIF (Golding et al. 2003; Wada et al. 2012) or laying supine (Golding et al. 1995). The strategy of supine position provides some protection of cruise ship passengers against sea sickness (Gahlinger 2000). Consistent with the general observation that reducing head movements can reduce motion sickness, movement restraint of head, shoulders, hips, and knees reduced motion sickness induced by playing a video game while standing (Chang et al. 2013). However, such protective postures and restriction of movement may be incompatible with task performance under many circumstances. It is usually better to be in active control, i.e. to be the driver or pilot rather than a passenger (Rolnick and Lubow 1991), a finding replicated in the laboratory (Golding et al. 2003). Similarly, enhanced perceptions of control and predictability appear to reduce motion-induced nausea (Levine et al. 2014). In a different context, exertion of control reduced motion sickness induced by playing video games on a tablet computer (Stoffregen et al. 2014).

Avoidance of tasks such as reading which enhance visuo–vestibular conflict is often recommended. The importance of this may be gauged by the observation that up to a quarter of co-drivers became motion sick in rally cars if they were reading a book or sitting in the back seat (Perrin et al. 2013). Stroboscopic illumination protected against motion sickness for back seat military helicopter personnel, per-haps because it reduces retinal slip and visual–vestibular conflicts (Webb et al. 2013). Obtaining a stable external horizon reference is helpful in preventing motion sickness (Turner and Griffin 1999b; Bos et al. 2005). However, although a direct view out of a car window reduced sickness, a real-time video display of the view ahead failed to reduce sickness in rear seat car passengers (Griffin and Newman 2004). Standing with a wider stance width and view of the horizon may reduce postural instability and motion sickness at sea (Stoffregen et al. 2013).

Controlled regular breathing has been shown to increase motion tolerance to provocative motion, being approximately half as effective as standard anti-motion sickness drugs yet rapid to implement and free of side effects (Yen-Pik-Sang et al. 2003a, 2005; Stromberg et al. 2015). See the case study at beginning of this Chapter. The mechanism by which controlled breathing has its protective effect is uncertain but may involve activation of the known protective inhibitory reflex between respiration and vomiting (Yen-Pik-Sang et al. 2003b). In other words, it is more than a simple placebo or distraction effect. Supplemental oxygen may be effective for reducing motion sickness in patients during ambulance transport. By contrast, it does not alleviate or prevent motion sickness in individuals who are otherwise healthy. This apparent paradox is explained by the suggestion that supplemental oxygen may work by ameliorating a variety of internal states in ill-patients that sensitize for motion sickness, rather than blocking motion sickness directly (Ziavra et al. 2003).

Anecdotally, modification of diet has been said to alter susceptibility to motion sickness. Unfortunately the evidence is contradictory; for example, one study suggested that protein-rich meals inhibit motion sickness (Levine et al. 2004), whereas another study drew the opposite conclusion that any meal of high-protein or dairy foods 3–6 h prior to flight should be avoided to reduce airsickness susceptibility (Lindseth and Lindseth 1995).

It has been suggested that ginger (main active agent gingerol) acts to calm gastrointestinal feedback (Lien et al. 2003), but conflicting reports of its effect on motion sickness indicate that any such effects are weak (Palatty et al. 2013). For habitual smokers, the temporary abstinence and consequent withdrawal from nicotine provides significant protection against motion sickness (Golding et al. 2011). Indeed, this finding may explain why habitual smokers are at reduced risk for PONV, whereas non-smokers have elevated risk, the other main PONV risk factors being female sex, greater motion sickness susceptibility, and previous episodes of PONV. The unavoidable temporary nicotine withdrawal perioperatively and the consequent increased tolerance to sickness may explain why smokers have reduced risk for PONV (Golding et al. 2011).

Placebo effects can be strong but very variable (Lackner 2014). Combining positive verbal instructions and placebo can promote reductions in motion sickness (Horing et al. 2013). High-frequency head vibration can provide some reduction in motion sickness (Bos 2015) but it is unclear if this is simply an additional placebo effect; moreover, its practicality outside of the laboratory is unproven. Providing pleasant (or unpleasant) scents had no effect on motion sickness sensitivity, although the reverse effect occurred since motion sickness enhanced sensitivity to odours (Paillard et al. 2014). By contrast, another study claimed pleasant smells alleviated motion sickness (Keshavarz et al. 2015). In an unpublished study, the present author used pleasant odours to prevent motion sickness during parabolic flights, at the initial stages of motion sickness some alleviation occurred but at higher levels of motion sickness the previously pleasant odour became aversive and exacerbated symptoms. Such findings suggest that the effect of pleasant odours is likely to be weak and of little practical use as a countermeasure for motion sickness. Listening to pleasant music can reduce motion sickness elicited by cross-coupled motion (Yen-Pik-Sang et al. 2003a), a finding replicated with visually induced motion sickness (Keshavarz and Hecht 2014). This may reflect a kind of distraction or placebo effect.

Although electrical stimulation of the vestibular apparatus, usually termed 'galvanic vestibular stimulation' (GVS), can cause vertigo and nausea, the opposite effect has been proposed, that it may provide a novel countermeasure for motion sickness. GVS synchronous with the visual field may normalize electrogastrographic and autonomic responses and reduce motion sickness during flight simulation (Cevette et al. 2012). The mechanism perhaps involves reducing visual–vestibular conflicts but it is uncertain if it is of practical use outside of the laboratory. Transcranial electrical stimulation has been shown to reduce motion sickness evoked by physical motion in the laboratory but this requires replication to prove its reliability (Arshad et al. 2015). Some report electroacupuncture, ordinary acupuncture, or acupressure to be effective against motion sickness (Bertalanffy et al. 2004). However, well-controlled trials find no evidence for their value (Bruce et al. 1990; Miller and Muth 2004); consequently it is probable that any specific protective actions are relatively small, over and above any placebo effects.

Pharmacological Countermeasures

Many of the drugs used against motion sickness were identified in the Second World War in research to reduce sea sickness and air sickness in military personnel. The most important were scopolamine and amphetamine. The antihistamine class of drugs were discovered shortly afterwards. It is noteworthy that nearly all the common drugs currently used against motion sickness had been identified and proven over 40 years ago (Wood and Graybiel 1969). They may be divided into the categories: antimuscarinics (e.g. scopolamine), H_1 antihistamines (e.g. dimenhydrinate), and sympathomimetics (e.g. amphetamine). Commonly used anti-motion sickness drugs are shown in Table 5. However, these drugs, alone or in combination, are only partially effective. Other classes of potent antiemetics are employed for treating nausea and vomiting due to a wide variety of causes, including emetic side effects of chemotherapy, but are not effective against motion sickness. These include D_2 dopamine receptor antagonists, $5HT_3$ antagonists (Levine et al. 2000), and neurokinin NK_1 receptor antagonists (Golding 2006b). This is probably because their sites of action may be at vagal afferent receptors or the brainstem chemoreceptor trigger zone (CTZ), whereas anti-motion sickness drugs act elsewhere. Additionally, in the case of neurokinin NK_1 receptor antagonists, although

Table 5 Common anti-motion sickness drugs (adapted from Benson 2002)

Drug	Route	Adult dose	Time of onset	Duration of action (h)
Scopolamine	Oral	0.3–0.6 mg	30 min	4
Scopolamine	Injection	0.1–0.2 mg:	15 min	4
Scopolamine	Transdermal patch	One	6–8 h	72
Promethazine	Oral	25–50 mg	2 h	15
Promethazine	Injection	25 mg	15 min	15
Promethazine	Suppository	25 mg	1 h	15
Dimenhydrinate	Oral	50–100 mg	2 h	8
Dimenhydrinate	Injection	50 mg	15 min	8
Cyclizine	Oral	50 mg	2 h	6
Cyclizine	Injection	50 mg	15 min	6
Meclizine	Oral	25–50 mg	2 h	8
Buclizine	Oral	50 mg	1 h	6
Cinnarizine	Oral	15–30 mg	4 h	8

Note the names given above are for the drug itself, the tradename of the formulation containing the particular drug may be different

they might stop vomiting from motion sickness in animals, it has been shown that they do not prevent motion sickness induced nausea in man.

Anti-motion sickness drugs often produce unwanted side effects, drowsiness being the most common. Promethazine is good example of an anti-motion sickness drug which is highly sedating (Cowings and Toscano 2000). Scopolamine may cause blurred vision in a minority of individuals, especially with repeated dosing. The combination Scopolamine + Dexamphetamine (so-called 'Scopdex') is highly effective since each drug acts through a different pathway, consequently their different anti-motion sickness properties are additive but their respective unwanted side effects of sedation and stimulation cancel each other out. For legal reasons (drug abuse potential of amphetamine) the Scopdex combination is no longer available, apart from specialized military use. Unfortunately new atypical stimulants such as Modafinil have been shown to be of no use as a replacement for amphetamine in motion sickness (Hoyt et al. 2009). Some medications such as transdermal scopolamine (i.e. scopolamine skin patch) or the calcium channel antagonist Cinnarizine are significantly less sedating than others (Gordon et al. 2001).

Well before more obvious symptoms such as nausea develop, motion sickness induces gastric stasis which prevents drug absorption by this route (Stewart et al. 2000). Consequently, oral administration must anticipate this and oral medications must be taken early. Injection of the drug overcomes the various problems of slow absorption kinetics of oral tablets and gastric stasis (or indeed expulsion of tablets by vomiting). Transdermal delivery offers the advantage of providing protection for up to 72 h with low constant concentration levels in the blood, thus reducing side effects. The slow onset time (6–8 h) of transdermal scopolamine can be offset by simultaneous administration of oral scopolamine, enabling protection from 30 min or so onwards (Nachum et al. 2001). Unfortunately, there may be variability in absorption via the transdermal route, which alters effectiveness between individuals (Gil et al. 2005). 'Chewing gum' formulations offer the prospect of motion sickness prophylaxis with reduced side effects compared to tablets, due to a more sustained release (Seibel et al. 2002). Buccal absorption (i.e. through the mucous membranes of the mouth and throat) is effective with scopolamine but an even faster route is via nasal scopolamine spray. Peak blood levels may be achieved in 9 min with nasal spray (Ahmed et al. 2000). This nasal route has been shown to be fast and effective against motion sickness (Simmons et al. 2010), although is not yet available for public use.

Research into new anti-motion sickness drugs includes re-examination of old drugs such as phenytoin, as well as the development of new agents. The range is wide, including phenytoin, betahistine, chlorpheniramine, cetirizine, fexofenadine, benzodiazepines and barbiturates, the antipsychotic droperidol, corticosteroids such as dexamethasone, tamoxifen, opioids such as the u-opiate receptor agonist loperamide, neurokinin NK_1 receptor antagonists, vasopressin V_{1a} receptor antagonists, NMDA antagonists, 3-hydroxypyridine derivatives, $5HT_{1a}$ receptor agonists such as the antimigraine triptan rizatriptan, selective muscarinic $M_3/m5$ receptor antagonists such as zamifenacin and darifenacin (for review see Golding 2006b). So far none of these drugs have proven to be of any major advantage over those currently available for motion sickness (Golding 2006b). The reasons are various and include relative lack of efficacy, or complex and variable pharmacokinetics, or in those that are effective, unacceptable side effects. A possible candidate for an effective anti-motion sickness drug with fewer side effects might be a selective antagonist for the m5 muscarinic receptor (Golding and Stott 1997b). The aim in the future should be to develop drugs with highly selective affinities to receptor subtypes relevant to motion sickness to produce an anti-motion sickness drug of high efficacy and with few side effects.

From a practical point of view, it is best for an individual to first of all try out any particular anti-motion sickness drug he or she proposes to use, in an undemanding motion-free environment. This enables them to check if they have any idiosyncratic sensitivities to unwanted side effects from that drug. If the person is a driver, they should be aware that side effects may persist for some time, which is especially important if driving a vehicle shortly after disembarking after having recently taken an anti-motion sickness drug. Also, it is sometimes forgotten that the usual mode of use of anti-motion sickness medication is to *prevent* motion sickness, not to *cure* sickness that has already started. The latter, so-called 'rescue' medication approach is very limited and is confined to the injection route of drugs such as promethazine or scopolamine, and then usually only when administered by a doctor or medical officer. Another factor which must always be borne in mind is to take any medication in good time, both because of gastric stasis with oral routes (see above) and because of the widely different times from administration of the drug to onset of motion protection, due to differing absorption rates and differing pharmacological mechanisms (see Table 5: Times to Onset). Finally, as can be seen in Table 5, the duration of protection provided varies widely between drugs.

Summary

As we have seen, the problem of motion sickness has been noted from very early written records; over two thousand years ago the Greek physician Hippocrates wrote, '... *sailing on the sea proves that motion disorders the body* ...'. It is almost certain that humans must have experienced motion sickness since they first travelled to sea with early boats, although written records do not exist from those prehistoric times. This chapter described the signs and symptoms of motion sickness and different types of provocative stimuli. The primary signs and symptoms of motion sickness are nausea and vomiting, additional symptoms may include drowsiness, especially during long-duration motion exposure often encountered at sea. Motion sickness can be provoked by a wide variety of transport environments, including land, sea, air, and space. The recent introduction of new visual technologies may expose more of the population to visually induced motion sickness. The 'how' of motion sickness (i.e. the mechanism) is generally accepted to involve sensory conflict or sensory mismatch between actual versus expected invariant patterns of vestibular, visual, and kinaesthetic inputs as predicted by an 'internal model'. New observations have concerned the identification of putative 'sensory conflict' neurones and the underlying brain mechanisms. In addition, there now seems to be greater understanding of why motions around 0.2 Hz should be so provocative of motion sickness. But what reason or purpose does motion sickness serve, if any? This is the 'why' of motion sickness, which we analyzed from both evolutionary and non-functional maladaptive theoretical perspectives. The most satisfactory explanation from this perspective is that motion sickness is simply the inadvertent activation by transportation environments of an ancient defence reflex against poisons. This so-called 'Toxin detector' hypothesis proposes that the vestibular system is thought to have evolved a secondary role in detecting toxins as a result of disruptions of its highly sensitive and accurate functioning. This toxin defence reflex evolved in vertebrate animals well before modes of transportation or moving visual displays were invented by humans. Individual differences in susceptibility are great in the normal population and recent studies would suggest a large degree of genetic basis. In more general terms the main predictors appear to be age (maximum susceptibility occurs around 9 years) and gender, females being somewhat more susceptible than males, although there is a large degree of overlap. Motion sickness susceptibility also varies dramatically between special groups of patients, including those with different types of vestibular diseases, and is elevated in migraineurs. Finally, the efficacy and relative advantages and disadvantages of various behavioural and pharmacological countermeasures have been evaluated. Habituation to motion is by far the most effective countermeasure but by definition is time consuming and can be very slow in some individuals. Habituation may also be specific to a particular type of motion, e.g. habituation to car sickness may not protect against seasickness, because the exact patterns of motion are not the same. Other behavioural countermeasures are only partially effective and sometimes may be prevented by circumstances or incompatible with requirements of work duties. These include obtaining a stable horizon reference, avoiding head movements, laying supine and avoiding close visual scanning. Controlled systematic breathing has been shown to provide some protection, albeit less than anti-motion sickness drugs. A possible new intervention involves applying very low electrical currents (not subjectively detectable) to the scalp in order to selectively stimulate and inhibit various cortical brain areas. This has been shown to be effective in the laboratory but needs to be shown to be of practical use in the field. Medication with various anti-motion sickness drugs remains a standby for those situations where habituation is not feasible (e.g. single trips or experiences of a provocative environment). The various types of medications were reviewed and their various advantages and disadvantages. They all have the limitations of side effects (e.g. drowsiness), drug absorption delays have to be factored in and they do not provide complete protection. Recently an intranasal scopolamine (hyoscine) dosing system has been developed by the military which provides absorption almost as fast as injection and avoids the limitations of oral tablet absorption. However, it is yet to be made available to the general public. Research continues with the aim of developing new anti-motion sickness drugs which would be highly selective for blocking those brain pathways involved in motion sickness but avoiding actions on other brain systems which would cause unwanted side effects.

References

Ahmed, S., Sileno, A. P., deMeireles, J. C., et al. (2000). Effects of pH and dose on nasal absorption of scopolamine hydrobromide in human subjects. *Pharmaceutical Research, 17,* 974–977.

Arshad, Q., Cerchiai, N., Goga, U., et al. (2015). Electro-cortical therapy for motion sickness. *Neurology* Sep 4. pii: 10.1212/WNL.0000000000001989. [Epub ahead of print]

Balaban, C. D. (1999). Vestibular autonomic regulation (including motion sickness and the mechanism of vomiting). *Current Opinion in Neurology, 12,* 29–33.

Balaban, C. D., Ogburn, S. W., Warshafsky, S. G., et al. (2014). Identification of neural networks that contribute to motion sickness through principal components analysis of fos labelling induced by galvanic vestibular stimulation. *PLoS ONE, 9*(1), e86730. doi:10.1371/journal.pone.0086730

Baloh, R. W. (1998). Advances in neuro-otology. *Current Opinion in Neurology, 11,* 1–3.

Benson, A. J. (1999). Motion sickness. In J. Ernsting, A. N. Nicholson, & D. S. Rainford (Eds.), *Aviation medicine* (pp. 318–338). Oxford, UK: Butterworth Ltd.

Benson, A. J. (2002). Motion sickness. In K. Pandolf & R. Burr (Eds.), *Medical aspects of harsh environments* (Vol. 2, pp. 1060–1094). Washington, DC: Walter Reed Army Medical Center.

Benson, P. W., Hooker, J. B., Koch, K. L., et al. (2012). Bitter taster status predicts susceptibility to vection-induced motion sickness and nausea. *Journal of Neurogastroenterology and Motility, 24,* 134–140.

Bertalanffy, P., Hoerauf, K., Fleischhackl, R., et al. (2004). Korean hand acupressure for motion sickness in prehospital trauma care: A prospective, randomized, double-blinded trial in a geriatric population. *Anesthesia and Analgesia, 98,* 220–223.

Bijveld, M. M., Bronstein, A. M., Golding, J. F., et al. (2008). Nauseogenicity of off-vertical-axis rotation versus equivalent visual motion. *Aviation, Space and Environmental Medicine, 79,* 661–665.

Boldingh, M. I., Ljostad, U., Mygland, A., et al. (2011). Vestibular sensitivity in vestibular migraine: VEMPs and motion sickness susceptibility. *Cephalalgia, 31*, 1211–1219.

Bos, J. E. (2015). Less sickness with more motion and/or mental distraction. *Journal of Vestibular Research, 25*, 23–33.

Bos, J. E., & Bles, W. (1998). Modelling motion sickness and subjective vertical mismatch detailed for vertical motions. *Brain Research Bulletin, 47*, 537–542.

Bos, J. E., MacKinnon, S. N., & Patterson, A. (2005). Motion sickness symptoms in a ship motion simulator: Effects of inside, outside, and no view. *Aviation, Space and Environmental Medicine, 76*, 1111–1118.

Bos, J. E., Ledegang, W. D., Lubeck, A. J., et al. (2013). Cinerama sickness and postural instability. *Ergonomics, 56*, 1430–1436.

Bosser, G., Caillet, G., Gauchard, G., et al. (2006). Relation between motion sickness susceptibility and vasovagal syncope susceptibility. *Brain Research Bulletin, 68*, 217–226.

Bowins, B. (2010). Motion sickness: A negative reinforcement model. *Brain Research Bulletin, 81*, 7–11.

Brey, R. L. (2005). Both migraine and motion sickness may be due to low brain levels of serotonin. *Neurology, 65*(4), E9–E10.

Bruce, D. G., Golding, J. F., & Pethybridge, R. J. (1990). Acupressure and motion sickness. *Aviation, Space and Environmental Medicine, 61*, 361–365.

Bubka, A., Bonato, F., Urmey, S., et al. (2006). Rotation velocity change and motion sickness in an optokinetic drum. *Aviation, Space and Environmental Medicine, 77*, 811–815.

Cevette, M. J., Stepanek, J., Cocco, D., et al. (2012). Oculo-vestibular recoupling using galvanic vestibular stimulation to mitigate simulator sickness. *Aviation, Space and Environmental Medicine, 83*, 549–555.

Cha, Y. H. (2009). Mal de debarquement. *Seminars in Neurology, 29*, 520–527.

Cha, Y. H., Cui, Y., & Baloh, R. W. (2013). Repetitive transcranial magnetic stimulation for mal de debarquement syndrome. *Otology & Neurotology, 34*, 175–179.

Chang, C. H., Pan, W. W., Chen, F. C., et al. (2013). Console video games, postural activity, and motion sickness during passive restraint. *Experimental Brain Research, 229*, 235–242.

Cheung, B., & Hofer, K. (2005). Desensitization to strong vestibular stimuli improves tolerance to simulated aircraft motion. *Aviation, Space and Environmental Medicine, 76*, 1099–1104.

Cheung, B., Nakashima, A. M., & Hofer, K. D. (2011). Various anti-motion sickness drugs and core body temperature changes. *Aviation, Space and Environmental Medicine, 82*, 409–415.

Cheung, B. S. K., Money, K. E., & Jacobs, I. (1990). Motion sickness susceptibility and aerobic fitness: A longitudinal study. *Aviation, Space and Environmental Medicine, 61*, 201–204.

Claremont, C. A. (1931). The psychology of sea-sickness. *Psyche, 11*, 86–90.

Clark, B. C., LePorte, A., Clark, S., et al. (2013). Effects of persistent Mal de debarquement syndrome on balance, psychological traits, and motor cortex excitability. *Journal of Clinical Neuroscience, 20*, 446–450.

Cohen, B., Dai, M., Yakushin, S. B., et al. (2008). Baclofen, motion sickness susceptibility and the neural basis for velocity storage. *Progress in Brain Research, 171*, 543–553.

Cowings, P. S., & Toscano, W. B. (2000). Autogenic-feedback training exercise is superior to promethazine for control of motion sickness symptoms. *Journal of Clinical Pharmacology, 40*, 1154–1165.

Cuomo-Granston, A., & Drummond, P. D. (2010). Migraine and motion sickness: What is the link? *Progress in Neurobiology, 91*, 300–312.

Dai, M., Raphan, T., & Cohen, B. (2011). Prolonged reduction of motion sickness sensitivity by visual-vestibular interaction. *Experimental Brain Research, 210*, 503–513.

Diamond, S. G., & Markham, C. H. (1991). Prediction of space motion sickness susceptibility by disconjugate eye torsion in parabolic flight. *Aviation, Space and Environmental Medicine, 62*, 201–205.

Diels, C., & Howarth, P. A. (2013). Frequency characteristics of visually induced motion sickness. *Human Factors, 55*, 595–604.

Dobie, T., McBride, D., Dobie, T., Jr., et al. (2001). The effects of age and sex on susceptibility to motion sickness. *Aviation, Space and Environmental Medicine, 72*, 13–20.

Drummond, P. D. (2005). Effect of tryptophan depletion on symptoms of motion sickness in migraineurs. *Neurology, 65*, 620–2.

Eversmann, T., Gottsmann, M., Uhlich, E., et al. (1978). Increased secretion of growth hormone, prolactin, antidiuretic hormone and cortisol induced by the stress of motion sickness. *Aviation, Space and Environmental Medicine, 49*, 55.

Farmer, A. D., Al Omran, Y., Aziz, Q., et al. (2014). The role of the parasympathetic nervous system in visually induced motion sickness: Systematic review and meta-analysis. *Experimental Brain Research, 232*, 2665–2673.

Finley, J. C., Jr., O'Leary, M., Wester, D., et al. (2004). A genetic polymorphism of the alpha2-adrenergic receptor increases autonomic responses to stress. *Journal of Applied Physiology, 96*, 2231–2239.

Flanagan, M. B., May, J. G., & Dobie, T. G. (2005). Sex differences in tolerance to visually-induced motion sickness. *Aviation, Space and Environmental Medicine, 76*, 642–646.

Furman, J. M., Marcus, D. A., & Balaban, C. D. (2011). Rizatriptan reduces vestibular-induced motion sickness in migraineurs. *Journal of Headache and Pain, 12*, 81–88.

Gahlinger, P. M. (2000). Cabin location and the likelihood of motion sickness in cruise ship passengers. *Journal of Travel Medicine, 7*, 120–124.

Gil, A., Nachum, Z., Dachir, S., et al. (2005). Scopolamine patch to prevent seasickness: clinical response vs. plasma concentration in sailors. *Aviation, Space and Environmental Medicine, 76*, 766–770.

Golding, J. F. (1992). Phasic skin conductance activity and motion sickness. *Aviation, Space and Environmental Medicine, 63*, 165–171.

Golding, J. F. (1998). Motion sickness susceptibility questionnaire revised and its relationship to other forms of sickness. *The Brain Research Bulletin, 47*, 507–516.

Golding, J. F. (2006a). Predicting individual differences in motion sickness susceptibility by questionnaire. *Personality and Individual Differences, 41*, 237–248.

Golding, J. F. (2006b). motion sickness susceptibility. *Autonomic Neuroscience, 30*, 67–76.

Golding, J. F., & Gresty, M. A. (2005). Motion sickness. *Current Opinion in Neurology, 18*, 29–34.

Golding, J. F., & Gresty, M. A. (2016). Biodynamic hypothesis for the frequency tuning of motion sickness. *Aerospace Medicine & Human Performance, 87*(1), 65–68.

Golding, J. F., Markey, H. M., & Stott, J. R. R. (1995). The effects of motion direction, body axis, and posture, on motion sickness induced by low frequency linear oscillation. *Aviation, Space and Environmental Medicine, 66*, 1046–1051.

Golding, J. F., Mueller, A. G., & Gresty, M. A. (2001). A motion sickness maximum around 0.2 Hz frequency range of horizontal translational oscillation. *Aviation, Space and Environmental Medicine, 72*, 188–192.

Golding, J. F., Kadzere, P. N., & Gresty, M. A. (2005). Motion sickness susceptibility fluctuates through the menstrual cycle. *Aviation, Space and Environmental Medicine, 76*, 970–973.

Golding, J. F., Paillard, A. C., & Denise, P. (2015). Motion sickness in zero-g parabolic flights. *Aerospace Medicine and Human Performance, 86*, 159.

Golding, J. F., & Stott, J. R. R. (1997a). Objective and subjective time courses of recovery from motion sickness assessed by repeated motion challenges. *Journal of Vestibular Research, 7*, 421–428.

Golding, J. F., & Stott, J. R. R. (1997b). Comparison of the effects of a selective muscarinic receptor antagonist and hyoscine (scopolamine) on motion sickness, skin conductance and heart rate. *British Journal of Clinical Pharmacology, 43*, 633–637.

Golding, J. F., & Tayyaba, S. A. (2014). Does motion sickness susceptibility relate to visceral disgust and bitter taste sensitivity? *Aviation, Space and Environmental Medicine, 85*, 344.

Golding, J. F., Bles, W., Bos, J. E., et al. (2003). Motion sickness and tilts of the inertial force environment: Active suspension systems versus active passengers. *Aviation, Space and Environmental Medicine, 74*, 220–227.

Golding, J. F., Prosyanikova, O., Flynn, M., et al. (2011). The effect of smoking nicotine tobacco versus smoking deprivation on motion sickness. *Autonomic Neuroscience: Basic and Clinical, 160*, 53–58.

Gordon, C. R., Ben-Aryeh, H., Spitzer, O., et al. (1994). Seasickness susceptibility, personality factors, and salivation. *Aviation, Space and Environmental Medicine, 65*, 610–614.

Gordon, C. R., Gonen, A., Nachum, Z., et al. (2001). The effects of dimenhydrinate, cinnarizine and transdermal scopolamine on performance. *Journal of Psychopharmacology, 15*, 167–172.

Graybiel, A. (1970). Susceptibility to acute motion sickness in blind persons. *Aerospace Medicine, 41*, 650–653.

Gresty, M. A., & Golding, J. F. (2009). Impact of vertigo and spatial disorientation on concurrent cognitive tasks. *Annals of the New York Academy of Sciences Journal, 1164*, 263–267.

Griffin, M. J., & Newman, M. M. (2004). Visual field effects on motion sickness in cars. *Aviation, Space and Environmental Medicine, 75*, 739–748.

Guedry, F. E., Rupert, A. R., & Reschke, M. F. (1998). Motion sickness and development of synergy within the spatial orientation system. A hypothetical unifying concept. *Brain Research Bulletin, 47*, 475–480.

Heer, M., & Paloski, W. H. (2006). Space motion sickness: Incidence, etiology, and countermeasures. *Autonomic Neuroscience, 129*, 77–79.

Henriques, I. F., Douglas de Oliveira, D. W., Oliveira-Ferreira, F., & Andrade, P. M. (2014). Motion sickness prevalence in school children. *European Journal of Pediatrics, 173*, 1473–1482.

Hettinger, L. J., Kennedy, R. S., & McCauley, M. E. (1990). Motion and human performance. In G. H. Crampton (Ed.), *Motion and space sickness* (pp. 412–441). Boca Raton, FL: CRC Press.

Horing, B., Weimer, K., Schrade, D., et al. (2013). Reduction of motion sickness with an enhanced placebo instruction: An experimental study with healthy participants. *Psychosomatic Medicine, 75*, 497–504.

Horn, C. C., Meyers, K., & Oberlies, N. (2014). Musk shrews selectively bred for motion sickness display increased anesthesia-induced vomiting. *Physiology & Behavior, 124*, 129–137.

Hoyt, R. E., Lawson, B. D., McGee, H. A., et al. (2009). Modafinil as a potential motion sickness countermeasure. *Aviation, Space and Environmental Medicine, 80*, 709–715.

Hromatka, B. S., Tung, J. Y., Kiefer, A. K., et al. (2015). Genetic variants associated with motion sickness point to roles for inner ear development, neurological processes and glucose homeostasis. *Human Molecular Genetics, 24*, 2700–2708.

International Organisation for Standardization 2631. (1997). *International Standard ISO 2631-1:1997(E). Mechanical vibration and shock. Evaluation of human exposure to whole-body vibration. Part 1: General Requirements* (2nd Edn.). Corrected and reprinted. Geneva: ISO.

Javid, F. A., & Naylor, R. J. (1999). Variables of movement amplitude and frequency in the development of motion sickness in Suncus murinus. *Pharmacology, Biochemistry and Behavior, 64*, 115–122.

Johnson, W. H., Sunahara, F. A., & Landolt, J. P. (1999). Importance of the vestibular system in visually induced nausea and self-vection. *Journal of Vestibular Research, 9*, 83–87.

Kaufman, G. D. (2005). Fos expression in the vestibular brainstem: What one marker can tell us about the network. *Brain Research Reviews, 50*, 200–211.

Kennedy, R. S., & Fowlkes, J. E. (1992). Simulator sickness is polygenic and polysymptomatic: Implications for research. *International Journal of Aviation Psychology, 2*, 23–38.

Kennedy, R. S., Lanham, D. S., Massey, C. J., et al. (1995). Gender differences in simulator sickness incidence: Implications for military virtual reality systems. *SAFE Journal, 25*, 69–76.

Keshavarz, B., & Hecht, H. (2014). Pleasant music as a countermeasure against visually induced motion sickness. *Applied Ergonomics, 45*, 521–527.

Keshavarz, B., Hettinger, L., Kennedy, R. S., et al. (2014). Demonstrating the potential for dynamic auditory stimulation to contribute to motion sickness. *Plos One 2014, 9*(1–9), e101016.

Keshavarz, B., Stelzmann, D., Paillard, A., et al. (2015). Visually induced motion sickness can be alleviated by pleasant odors. *Experimental Brain Research, 233*, 1353–1364.

Klosterhalfen, S., Kellermann, S., Pan, F., et al. (2005). Effects of ethnicity and gender on motion sickness susceptibility. *Aviation, Space and Environmental Medicine, 76*, 1051–1057.

Knox, G. W. (2014). Motion sickness: an evolutionary and genetic basis for the negative reinforcement model. *Aviation, Space and Environmental Medicine, 85*, 46–49.

Koch, K. L. (2014). Gastric dysrhythmias: A potential objective measure of nausea. *Experimental Brain Research, 232*, 2553–2561.

Lackner, J. R. (2014). Motion sickness: More than nausea and vomiting. *Experimental Brain Research, 232*, 2493–2510.

Lackner, J. R., & Graybiel, A. (1994). Use of promethazine to hasten adaptation to provocative motion. *Journal of Clinical Pharmacology, 34*, 644–648.

Lamb, S., Kwok, K. C. S., & Walton, D. (2014). A longitudinal field study of the effects of wind-induced building motion on occupant wellbeing and work performance. *Journal of Wind Engineering and Industrial Aerodynamics, 133*, 39–51.

Lawson, B. D., Graeber, D. A., Mead, A. M., & Muth, E. R. (2002). Signs and symptoms of human syndromes associated with synthetic experiences. Chapter 30. In K.M. Stanney (Ed.), *Handbook of virtual environments* (pp. 589–618). Mahwah, NJ: Lawrence Erlbaum Associates, Inc.

Lawther, A., & Griffin, M. J. (1988). A survey of the occurrence of motion sickness amongst passengers at sea. *Aviation, Space and Environmental Medicine, 59*, 399–406.

Lentz, J. M. (1984). Laboratory tests of motion sickness susceptibility. In: *Motion Sickness: Mechanisms, Prediction, Prevention and Treatment* (pp 29–1 to 29–9). AGARD Conference Proceedings No. 372.

Levine, M. E., Chillas, J. C., Stern, R. M., et al. (2000). The effects of serotonin (5-HT3) receptor antagonists on gastric tachyarrhythmia and the symptoms of motion sickness. *Aviation, Space and Environmental Medicine, 71*, 1111–1114.

Levine, M. E., Stern, R. M., & Koch, K. L. (2014). Enhanced perceptions of control and predictability reduce motion-induced nausea and gastric dysrhythmia. *Experimental Brain Research, 232*, 2675–2684.

Levine, M. E., Muth, E. R., Williamson, M. J., et al. (2004). Protein-predominant meals inhibit the development of gastric tachyarrhythmia, nausea and the symptoms of motion sickness. *Alimentary Pharmacology & Therapeutics, 19*, 583–590.

Lien, H. C., Sun, W. M., Chen, Y. H., et al. (2003). Effects of ginger on motion sickness and gastric slow-wave dysrhythmias induced by circular vection. *American Journal of Physiology-Gastrointestinal and Liver Physiology, 284*, G481–G489.

Lindseth, G., & Lindseth, P. D. (1995). The relationship of diet to airsickness. *Aviation, Space and Environmental Medicine, 66*, 537–541.

Lubeck, A. J. A., Bos, J. E., & Stins, J. F. (2015). Motion in images is essential to cause motion sickness symptoms, but not to increase postural sway. *Displays, 38*, 55–61.

Lucertini, M., Verde, P., & Trivelloni, P. (2013). Rehabilitation from airsickness in military pilots: Long-term treatment effectiveness. *Aviation, Space and Environmental Medicine, 84*, 1196–1200.

Matsangas, P., & McCauley, M. E. (2014). Yawning as a behavioral marker of mild motion sickness and sopite syndrome. *Aviation, Space and Environmental Medicine, 85*, 658–661.

Miller, K. E., & Muth, E. R. (2004). Efficacy of acupressure and acustimulation bands for the prevention of motion sickness. *Aviation, Space and Environmental Medicine, 75*, 227–234.

Money, K. E., & Cheung, B. S. (1983). Another function of the inner ear: Facilitation of the emetic response to poisons. *Aviation, Space and Environmental Medicine, 54*, 208–211.

Morrow, G. R. (1985). The effect of a susceptibility to motion sickness on the side effects of cancer chemotherapy. *Cancer, 55*, 2766–2770.

Murdin, L., Golding, J., & Bronstein, A. (2011). Managing motion sickness. *British Medical Journal, 343*, 1213–1217.

Murdin, L., Chamberlain, F., Cheema, S., et al. (2015). Motion sickness susceptibility in vestibular disease. *Journal of Neurology, Neurosurgery and Psychiatry, 86*, 585–587.

Nachum, Z., Shahal, B., Shupak, A., et al. (2001). Scopolamine bioavailability in combined oral and transdermal delivery. *Journal of Pharmacology and Experimental Therapeutics, 296*, 121–123.

Nachum, Z., Shupak, A., Letichevsky, V., et al. (2004). Mal de debarquement and posture: Reduced reliance on vestibular and visual cues. *Laryngoscope, 114*, 1581–6.

Nalivaiko, E., Rudd, J. A., & So, R. H. Y. (2014). Motion sickness, nausea and thermoregulation: The "toxic" hypothesis. *Temperature, 1*(3), 164–171.

Nakagawa, A., Uno, A., Horii, A., et al. (2003). Fos induction in the amygdala by vestibular information during hypergravity stimulation. *Brain Research, 986*, 114–123.

Napadow, V., Sheehan, J. D., Kim, J., et al. (2013a). The brain circuitry underlying the temporal evolution of nausea in humans. *Cerebral Cortex, 23*, 806–813.

Napadow, V., Sheehan, J., Kim, J., et al. (2013b). Brain white matter microstructure is associated with susceptibility to motion-induced nausea. *Journal of Neurogastroenterology and Motility, 25*, 448–450.

Naqvi, S. A., Badruddin, N., Malik, A. S., Hazabbah, W., & Abdullah, B. (2013). Does 3D produce more symptoms of visually induced motion sickness? *Conference Proceedings IEEE Engineering in Medicine and Biology Society* (pp. 6405–6408).

Nunn, P. W. G. (1881). Seasickness, its causes and treatment. *Lancet ii*, 1151–1152.

O'Hanlon, J. F., & McCauley, M. E. (1974). Motion sickness incidence as a function of the frequency and acceleration of vertical sinusoidal motion. *Aviation, Space and Environmental Medicine, 45*, 366–369.

Oman, C. M. (1990). Motion sickness: A synthesis and evaluation of the sensory conflict theory. *Comparative Biochemistry and Physiology, 68*, 294–303.

Oman, C. M. (2012). Are evolutionary hypotheses for motion sickness "just-so" stories? *Journal of Vestibular Research, 22*, 117–127.

Oman, C. M., & Cullen, K. E. (2014). Brainstem processing of vestibular sensory exafference: Implications for motion sickness etiology. *Experimental Brain Research, 232*, 2483–2492.

Paillard, A. C., Quarck, G., Paolino, F., et al. (2013). Motion sickness susceptibility in healthy subjects and vestibular patients: Effects of gender, age and trait-anxiety. *Journal of Vestibular Research, 23*, 203–210.

Paillard, A. C., Lamôré, M., Etard, O., et al. (2014). Is there a relationship between odours and motion sickness? *Neuroscience Letters, 566*, 326–30.

Palatty, P. L., Haniadka, R., Valder, B., et al. (2013). Ginger in the prevention of nausea and vomiting: A review. *Critical Reviews in Food Science and Nutrition, 53*, 659–669.

Perrin, P., Lion, A., Bosser, G., et al. (2013). Motion sickness in rally car co-drivers. *Aviation, Space and Environmental Medicine, 84*, 473–477.

Pethybridge, R. J. (1982). *Sea sickness incidence in Royal Navy ships.* (Report No. INM 37/82). Gosport, England: Institute of Naval Medicine.

Pompeiano, O., d'Ascanio, P., Balaban, E., et al. (2004). Gene expression in autonomic areas of the medulla and the central nucleus of the amygdala in rats during and after space flight. *Neuroscience, 124*, 153–69.

Radtke, A., Popov, K., Bronstein, A. M., et al. (2003). Vestibular-autonomic control in man: short- and long-latency effects on cardiovascular function. *Journal of Vestibular Research, 13*, 25–37.

Reason, J. T., & Brand, J. J. (1975). *Motion sickness.* London: Academic Press.

Reavley, C. M., Golding, J. F., Cherkas, L. F., et al. (2006). Genetic influences on motion sickness susceptibility in adult females: A classical twin study. *Aviation, Space and Environmental Medicine, 77*, 1148–1152.

Ressiot, E., Dolz, M., Bonne, L., & Marianowski, R. (2013). Prospective study on the efficacy of optokinetic training in the treatment of sea sickness. *European Annals of Otorhinolaryngology, Head and Neck Diseases, 130*, 263–268.

Riccio, G. E., & Stoffregen, T. A. (1991). An ecological theory of motion sickness and postural instability. *Ecological Psychology Journal, 3*, 195–240.

Rolnick, A., & Lubow, R. E. (1991). Why is the driver rarely sick? The role of controllability in motion sickness. *Ergonomics, 34*, 867–879.

Schaub, N., Ng, K., Kuo, P., et al. (2014). Gastric and lower esophageal sphincter pressures during nausea: A study using visual motion-induced nausea and high-resolution manometry. *American Journal of Physiology-Gastrointestinal and Liver Physiology, 306*, G741–G747.

Schelgel, T. T., Brown, T. E., Wood, S. J., et al. (2001). Orthostatic intolerance and motion sickness after parabolic flight. *Journal of Applied Physiology, 90*, 67–82.

Schutz, L., Zak, D., & Holmes, J. F. (2014). Pattern of passenger injury and illness on expedition cruise ships to Antarctica. *Journal of Travel Medicine, 21*, 228–234.

Seibel, K., Schaffler, K., & Reitmeir, P. (2002). A randomised, placebo-controlled study comparing two formulations of dimenhydrinate with respect to efficacy in motion sickness and sedation. *Arzneimittel-Forschung, 52*, 529–536.

Serrador, J. M., Schlegel, T. T., Black, F. O., et al. (2005). Cerebral hypoperfusion precedes nausea during centrifugation. *Aviation, Space and Environmental Medicine, 76*, 91–96.

Sharma, K., Sharma, P., Sharma, A., et al. (2008). Phenylthiocarbamide taste perception and susceptibility to motion sickness: Linking higher susceptibility with higher phenylthiocarbamide taste acuity. *Journal of Laryngology and Otology, 122*, 1064–1073.

Sharon, J. D., & Hullar, T. E. (2014). Motion sensitivity and caloric responsiveness in vestibular migraine and Meniere's disease. *Laryngoscope, 124*, 969–973.

Simmons, R. G., Phillips, J. B., Lojewski, R. A., et al. (2010). The efficacy of low-dose intranasal scopolamine for motion sickness. *Aviation, Space and Environmental Medicine, 81*, 405–412.

Solimini, A. G. (2013). Are there side effects to watching 3D movies? A prospective crossover observational study on visually induced motion sickness. *PLoS One. 8*(2), e56160. doi: 10.1371/journal.pone.0056160. [Epub 2013 Feb 13]

Stern, R. M., Koch, K. L., Leibowitz, H. W., et al. (1985). Tachygastria and motion sickness. *Aviation, Space and Environmental Medicine, 56*, 1074–1077.

Stern, R. M., Hu, S., LeBlanc, R., et al. (1993). Chinese hyper-susceptibility to vection-induced motion sickness. *Aviation, Space and Environmental Medicine, 64*, 827–830.

Stewart, J. J., Wood, M. J., Parish, R. C., et al. (2000). Prokinetic effects of erythromycin after antimotion sickness drugs. *Journal of Clinical Pharmacology, 40*, 347–353.

Stoffregen, T. A., Chen, Y. C., & Koslucher, F. C. (2014). Motion control, motion sickness, and the postural dynamics of mobile devices. *Experimental Brain Research, 232*, 1389–1397.

Stoffregen, T. A., Chen, F. C., Varlet, M., et al. (2013). 2013. *Getting Your Sea Legs. PLoS One., 8* (6), e66949.

Stott, J. R. R. (1986). Mechanisms and treatment of motion illness. In C. J. Davis, G. V. Lake-Bakaar, & D. G. Grahame-Smith (Eds.), *Nausea and vomiting: mechanisms and treatment* (pp. 110–129). Berlin: Springer.

Stromberg, S. E., Russell, M. E., & Carlson, C. R. (2015). Diaphragmatic breathing and its effectiveness for the management of motion sickness. *Aerospace Medicine and Human Performance, 86*, 452–457.

Stroud, K. J., Harm, D. L., & Klaus, D. M. (2005). Preflight virtual reality training as a countermeasure for space motion sickness and disorientation. *Aviation, Space and Environmental Medicine, 76*, 352–356.

Tal, D., Hershkovitz, D., Kaminski-Graif, G., et al. (2013). Vestibular evoked myogenic potentials and habituation to seasickness. *Clinical Neurophysiology, 124*, 2445–2449.

Tal, D., Wiener, G., & Shupak, A. (2014). Mal de debarquement, motion sickness and the effect of an artificial horizon. *Journal of Vestibular Research, 24*, 17–23.

Thornton, W. E., & Bonato, F. (2013). Space motion sickness and motion sickness: Symptoms and etiology. *Aviation, Space and Environmental Medicine, 84*, 716–721.

Treisman, M. (1977). Motion sickness: An evolutionary hypothesis. *Science, 197*, 493–495.

Turner, M., & Griffin, M. J. (1999a). Motion sickness in public road transport: Passenger behaviour and susceptibility. *Ergonomics, 42*, 444–461.

Turner, M., & Griffin, M. J. (1999b). Motion sickness in public road transport: the relative importance of motion, vision and individual differences. *British Journal of Psychology, 90,* 519–530.

van Marion, W. F., Bongaerts, M. C., Christiaanse, J. C., et al. (1985). Influence of transdermal scopolamine on motion sickness during 7 days' exposure to heavy seas. *Clinical Pharmacology and Therapeutics, 38,* 301–305.

Von Gierke, H. E., & Parker, D. E. (1994). Differences in otolith and abdominal viscera graviceptor dynamics: implications for motion sickness and perceived body position. *Aviation, Space and Environmental Medicine, 65,* 747–751.

Wada, T., Konno, H., Fujisawa, S., et al. (2012). Can passengers' active head tilt decrease the severity of carsickness? Effect of head tilt on severity of motion sickness in a lateral acceleration environment. *Human Factors, 54,* 226–234.

Webb, C. M., Estrada, A., & Athy, J. R. (2013). Motion sickness prevention by an 8-Hz stroboscopic environment during air transport. *Aviation, Space and Environmental Medicine, 84,* 177–183.

Whittle, J. (1689) An exact diary of the late expedition of His Illustrious Highness the Prince of Orange, 1689. In: J. Pike (Ed.) (1986). *Tall Ships in Torbay a Brief Maritime History* (p. 35). Bradford on Avon, UK: Ex Libris Press.

Wood, C. D., & Graybiel, A. (1969). Evaluation of 16 antimotion sickness drugs under controlled laboratory conditions. *Aerospace Medicine, 39,* 1341–1344.

Wood, C. D., Manno, J. E., Manno, B. R., et al. (1986). The effect of anti-motion sickness drugs on habituation to motion. *Aviation, Space and Environmental Medicine, 57,* 539–542.

Yates, B. J., Miller, A. D., & Lucot, J. B. (1998). Physiological basis and pharmacology of motion sickness: an update. *Brain Research Bulletin, 47,* 395–406.

Yates, B. J., Catanzaro, M. F., Miller, D. J., et al. (2014). Integration of vestibular and emetic gastrointestinal signals that produce nausea and vomiting: Potential contributions to motion sickness. *Experimental Brain Research, 232,* 2455–2469.

Yen-Pik-Sang, F., Billar, J. P., Golding, J. F., et al. (2003a). Behavioral methods of alleviating motion sickness: Effectiveness of controlled breathing and music audiotape. *Journal of Travel Medicine, 10,* 108–112.

Yen-Pik-Sang, F., Golding, J. F., & Gresty, M. A. (2003b). Suppression of sickness by controlled breathing during mild nauseogenic motion. *Aviation, Space and Environmental Medicine, 74,* 998–1002.

Yen-Pik-Sang, F., Billar, J., Gresty, M. A., et al. (2005). Effect of a novel motion desensitization training regime and controlled breathing on habituation to motion sickness. *Perceptual and Motor Skills, 101,* 244–256.

Young, L. R., Sienko, K. H., Lyne, L. E., et al. (2003). Adaptation of the vestibulo-ocular reflex, subjective tilt, and motion sickness to head movements during short-radius centrifugation. *Journal of Vestibular Research, 13,* 65–77.

Ziavra, N. V., Yen-Pik-Sang, F. D., Golding, J. F., et al. (2003). Effect of breathing supplemental oxygen on motion sickness in healthy adults. *Mayo Clinic Proceedings, 78,* 574–578.

Risk Communication: Following a Maritime Disaster

Ian de Terte and Elspeth Tilley

Case Study

On 5 October 2011, a container ship *Rena* ran aground on Astrolabe Reef in the entrance to Tauranga Harbour, New Zealand. The ship damaged its hull and approximately 350 tonnes of heavy fuel oil spilled into the environment and subsequently washed up on the shores of Bay of Plenty, New Zealand. In addition, the ship lost the majority of its containers and was deemed to be a total loss (Transport Accident Investigation Commission 2014). Although there was no loss of human life, the crew and cleanup workers, particularly those dealing with injured wildlife, reported a range of signs and symptoms of trauma. Maritime New Zealand national scene commander Nick Quinn commented in the media on the "unbelievably huge emotional aspect to it all" (Fairfax 2011, para. 19), and counsellors were called into assist.

Later, charges were laid against *Rena*'s captain and navigator under New Zealand's Maritime Transport Act, Resource Management Act, and Crimes Act, and they were found guilty of operating a vessel in a manner likely to cause danger (Daly 2012). Part of the issue, according to the judgement in the case, was a single-minded focus on reaching the pilot station by a particular deadline, to the detriment of focus on other navigational principles (Bowen and Migone 2012). The judge concluded that the crew had failed to follow "basic navigation practices" before the ship ran aground, cutting corners and sailing hazardously (Bowen and Migone 2012). A defence lawyer for one of the men pointed out that the men were

I. de Terte (✉)
School of Psychology—Te Kura Hinengaro Tangata, Massey University,
Wellington 6140, New Zealand
e-mail: i.deterte@massey.ac.nz

E. Tilley
School of English and Media Stuides, Massey University, Wellington 6140,
New Zealand

© Springer International Publishing Switzerland 2017
M. MacLachlan (ed.), *Maritime Psychology*, DOI 10.1007/978-3-319-45430-6_8

not thinking clearly at the time—they knew that all their discussions on the bridge were recorded by the black box, yet held an audible conversation about falsifying navigation records: "That gives an idea of their state of mind" (Bowen and Migone 2012).

The *Rena* incident, while foremost in damage to property and environment, was not an isolated case for New Zealand, where the combination of rocky coastline and extreme weather mean there have been major incidents of both environmental impact and lives lost, as well as frequent "near misses." Just some of the major incidents in New Zealand waters include the 1863 loss of the Royal Navy steam ship HMS *Orpheus*, which was wrecked at the entrance to Auckland's Manukau Harbour, killing 189 men; the 1881 *Tararua* shipwreck in which 131 passengers and crew were lost; the 1909 Cook Strait ferry *Penguin* shipwreck off Cape Terawhiti with the loss of 72 lives; the sinking of the ferry *Wahine* in 1968 which killed 53 people; the *Mikhail Lermontov* cruise ship which sank in 1986, killing a crew member; the 1998 grounding of the *Don Wong 529* with 400 tonnes of automotive gas oil spilled; and the *Jody F Millennium*, which spilled 25 tonnes of fuel oil in 2002 (see Maritime New Zealand N.d.; Ministry for Culture and Heritage 2014 for these and more incidents). While these are the worst cases, they illustrate the outer extent of risks that maritime workers live with on a regular basis. Globally, maritime professions have long been recognized as inherently dangerous, with fatality rates fluctuating, but ranging from peaks of 18 times the national work-fatality average in Australia to more than 50 times higher than the national average in the United Kingdom, and 25–30 times higher in Denmark (Lindøe 2007).

While some of the industry-level costs of this risk have been well researched, the practical implications for effective interpersonal and group communication practices during both everyday maritime work and before, during and after a high-risk or crisis situation have not previously been well documented. Complicating this is the fact that, as Pomeroy (2014) and Bailey (2006) report, these risks are not always accurately perceived or acknowledged by maritime professionals. Pomeroy believes divergence between actual and perceived risks "may explain some of the maritime incidents that appear to be the consequence of apparently inexplicable acts" (2014, p. 50). Such a divergence also has important communication implications. First, it indicates the need for circulation of clear, accurate, meaningful information right throughout the industry as to real levels of risk. Preparing to face risk with responses that ensure resilience takes effort, and one of the key motivators for expending such effort is realistic appreciation of the personal consequences of the risk. Second, living with daily risk as occurs in maritime industries will certainly impact on the design and delivery required for effective risk communication. Hence in this chapter, we outline both the psychological impacts of a crisis and how best to communicate with people who are living with heightened daily risk.

Review of State of the Knowledge

The impact of disasters such as those outlined previously is far reaching and may have psychological consequences for some of the people involved. Disasters have been categorized into two separate domains, natural disasters and human-made disasters (Galea et al. 2005). Sometimes human-made disasters have been further divided into human-made and technological disasters. Natural disasters are events that occur because of acts of nature, for example, earthquakes. Human-made disasters are events that are the result of some act by human beings, such as terrorism. Technological disasters are events that occur because of some malfunction in technology, such as factory explosions (Neria et al. 2008). Scientific research has found that individuals have more difficulty psychologically recovering from a human-made disaster or a technological disaster than a natural disaster (Norris et al. 2002). However, there is some scientific debate about the simplistic nature of this categorization of disasters (Grimm et al. 2012). The *Rena* disaster would be characterized as a human-made disaster because it was an event that could have been avoided by better human decision-making. There are some common reactions to such events or situations that can be directly transferable to other marine disasters. There are some other psychological phenomena that may have impacted on this marine catastrophe such as crew fatigue and cognitive performance. However, this chapter will focus on the psychological consequences of such an event and how these consequences impact on communication processes.

The psychological reactions to such an event may be plotted on a continuum. This continuum would include posttraumatic stress disorder (PTSD), psychological distress, secondary traumatic stress, and no reaction. At one end of the continuum people may have a reaction like PTSD. For an individual to be diagnosed with PTSD, according to the *fifth edition of the Diagnostic and Statistical Manual of Mental Disorders* (DSM-5; American Psychiatric Association 2013), they need to be exposed to a traumatic event. Then the individual concerned must have the following reaction to the traumatic event: intrusion symptoms, avoidance symptoms, negative alterations in cognitions and mood, and marked alterations in arousal and reactivity. There are a number of symptoms under each sub-construct that stipulate when an individual meets the relevant criterion. For a full description of the diagnostic criteria the reader is referred to the DSM5 (American Psychiatric Association 2013). It should be noted that in some jurisdictions only psychiatrists or clinical psychologists are able to diagnose people with such a clinical phenomenon. The second stage of the continuum is where people may not meet the first diagnostic criteria for PTSD, which relates to being exposed to the traumatic event, but they may still have some of the reactive symptomatology of PTSD (e.g. avoidance). In addition, some people may have other psychological phenomena, such as stress, fear, anxiety, blaming, anger, fatigue or dissociation. This is not an exhaustive list, but notes some of the psychological difficulties that some people who are exposed to a traumatic event may exhibit.

Some people who are exposed to an event like the grounding of the *Rena* may not meet the criterion stipulated by the DSM5 regarding what constitutes exposure to a traumatic event. However, they may still exhibit psychological difficulties. The third stage of the continuum is when an individual may have secondary traumatic stress. Secondary traumatic stress is where the individual does not directly experience the traumatic event, but hears about the event via a third party and mimics the reactive symptoms of PTSD. Finally, some people may have no reaction to such an event whatsoever. To summarize, people who are exposed to such an event may have a diverse range of reactions.

An alternative phenomenon is that people may begin to problem-solve the issue. In the case of the *Rena*'s grounding, the crude oil that leaked from the container ship washed up on the Bay of Plenty shores. An example of the problem solving of local people is that in this incident they began to clean their foreshore of oil residue. However, this modus operandi displayed by the helpers was not considered to be the best option because of their physical safety (Goldstein et al. 2011), further environmental contamination, or the correct disposal of oil residue (K. Manch, personal communication, April 28 2015). However, the people who were cleaning up the beach believed that they were providing an appropriate response.

There are two matters to consider here. On the one hand, some people may have a psychological response to a crisis event and are not sure if this is a normal reaction or how this response should be dealt with. On the other hand, some people may commence problem solving without full knowledge of how they should respond to such a marine disaster. Both matters require some expertise and knowledge on the subjects as to how to deal with them. In addition, after an event like the *Rena* there are multiple impacts that need to be dealt with, so human reactions may be low on the list of priorities for some individuals. However, we believe that people should be informed about how these subjects should be dealt with. These messages need to be communicated to the people involved, but how should such a message be communicated so that the recipients engage with the message? Unless psychological factors are addressed in the design of risk communication not only during an incident, but also before and after, understanding and compliance will be hard to obtain and harm can be exacerbated (Mehta et al. 2014).

The Implications for Communication Practice

There are many communication guidelines that can help, but one highly relevant one is the elaboration likelihood model (ELM). Developed by social psychologists Petty and Cacioppo (1986), ELM investigates the different ways that people process communication messages, and the different results for communication effectiveness, including changes in attitude or behaviour, such as compliance or rejection. Elaboration refers to mental processing, or the effort spent considering and evaluating arguments and context.

Petty and Cacioppo's (1986) research led them to group people's communication processing into two main categories: central processing, in which attitudes are formed as a result of careful assessment of a range of information; and peripheral processing, in which attitudes are adopted more rapidly and in a less considered way. Both can result in effective communication, but the central route requires more intensive message elaboration, meaning higher levels of mental effort are involved, while the peripheral route involves low message elaboration, offering a short-hand or intuitive way to accept or reject a message. The two are not mutually exclusive and a combination anywhere along a spectrum may be used.

ELM studies have suggested that attitudes adopted after lower elaboration are vulnerable to subsequent counter-persuasion, but also that few people regularly have time, ability and inclination to conduct a lot of central processing other than for particular issues in which they have a deep personal emotional investment, and therefore most everyday attitudes are predominately peripherally formed rather than deeply researched and considered (Petty and Cacioppo 1986; Petty and Wegener 1999). Additionally, some people are in a better position to elaborate either generally or on particular topics than others—plus at different times and in different circumstances we may shift on the spectrum in terms of our processing. For example, children will typically process differently than adults, as will experts versus novices, as will anyone who is feeling too busy and tired to elaborate, or who is in a highly distracting situation (hence why expensive fashion boutiques often play distracting music, to encourage a quick and emotive rather than thoughtful and cognitive purchasing decision). In particular, stressed or traumatized audiences are very unlikely to be able to devote much cognitive effort to central processing and will typically make highly intuitive, peripherally processed decisions. So in times of crisis, such as a ship heading for a reef, we are often reliant on our "gut instinct" and may ignore things we would "know" to do, based on evidence or prior learning, in calmer times. On the flip side of this, if we spend time developing and practising centrally developed attitudes and behaviours during calm times, those attitudes will be more likely to withstand counter-pressures even during times of stress.

People using either communication processing route as the dominant one to deal with incoming information will typically seek different things to aid their decision. Those primarily using central processing at any given time seek out facts, statistics and "hard data." They want reasoned, logical arguments with supporting examples and evidence. For example, if we are grocery shopping and we are not in a hurry, and we want to make some dietary or budgetary decisions with particular outcomes, we might process our shopping selections centrally. We may scrutinize nutritional and ingredient information, calculate price per kilogramme and compare with other package sizes or brands, read the fine print of environmental information and look carefully at brands we have never bought before to see if they better meet our goals than our regular brand. Then we make a considered, and likely quite lasting, decision.

By contrast, if we are processing the shopping choices peripherally, perhaps because we are in a hurry, tired, stressed or just do not have the inclination to elaborate today, we will seek a different set of cues for our decision-making. These may include cognitive heuristics or mental shortcuts such as a trusted recommendation: "Mum used this brand so it must be good." Familiarity also works as a mental shortcut, such as recognizing the package or logo from advertising. Prior experience can also provide a mental shortcut ("this is the brand I got last time" or "this is the way we've always done it"), as can an endorsement from a celebrity, expert, person we look up to (for example in a maritime context "the best captain I ever sailed with always did it this way") or a person we like ("my friends do it this way"). In a peripheral context, we also place value on visual elements (photos, simple graphics and diagrams, using clearly differentiated bright colours) and what could be called "window dressing" of the communication rather than the information itself (e.g., for a product that could mean glossy packaging, a price reduction, a giveaway or contest, or a photo of a celebrity on the box, while on a ship that may mean the brightest coloured signage placed most prominently at eye level at the precise moment when we have to make a decision). When processing peripherally we seek very simple information messages, and are also quite susceptible to directive messages that tell us what to do, provided they come from a source we trust and like. An entertainment element to the message, not just purely information, is also effective in peripheral processing—so if your audience is likely to process at least part of your communication peripherally, your message can potentially be delivered with (appropriate) humour, or delivered in the context of other entertainment values, such as being part of a day of fun activities or simulation games that "embed" serious learning messages about managing risk or achieving safety outcomes in an entertaining format.

What Happens During Message Processing?

Messages processed by the central route usually result in long-lasting attitude or behavioural change if arguments are well presented and credible and particularly if "inoculation" against opposing arguments is provided—that is, you let your audience know what counterarguments exist and actually take them through those arguments to evaluate their validity (Banas and Rains 2010). This all takes time, so cannot be done in the heat of the moment of crisis. It can, however, be done beforehand—and so in the context of maritime risk, preparation in advance of the attitudes and behaviours that will help when a typical maritime crisis hits is crucial. This includes running regular crisis training in which both common and uncommon disasters are simulated, debriefing everyone afterwards, and evaluating and updating communication materials after every crisis test. Important aspects include getting all levels of staff involved in planning these crisis simulations and creating an atmosphere of co-operation and trust in which people are happy to talk about the risks they perceive and areas where safety problems could arise (Moats et al. 2008). Effective crisis simulations can include both computer-game-based simulations and live-action rehearsals (Boin et al. 2004).

An important communication-related element of preparation is ensuring that those who will lead a real crisis response have plenty of positive contact with all staff during non-crisis times, and are well-known faces and personalities. Because trust, familiarity, likeability and status are important peripheral cues when people are stressed, it is also extremely important to build those kinds of relationships with your audience beforehand too. This preparation phase when efforts are being made to inculcate the kinds of attitudes and behaviours that reduce risk and increase safety or that prepare people to know their role and responsibility should a crisis occur is also the most appropriate time to include entertainment value. When audiences are conscious of a persuasive intent, they are more likely to resist a message through reactance (a "boomerang" or push-back attitude against authority that involves resisting perceived pressure to change; Brehm and Brehm 1981) and counterarguing (actively thinking up reasons to contradict or undermine a persuasive message; Eveland and Cooper 2013). Antiauthoritarian sentiment has been shown to be increasing over the last three generations in many cultures, so there will be age-related differences in resistance to authority (McCrindle and Wolfinger 2009). Eveland and Cooper note that "Entertainment media that contain persuasive messages can reduce these forms of resistance through greater involvement with the narrative. This involvement facilitates the development of message-consistent beliefs, especially in audiences otherwise predisposed to disagree with the message" (2013, p. 14091) Entertainment-based communication methods, such as skits, songs, dance, comedy, television drama or multimedia including animations and dramatized scenes, are all methods that may assist with overcoming barriers to message processing (Edmond and Tilley 2002). An added bonus is that these are often non-print channels and therefore accessible to audiences with widely different levels of print literacy. An example of this is an African mining company that found a 30 % reduction in workplace accidents 18 months after introducing a series of short performance pieces dramatizing safety issues through oral storytelling, song, dance, chanting, music and metaphor (Edmond and Tilley 2002).

The peripheral route usually results in only a temporary shift of attitudes or behaviour, so you cannot predict long-term results and need to keep repeating your message (even top brands need to keep advertising to maintain buyer purchasing behaviour). However, if all you need is a quick response of compliance, by traumatized people who cannot think things through, then peripheral cues such as likeability are very powerful—so in a maritime crisis, ask the most liked and trusted leader on the ship to deliver short, simple, directive messages, but to do so in a way that is humanized and empathetic. This should help provide the necessary peripheral cues for compliance.

In life and work, most messages are in fact processed peripherally. And the most effective peripheral messages are those that emphasize tangible, immediate, personal rewards ("Together we will make this ship as safe as we can, for everyone. I trust you with this important responsibility—to check every lifeboat has stores— because I know you won't let me down"). Alongside personal benefits, design peripheral messages to emphasize the positive characteristics of whomever is delivering the message, including their credibility and expertise ("We have trained many times for this, we know exactly what to do"), likeability (be human), and familiarity (messages before, during and after crises should come from one of the ship's own, not from an external body or stranger, and most definitely not from an officious-sounding bureaucratic organizational title that is not actually a person with a name and identity as a human).

These kinds of noncognitive cues are particularly important for unmotivated, incapable, stressed audiences. If peripheral cues are not present, stressed audiences may simply "not hear." Peripheral attitude change is typically short term (messages need to be repeated, and repeated and repeated during a crisis). Celebrity endorsements provide one of the strongest peripheral cues yet discovered, yet even then the change is small and transitory (Chaudhuri and Buck 1995). Expert testimonials are also effective, with high-credibility sources producing more attitude change (hence the Captain should speak in times of stress), but even high-credibility sources typically convince less than half of an audience if the audience is not predisposed to agree with their message through likeability cues (Chaiken et al. 1989). Maintaining consistently good relations between ships' officers and crew, then, has psychological and communication consequences for mitigating a maritime disaster—as does ensuring senior crew are sober and ready to take command during a crisis. Because crew look first and foremost to their most trusted expert to lead crisis communication, the absence or incapacity of a senior officer whom crew respect and like may have far more wide-reaching negative consequences during a crisis than the simple absence of any one person among many may logically be expected to cause.

How Does This Relate to More Typical Everyday Maritime Risk Communication?

The maritime audience, which refers to those people who are in the maritime industry either in a professional or social capacity, is always slightly aroused (in the psychological sense of heightened alertness, and higher-than-average vigilance to risk in the surrounding environment). Factors that may exacerbate that arousal along a continuum that leads ultimately to a state of trauma in which communication is difficult to hear and process include: shift work, particularly night shifts (disruption to circadian rhythms increases adrenal strain), long shifts or repeated long shifts over several days (fatigue and lack of concentration build up both over a shift and cumulatively across several days of long shifts; Rosa and Colligan 1997); build-up of residual stress from prior incidents (e.g., prolonged sequential periods of bad weather); alcohol and drugs; relationship difficulties (personal or work); changes in life circumstances (divorce, death of a loved one, moving house); culture shock (transition from one cultural group or context to another or, as can be the situation on commercial maritime vessels, hiring cross-cultural labour, teams from different cultures working together or groups from different cultures working at different organizational levels of the ship hierarchy); and illness (Bailey 2006, reports higher than average levels of illness and mental illness among seafaring workers). Additional maritime-specific factors contributing to heightened adrenal stress and, consequently, fatigue, may include jobs with strenuous physical labour, using heavy or dangerous machinery, and handling dangerous goods or volatile cargo and equipment. In New Zealand, the Maritime Union has also raised the casualization of the industry and irregular short-contract work patterns as contributing to worker stress, reduced skills and safety issues in parts of the industry (Maritime Union of New Zealand 2015). And in maritime workplaces, as in many workplaces globally, there may be multiple languages, plus print literacy levels may also be an issue for written communication processing. In general with increasing global access to cheap audiovisual technologies, many younger populations are shifting towards a more heavily oral and visual skillset, with a concomitant reduction in print-processing literacy (Ong 2002). Literacy levels may particularly be of issue for some kinds of maritime workers because of the limited access to print materials on board ship, cultural preferences for orality and/or background education levels. Loading a worker who struggles with print literacy with frequent or crucial written communication material has been shown to be a factor in worker stress and feelings of depression and inadequacy (Tilley et al. 2006). This again causes heightened adrenal arousal, which means when an individual has an increased level of biological reactivity in their body, including an increase in the release of adrenaline in their body (Friedman and McEwen 2004), that can in turn lead to fatigue and inability to concentrate, in what can only be described as a vicious cycle.

Factors that may alleviate that arousal and keep it at levels that are less likely to impede the processing of risk communication include preparation and planning; risk and crisis scenario forecasting; crisis response rehearsal; sense of personal control (such as over a specific response task); sense of accountability for outcomes of tasks in an individual's control (if I do this task well, I personally can help save lives); general health and safety practices (sleep, diet, opportunities to talk formally, opportunities to socialize informally); and sense of values alignment with the organization (this ship is run in a way that aligns with the things I care about, such as safety—and when it is not, I have opportunities to speak up and be listened to, and my input is valued). Good management practices generally are important to creating a crew that can communicate well under pressure.

Even with good health and safety practices, however, seafaring is an inherently high-arousal state. These arousal factors mean that while at sea, messages will need to be largely peripheral. They should be reminder messages, not new information. Simple, one-sided messages will be most effective on audiences who already agree with the gist of what you are saying. The peripheral messages should provide a prompt or reminder of what to do—meaning the careful elaboration through the central route that establishes compliance attitudes must have been completed prior. Simple messages are also most effective on audiences with lower standards of education, limited knowledge of the topic and less sense of personal involvement in the topic—this kind of audience is generally less sceptical than an audience that sees itself as expert and involved. On a ship, it will often be necessary to differentiate between levels of central and peripheral messaging for different segments of the audience, rather than try to use one message for everyone on board. When the entire audience has no ability to elaborate, however, one-sided messages will best meet everyone's needs.

Two-sided messages are most effective if the audience disagree with you, have a high standard of education, knowledge and involvement with the topic, and have time and ability to elaborate. Again, strategies may need to be adjusted for different groups at different times. And at any one time, people are both rational and irrational—meaning a mix of communication styles is usually needed but the balance shifts.

In General

- If your audience is tired, stressed, busy, distracted or traumatized, you need to include lots of peripheral route cues.
- Avoid print-heavy communication for any audience other than one specifically accustomed to dealing with large quantities of print, but particularly avoid it for stressed and traumatized audiences.
- You cannot tell accurately if anyone in your audience is traumatized, so just in case they are, include plenty of peripheral route cues such as simple, personalized messages from a speaker they like and trust, verbal, visual and audio-visual communication and repetition of prior key messages on the same topic.
- Repetition may increase elaboration—the more you repeat, the more you can start to add central cues to the communication, for example as the time after a crisis event increases, people can start to process more detailed information.

Back to the Maritime Case Study

After a crisis has been weathered people may experience traumatic symptoms including replaying the event, intrusive images or thoughts about the event, or nightmares. A judge hearing the *Rena* case commented that "an entire community was sent into shock" by the large scale of environmental oil-spill devastation (Bowen and Migone 2012). For traumatized people, whether on ship or off, helpful responses include providing opportunities to discuss the event—if they are motivated to engage with a health professional—plus remembering the importance of relaxation, enjoyment and social activities. Ensure referral to a specialist for anyone who has a noticeable change in behaviour, difficulty with their normal routine, relationship issues, overuse of substances, disturbed sleep or withdrawal from social activities.

All people may be affected by a crisis in ways that reduce their cognitive processing and all messaging should tend more towards peripheral reiteration of well-established ideas, and only gradually reintroduce central elements after a crisis. However, the possibility of people becoming traumatized by an incident may be reduced if those responsible for communicating about risk and crisis understand some of the science of communication processing and are able to target message content, style and delivery to the time, place and conditions of their audience.

Good crisis preparation including systematic pre-inculcation of lasting attitudes and behaviours for appropriate response, along with apt communication modes during a crisis, may empower maritime workers to feel more in control, recognize the style of their own responses under stress, and consequently be more successful in handling whatever their risky profession throws at them. In the case of the *Rena*, indigenous New Zealanders who were affected by the oil spill devastating their customary fishing grounds recognized that while two men, the captain and navigator, took personal responsibility for the crisis, there were also issues that were larger than individuals. Colin Reeder, chairman of the Te Moana a Toi iwi leaders' forum, read out a victim impact statement in court: "Through restorative justice, Tangata whenua (indigenous owners of the seabed and foreshore) have forgiven the defendants, who were able to apologise to the community. That apology has been accepted. We do not, however, forgive the system that may allow this to happen". This perceptive statement pointed to the wider systemic issues that create or prevent conditions for individual failures of decision-making—but also signalled the opportunity for maritime operators to address crisis preparation systemically, through understanding and implementing appropriate risk communication designs before, during and after a crisis, to reduce the likelihood that crew will abandon cognitive processing and resort to "gut instinct" just when it is least appropriate.

Summary

- There are some visible signs of severe trauma—if you notice these, refer to a health professional.
- However, you cannot necessarily tell if your audience is traumatized. And in a maritime situation, your audience is likely to be somewhat aroused *all the time*.
- The more aroused the audience, the less capable they are of elaborating (processing messages cognitively) and the more likely they are to process messages with an instinctual, emotive reaction. A traumatized audience has almost no ability to elaborate at all and may simply "not hear'" or "not see" the communication.
- Before going to sea, use a mix of central processing (data, explanations, pros and cons, evidence, background context, numbers or statistics) and some peripheral (colour, charts, photos and multimedia including entertaining elements) to build the audience's cognitive engagement with your most important

messages, and inculcate strong learned behaviours and attitudes of crisis best practice.

- Before going to sea, create relationships between the audience and information sources by providing evidence that the source is credible, human, has similar values to the audience, and can be trusted.
- At sea, use predominantly peripheral messaging (simple, directive, visual, colourful, repetition, using pre-established familiar and likeable sources and expert testimonial).
- The peripheral effect is temporary; so repeat key information regularly, and as time from an incident elapses complement increasingly with central cues (more data, less directed needed over time, more ability to use other spokespeople and bring in multiple perspectives over time).

Key Research Questions and Rationale for Future Research in the Area

While the persuasive efficacy of ELM communication design has been tested with experimental research in a range of risk communication situations such as food safety risk (Frewer et al. 1997), and exercise promotion (Jones et al. 2003), our extensive literature searching could find no experimental research testing ELM-based message design in maritime situations. The literature also contains ELM model designs for such diverse contexts as marketing products online (Sher and Lee 2009), public health campaigns communicating the health risks of tobacco, alcohol, unprotected sex and not wearing a seatbelt (Rucker and Petty 2006), and for communicating the risk of not immunizing infants (Tilley et al. 2014). The latter research also included the development of a specific ELM-based communication messaging tool for use with immunization decision-makers. An extensive search of published research, however, found no communication modelling for maritime risk communication, with this chapter being the first publication to link the established efficacy of ELM-informed approaches for risk communication generally to the specific high-arousal situation of maritime professionals.

ELM is only one of a number of communication models that might potentially assist in strengthening risk communication design for maritime situations. Others that could be investigated include social judgement theory, which identifies existing attitudes on a topic before determining the ideal way to pitch an attitude-changing message (see further Hovland and Sherif 1980); narrative transportation theory (which uses storytelling techniques to help people visualize themselves engaging in particular behaviours—see further Green and Brock 2002); and, as noted earlier, inoculation theory (which prepares people to resist counterarguments by ensuring they have already thought through all the positions opposed to the attitude you want them to adopt—see further McGuire 1964).

ELM has strengths and weaknesses—in particular it has been critiqued for being difficult to test and falsify, and for failing to produce clear guidelines as to what makes a strong or weak argument (e.g., Mongeau and Stiff 1993). Despite this, it has been one of the most influential theories of attitude change in the last 30 years, providing a practical synthesis of many diverse aspects of persuasion research. The particular strength of ELM in the maritime context is that it offers specific guidance for communicating with people who are not in a position to carefully consider long or detailed information, but need to make "snap decisions." For this reason we believe it offers more potential for primary investigation as a maritime risk communication approach than other theories at this point in time.

Future research therefore should proceed on two fronts: first, to develop specific prototype maritime risk communication messaging, ideally based on participative action research approaches that involve maritime professionals collaboratively in their development for known maritime situations yet also draws on the vast repository of research in the communication discipline in extant models, particularly ELM. Second, to conduct experimental research to refine and validate the prototypes to develop an evidence-based set of risk communication tools that are uniquely adapted to the differing cognitive and emotional functioning states of maritime workers before, during and after a crisis, and during everyday heightened-risk maritime contexts.

References

American Psychiatric Association. (2013). *Diagnostic and statistical manual of mental disorders* (5th ed.). Arlington, VA: American Psychiatric Association.

Bailey, N. (2006). Risk perception and safety management systems in the global maritime industry. *Policy and Practice in Health and Safety, 2*, 59–75.

Banas, J., & Rains, S. A. (2010). A meta-analysis of research on inoculation theory. *Communication Monographs, 77*(3), 281–311.

Boin, A., Kofman-Bos, C., & Overdijk, W. (2004). Crisis simulations: Exploring tomorrow's vulnerabilities and threats. *Simulation & Gaming, 35*(3), 378–393.

Bowen, M., & Migone, P. (2012, May 25). *Rena* captain and officer sent to jail. Retrieved from http://www.stuff.co.nz/national/crime/6984980/Rena-captain-and-officer-sent-to-jail. Accessed 10 April 2015.

Brehm, S. S., & Brehm, J. W. (1981). *Psychological reactance: A theory of freedom and control.* New York, NY: Academic Press.

Chaiken, S. A., Liberman, A., & Eagly, A. H. (1989). Heuristic and systematic information processing within and beyond the persuasion context. In J. S. Uleman & J. A. Bargh (Eds.), *Unintended thought* (pp. 212–252). New York: Guilford.

Chaudhuri, A., & Buck, R. (1995). Affect, reason, and persuasion: Advertising strategies that predict affective and analytic-cognitive responses. *Human Communication Research, 21*, 422–441.

Daly, M. (2012, September 6). *Rena* captain, officer keep employment. Retrieved from http://www.stuff.co.nz/national/crime/7626587/Rena-captain-officer-keep-employment. Accessed 08 April 2015

Edmond, G., & Tilley, E. (2002, July 10–12). Beyond role play: Workplace theatre and employee relations. In *Australian & New Zealand Communication Association Conference, July 10–12, Gold Coast, 2002: Refereed Proceedings*. Retrieved from http://hdl.handle.net/123456789/175

Eveland, W. P., & Cooper, K. E. (2013). An integrated model of communication influence on beliefs. In B. Fischhoff & D. A. Scheufele (Eds.) *The Science of Science Communication* (pp. 14088–14095). Proceedings of the Arthur M. Sackler Colloquium of the National Academy of Sciences of the United States of America, August 20, 2013, Vol. 110 (supplement 3). Washington, DC: National Academy of Sciences. Retrieved from www.pnas.org/cgi/doi/10.1073/pnas.1212742110

Fairfax. (2011). Rena only just holding together. Retrieved from http://www.stuff.co.nz/environment/rena-crisis/5789177/Rena-only-just-holding-together. Accessed 03 February 2015.

Frewer, L., Howard, C., Hedderley, D., & Shepherd, R. (1997). The elaboration likelihood model and communication about food risks. *Risk Analysis, 17*(6), 759–770.

Friedman, M. J., & McEwen, B. S. (2004). Posttraumatic stress disorder, allostatic load, and medical illness. In P. P. Schnurr & B. L. Green (Eds.), *Trauma and health: Physical health consequences to extreme stress* (pp. 157–188). Washington, DC: American Psychological Association.

Galea, S., Nandi, A., & Vlahov, D. (2005). The epidemiology of post-traumatic stress disorder after disasters. *Epidemiologic Reviews, 27*, 78–91. doi:10.1093/epirev/mxi003

Goldstein, B. D., Osofsky, H. J., & Lichtveld, M. Y. (2011). The Gulf oil spill. *The New England Journal of Medicine, 364*, 1334–1348. doi:10.1056/NEJMra1007197

Green, M. C., & Brock, T. C. (2002). In the mind's eye: Transportation-imagery model of narrative persuasion. In M. C. Green, J. J. Strange, & T. C. Brock (Eds.), *Narrative impact: Social and cognitive foundations* (pp. 315–341). Mahwah, NJ: Lawrence Erlbaum.

Grimm, A., Hulse, L., Preiss, M., & Schmidt, S. (2012). Post- and peritraumatic stress in disaster survivors: An explorative study about the influence of individual and event characterisitics across different types of disasters. *European Journal of Psychotraumatology*, 1–10.

Hovland, C. I., & Sherif, M. (1980). *Social judgment: Assimilation and contrast effects in communication and attitude change*. Westport: Greenwood.

Jones, L. W., Sinclair, R. C., & Courneya, K. S. (2003). The effects of source credibility and message framing on exercise intentions, behaviors, and attitudes: An integration of the elaboration likelihood model and prospect theory. *Journal of Applied Social Psychology, 33*(1), 179–196.

Lindøe, P. H. (2007). Safe offshore workers and unsafe fishermen—A system failure? *Policy and Practice in Health and Safety, 5*(2), 25–39.

Maritime New Zealand. (N.d.). Major oil spills around New Zealand. Retrieved from http://www.maritimenz.govt.nz/Environmental/Responding-to-spills-and-pollution/Past-spill-responses/Past-spill-responses.asp. Accessed 01 March 2015.

Maritime Union of New Zealand. (2015). Maritime industry inquiry into health and safety required to "shine a light on dark places". Retrieved from http://www.munz.org.nz/2015/03/03/maritime-industry-inquiry-into-health-and-safety-required-to-shine-a-light-on-dark-places/. Accessed 03 March 2015.

McCrindle, M., & Wolfinger, E. (2009). *The ABC of XYZ: Understanding the global generations*. Sydney: UNSW Press.

McGuire, W. J. (1964). Inducing resistance to persuasion: Some contemporary approaches. In L. Berkowitz (Ed.), *Advances in experimental social psychology* (pp. 191–229). New York: Academic Press.

Mehta, A., Greer, D., Dootson, P., Christensen, S.A., Duncan, B., & Stickley, A., et al. (2014, October 1–3). Making smart decisions: Key steps towards a typology for emergency communication during natural hazards. In *International Communication Association 2014: Digital Transformations, Social Media Engagement and the Asian Century*, 1–3 October 2014, Brisbane, QLD.

Ministry for Culture and Heritage. (2014). New Zealand disasters timeline. Retrieved from http://
www.nzhistory.net.nz/culture/new-zealand-disasters/timeline. Accessed 14 March 2015

Moats, J. B., Chermack, T. J., & Dooley, L. M. (2008). Using scenarios to develop crisis
managers: Applications of scenario planning and scenario-based training. *Advances in
Developing Human Resources, 10*(3), 397–424.

Mongeau, P. A., & Stiff, J. B. (1993). Specifying causal relationships in the Elaboration
Likelihood Model. *Communication Theory, 3*(1), 65–72.

Neria, Y., Nandi, A., & Galea, S. (2008). Post-traumatic stress disorder following disasters: A
systematic review. *Psychological Medicine, 38*, 467–480. doi:10.1017/S0033291707001353

Norris, F. H., Friedman, M. J., Watson, P. J., Byrne, C. M., Diaz, E., & Kaniasty, K. (2002).
60,000 disaster victims speak: Part I. An empirical review of the empirical literature, 1981–
2001. *Psychiatry: Interpersonal and Biological Processes, 65*(3), 207–239. doi:10.1521/psyc.
65.3.207.20173

Ong, W. J. (2002). *Orality and literacy: The technologizing of the word* (2nd ed.). New York:
Methuen.

Petty, R. E., & Cacioppo, J. T. (1986). *Communication and persuasion: Central and peripheral
routes to attitude change*. New York: Springer-Verlag.

Petty, R. E., & Wegener, D. T. (1999). The elaboration likelihood model: Current status and
controversies. In S. Chaiken & Y. Trope (Eds.), *Dual process theories in social psychology*
(pp. 41–72). New York: Guilford.

Pomeroy, V. (2014). On future ship safety—People, complexity and systems. *Journal of Marine
Engineering & Technology, 13*(2), 50–61.

Rosa, R. R., & Colligan, M. J. (1997). *Plain language about shiftwork: Public health summary*.
Cincinnati, Ohio: Department of Health and Human Services.

Rucker, D. D., & Petty, R. E. (2006). Increasing the effectiveness of communications to
consumers: Recommendations based on elaboration likelihood and attitude certainty perspectives. *Journal of Public Policy & Marketing, 25*(1), 39–52.

Sher, P. J., & Lee, S. H. (2009). Consumer skepticism and online reviews: An elaboration
likelihood model perspective. *Social Behavior and Personality, 37*(1), 137–143.

Tilley, E., Murray, N., Watson, B., & Comrie, M. A. (2014). New views on a 'stuck' issue:
Communicating about childhood immunisation in Aotearoa New Zealand. *Media International
Australia, 152*, 40–56.

Tilley, E., Sligo, F., Shearer, F., Comrie, M., Murray, N., & Franklin, J., et al. (2006). *Voices:
First-hand experiences of adult literacy learning and employment in Wanganui*. Palmerston
North, New Zealand: Department of Communication & Journalism, Massey University. ISBN
978-0-9582646-5-5. Series: Adult Literacy and Employment in Wanganui 0605. ISSN 1176-
9807.

Transport Accident Investigation Commission. (2014). Final report on grounding of MV *Rena*.
Retrieved from http://img.scoop.co.nz/media/pdfs/1412/11204.pdf

Psychometric Assessment: A Case Study of Greek Merchant Marine Officers Using the MMPI-2

Yannis Zolotas, Maria Kalafati, Ernestos Tzannatos
and Dionysios Rassias

Introduction

Psychometric assessment was officially introduced in the maritime industry through the Oil Companies International Marine Forum's (OCIMF) Tanker Management and Self Assessment (TMSA) in 2004, which was addressed to tanker operators and managers in an effort to enhance the implementation of the International Safety Management (ISM) Code. The objective of TMSA is to exhort managers to assess, measure and improve their Safety Management Systems (SMS) through Key Performance Indicators (KPIs) and best practice guidance. In respect of "the recruitment and management of vessel personnel", TMSA points out that managers and/or operators must "ensure that all ships in the fleet have competent crew who fully understand their roles and responsibilities and who are capable of working as a team". As a KPI to this requirement, TMSA suggests that "the company conducts pre-employment assessment for job competence and training for officers and ratings" and considers as "best practice guidance" that "techniques such as simulator training and computer-based or psychometric assessment should be used to confirm competence before confirmation of employment" (OCIMF 2008, p. 28). The ambiguity of this formulation leaves room for interpretation for the shipping companies and

Y. Zolotas (✉)
Dromokaiteio Hospital, Athens, Greece
e-mail: yzolotas@gmail.com

M. Kalafati
Faculty of Nursing, School of Health Sciences, National and Kapodistrian
University of Athens, Athens, Greece

E. Tzannatos
University of Piraeus, Piraeus, Greece

D. Rassias
Merchant Marine Academy of Ionian Islands, Argostoli, Greece

© Springer International Publishing Switzerland 2017
M. MacLachlan (ed.), *Maritime Psychology*, DOI 10.1007/978-3-319-45430-6_9

manning agents to decide on a number of issues. Psychometric assessment is a large area of psychological endeavour which tries to quantify in a standardized way aspects of human behaviour. Occupational psychometric assessment can take several forms and focus on cognitive abilities, the aptitudes considered necessary for a particular job, the personality characteristics that enhance or hinder performance, safety etc., the appropriate attitudinal or motivational characteristics, the clinical assessment of an employee (if safety-critical positions are to be evaluated) or a combination of these.

The notion of "competence" in the maritime profession has evolved and changed rapidly, as has the profession itself, in the last few decades. It comprises, as in most jobs, technical knowledge and skills and non-technical skills. While the technical skills of the mariner have been under scrutiny for quite a long time and have evolved in conjunction with technical advancements and regulatory requirements, there is considerable lack of proportionate research and agreement in respect of non-technical competence with which we are concerned.

As Sanden et al. (2014) state, "a large body of evidence has shown that working on board merchant ships is one of the most mentally and physically demanding professions, with a potential for severe somatic and psychological distress" (p. 93). Working conditions are often physically adverse—ship motion and vibration, noise, heat, cold, humidity, weather conditions etc. Haka et al. (2011), in a study of Danish seafarers, found that the best and worst aspects of the job were perceived to be of a psychosocial nature. Psychosocial stressors are ever present due to the peculiarities of the profession—social and familial isolation, loneliness, lack of shore leave, lack of leisure time and recreational activities, security threats, intermittent sleep, fatigue, disturbed sexual life, language difficulties, living and working in the confined space of the ship with the same people 24/7, the organizational hierarchy of the ship, harassment and bullying, emotional labour ("the effort, planning and control needed to express organizationally desired emotion during interpersonal transactions;" Morris and Feldman 1996, p. 987) and the need for containment of emotions and conflicts, excessive workload, paperwork and time pressure, boredom, the "Damocles' sword" of contemporary regulations and criminalization, cross-cultural communication and relationships, ship-office relationships and commercial demands, and so on. Consequently, psychological health is a prerequisite for the mariners' competence. Furthermore, imperfections of the human-machine interface attributed to the frequently observed mismatch between the quality of crews and new technologies can increase the operator's mental workload, whilst the withdrawal of the operator from highly automated onboard systems reduces his awareness and subsequently his readiness to intervene effectively (and preferably without panic) when automation fails (Goulielmos and Tzannatos 1997).

The Manila Amendments to the Standards of Training, Certification and Watchkeeping for Seafarers (IMO 2011) describe some seafarers' occupational competencies at the management and operational level, like leadership, teamworking and managerial skills, including: bridge and engine resource management, shipboard personnel management and training, task and workload management, decision making, situational awareness, contribution to good human and working conditions, effective communication in individual and team work, assertiveness, reflective consideration of team experience, conflict resolution, motivation, and so on.

Lastly, legal issues pertaining to the improper discrimination of applicants in pre-employment screening can also pose a problem. In some countries this option is rendered invalid since "an employer may ask disability-related questions and require medical examinations of an applicant only after the applicant has been given a conditional job offer" (Equal Employment Opportunity Commission [EEOC] 1995).

Selecting psychometric assessment instruments in an occupationally safety-critical setting like the shipping industry—where the lives of people, the safety and security of the ship, goods worth millions of USD, inestimable potential environmental consequences and the reputation of a company are all at stake due to a person's behaviour and performance—is a task which has to be based on validity and reliability. The aforementioned ambiguity of TMSA may also lead to the use of psychometrically unsound instruments for reasons of cost, short administration time, and lack of appropriate standardized tests in a particular language, etc.

Personality Assessment and the MMPI-2 in the Maritime Industry

In this chapter we describe the personality profile of officers of a major Greek shipping company, using the MMPI-2 in the context of the routine psychometric assessment procedures of this company. Research regarding the personality of the modern seafarer is limited. Lipowski et al. (2014) studied the relationship of merchant marine officers' personality, as it is portrayed by the NEO-Five Factor Inventory (NEO-FFI, Costa and MacCrae 1992), with health behaviours and physical activity. Jeżewska et al. (2013) studied the work-related quality of life of Polish seafarers and its relationship with personality traits and temperamental features and among other questionnaires they also used the NEO-FFI. A research by Elo (1985) showed that personality factors were significant predictors of perceived health status and stress. Jeżewska, in another study (Jeżewska and Leszczyńska 2004), explored the possible relation of certain personality factors in predicting successful career development of Polish Maritime Academy students. Jeżewska (2003) has also used a "Consciousness, Intuition, Anticipation" test for the psychological evaluation of Filipino seafarers.

The MMPI and MMPI-2 are two of the most widely used and empirically researched psychometric instruments of adult personality and psychopathology in the world. The MMPI was developed in the 1940s (Hathaway and McKinley 1943) in the USA, initially as a clinical instrument to be used with adults facing psychological problems. In 1989, a major re-standardization and revision of the inventory produced the MMPI-2 (Butcher et al. 1989, 2001). It is considered one of the main assessment tools of psychologists in clinical settings but it has also been utilized in occupational assessments since 1944 (Butcher 2012).

MMPI-2 is a self-report questionnaire with 567 items and is addressed to adults 18 years old onwards. It requires at least a sixth-grade educational level (Butcher et al. 2001) and it takes around 90 min to be administered. It has been translated into many languages and used in many countries (Butcher 1996). One of the advantages of MMPI-2 is the extensive set of Validity Scales it contains, which have also been applied and researched in various different settings. These scales can measure the respondent's "attitude" towards the test and when used in occupational assessment identify quite distinctly potential underreporting (of possible psychological problems or symptoms), either intentional ("positive impression management") or unintentional ("self deception") in the applicants' effort to "put their best foot forward" (Bagby et al. 2006).

MMPI-2 has been used in many occupational contexts in various ways (Butcher et al. 2009). Considerable research has focused on police officers (Weiss and Weiss 2010) and their pre-employment screening (Dantzker 2011; Laguna et al. 2013; Gamez 2010), predicting performance problems (Weiss et al. 2013; Aamodt 2004; Enright 2004; Matyas 2004), employment outcomes (Caillouet et al. 2010; Davis and Rostow 2004), brutality (Campion 2006), misconduct (Macintyre et al. 2005; French 2002), supervisors' performance ratings (Brewster and Stoloff 2004), intercultural sensitivity (Hamill 2004), police academy performance (Chibnall and Detrick 2003) and other occupational issues (Lijewski et al. 2013; Laguna et al. 2009; Detrick and Chibnall 2008; Devan 2004).

The Federal Aviation Administration (FAA) has used MMPI-2 as part of the psychopathology screening process for hiring air traffic control specialists (FAA 2008, 2010). It has also been used in the assessment of airline pilots (King 2014; Butcher 1994), in military personnel assessment (Kennedy and Zillmer 2006; Cigrang and Staal 2001), in personnel selection of federal law enforcement and intelligence candidates (Sheneman 2004), in the assessment of international organizations' expatriates for successful assignments (Branton 2004), in cross-cultural occupational comparisons (Zapata et al. 2009), in the clergy (Gamino et al. 2007; Gafford 2001; Perri 2001), and elsewhere (Butcher 2012). The validity scales of the MMPI-2, when the test is administered as part of a battery, have been used as an indicator of the general response style of a job applicant to inform results from other tests that do not contain Validity Scales (King 2014).

Considering the use of the MMPI with seafarers there are two studies by Dolmierski et al. (1988, 1990) concerning the evaluation of "psychical state" and "psychic parameters" of seamen and fishermen with a long period of employment at sea. In the first of these studies the authors report a high prevalence of "psychosomatic neurosis". Also, a study by Xiao et al. (2006) explored the mental health of 2272 seamen with the MMPI. However, from our search we could not find any study of seafarers with the MMPI-2.

The Greek version of the MMPI-2 (Karaminas et al. 2007) consists of the 8 Validity Scales, the 10 Standard Clinical Scales, the 9 Restructured Clinical Scales, the 31 Harris–Lingoes Clinical and Si Subscales, the 42 Content and Content Component Scales, the Personality Psychopathology Five Scales (PSY-5), the 15 Supplementary Scales and the Lachar–Wrobel Critical Items. In this chapter we explore the application of MMPI-2 as a psychometric tool in order to assess the personality characteristics of Greek merchant marine officers.

Method

Sample

The participants in this study were Greek merchant marine officers of a major Greek shipping company to whom the MMPI-2 was administered from January 2012 until December 2013. All officers of the sample had at least 16 years of education (12 years of formal education plus 4 years in the Merchant Marine Academy and 2 more years of further education before they reach the rank of the Master or Chief Engineer. Most of our participants were men (5.5 % females $N = 11$).

Of the 198 officers who completed the MMPI-2 in the study, 15 protocols were considered invalid as having T-Scores on the (inconsistency) VRIN or TRIN scales greater than 80, but there were no protocols with a substantial number of missing items (Butcher et al. 2001). Following the suggestion by Butcher (1994, 2006), 55 profiles with T-Scores on the L or K greater than 65 and 70 respectively were also excluded from the sample as being overtly defensive. All the remaining protocols had T-scores of 65 or less on the S scale, except for one having a score of 67. The number of excluded protocols in the current study is close to those reported by other researchers in other personnel assessment settings (Baer and Miller 2002). The total sample included in the study was therefore 128 officers (female 2.3 %, $N = 3$).

The demographic and professional characteristics of the participants are presented in Table 1. The officers enrolled in two subsets/groups according to their working position. There were 58.6 % ($N = 75$) deck officers and 41.4 % ($N = 53$) engine officers. The mean age of the sample was 35 years (SD = 11.11), ranging from 22 to 68 years.

For the purposes of the study six age groups were created. In our effort to establish appropriate age groups, especially for the younger ages of the sample, we consulted the shipping company's crew department and we arrived at an estimate of the mean age when the Greek officers at this company are promoted to the three stages of their career: Apprentices 22–25 years old; second officers (deck) and third officers (engine) 26–29 years old; chief officers (deck) and second officers (engine) 30–34 years old; and masters and chief engineers 35 years old and over.

Table 1 Demographic characteristics of the participants

Variables		Percentage (frequency)
Gender	Male	97.7 (125)
	Female	2.3 (3)
Work position	Deck officers	58.6 (75)
	• Master	• 14.8 (19)
	• C/O	• 10.2 (13)
	• 2nd Officer	• 33.6 (43)
	Engine officers	• 41.4 (53)
	• Chief Engineer	• 17.2 (22)
	• 2nd Engineer	• 10.9 (14)
	• 3rd Engineer	• 13.3 (17)
Age groups (years)	1 = 22–25	22.7 (29)
	2 = 26–29	21.1 (27)
	3 = 30–34	13.3 (17)
	4 = 35–40	16.4 (21)
	5 = 41–50	15.6 (20)
	6 = 51>	15.6 (20)
Age mean = 35 years (min = 22 years, max = 68 years)		

Ethical Considerations

The researchers requested permission to use the officers' MMPI-2 data from the shipping company. The formal application was accompanied by a consent form that explained the aim of the study, and guaranteed confidentiality and anonymity for the officers and the company. This study therefore used secondary data analysis of anonymous data.

Assessment and Analysis Procedures

The test was administered to the officers in small groups during the period the officers were assembling their medical certificates prior to embarkation and after a conditional offer of employment by the company. The MMPI-2 was chosen as an appropriate psychometric instrument due to the validity and reliability of the test, the extensive research base in occupational settings, its standardization in the Greek language and the inclusion of the validity scales, since it was assumed that a certain degree of defensive style of responding (intentional and/or unintentional) was expected to be adopted by the officers in an employment assessment context.

   A licensed psychologist administered the test and gave standard formal instructions to the officers. Answer sheets were scanned, and the appropriate computer program produced the results. Feedback of the test results to the officers was optional and available to whoever wished for it. Data analysis was performed using the Statistical Package for Social Sciences (SPSS 22). Descriptive statistics of all variables were explored and mean values and SDs were reported. Mean and median values and parametric comparisons were used to assess the differences between groups.

Results

Descriptive statistics for MMPI-2 of Merchant Marine Officers' (MMOs) profiles (means and standard deviation of T-Scores) and the comparison with the MMPI-2 of the Greek normative sample ($T = 50$) are shown in Table 2.

Most of the MMPI-2 scales scores of MMOs' profiles are not close to the mean of the MMPI-2 scores of the Greek normative sample (Fig. 1, Table 2). The highest elevation difference on means of T-Scores occurs to RC3 (Cynicism), RC6 (Ideas of Persecution), CYN (Cynicism) and R (Repression) scales and the highest reduction to F (Infrequency), 1 (Hypochondriasis), 2 (Depression), 0 (Social Introversion), RC4 (Antisocial Behaviour), DISC (Disconstraint), AAS (Addiction Acknowledgment) and APS (Addiction Potential) scales (these scale scores are plotted relative to general population norms in Fig. 1).

In Table 2, statistically significant difference was observed between the T-Scores of the normative sample and MMOs' profiles in most of the Validity, Standard Clinical, Restructured Clinical, Content, PSY-5 and Supplementary Scales ($p < 0.05$).

In addition, high mean elevations were obtained on both RC3 and RC6 scales (Restructured Scales), with 19.5 and 20.3 % of the MMOs sample producing RC3 and RC6 scores respectively greater than or equal to $65T$ and on the CYN scale (Content Scales) with 30.5 % of the MMOs sample producing CYN scores greater than or equal to 60 (Table 2).

No statistically significant differences were observed between the T-Scores of Deck and Engine groups, although there are differences in means of T-scores in some scales (Fig. 2).

Although there are differences on means in T-Scores between the age groups (Fig. 3), Table 3 provides the statistically significant differences between T-Scores of MMOs and age groups ($p < 0.05$).

A statistically significant difference in T-Score of K scale ($F_{5,\,128} = 4.78$, $p = 0.001$) between age groups can be seen. The age group 26-29 years has a negative statistically significant difference ($t = -9.914$, $p = 0.001$) with the 22–25 years age group and positive statistically significant difference ($t = 9.659$, $p = 0.006$) with MMOs >50 years.

In Clinical Scales, only scale 7 can be seen to have a statistically significant difference ($F_{5,\,128} = 3.25$, $p = 0.009$) between age groups, with 35-40 years showing a negative statistically significant difference with 22–25 years (t = -5.45, $p = 0.019$) and 26–29 years ($t = -5.56$, $p = 0.018$).

Table 2 Descriptive Scales, mean differences, comparison statistics with Greek general population/normative sample and percentage above 65 or 60

	Scales	N	Mean	SD	t-test with Greek normative sample (Test value = 50)		Percent (%) ≥ 65(mean) ≥ 60(mean) (Content Scales)
					t value	p-value	
Validity Scales	L	128	49.27	9.30	−0.9	0.374	
	F	128	44.47	5.25	−11.9	0.001*	
	Fb	128	47.34	6.41	−4.68	0.001*	
	K	128	54.32	9.58	5.1	0.001*	
	S	128	52.20	6.84	3.6	0.001*	
Standard Clinical Scales	1 (Hs)	128	43.78	7.15	−9.84	0.001*	0.8
	2 (D)	128	43.15	6.53	−11.86	0.001*	–
	3 (Hy)	128	49.73	7.06	−0.44	0.662	2.3
	4 (Pd)	128	48.79	7.36	−1.86	0.065	2.3
	5ᵃ (Mf)	125	45.09	9.23	−5.95	0.001*	1.6
	6 (Pa)	128	45.12	6.60	−8.37	0.001*	1.6
	7 (Pt)	128	46.33	6.01	−6.90	0.001*	0.8
	8 (Sc)	128	44.91	5.66	−10.18	0.001*	–
	9 (Ma)	128	50.36	9.11	0.446	0.656	5.5
	0 (Si)	128	41.64	8.90	−10.63	0.001*	–
Restructured Scales	RCD	128	47.79	6.65	−3.76	0.001*	0.8
	RC1	128	49.88	7.50	−0.18	0.860	4.7
	RC2	128	46.78	6.65	−5.49	0.001*	–
	RC3	128	58.41	8.60	11.07	0.001*	19.5
	RC4	128	43.34	6.50	−11.60	0.001*	0.8
	RC6	128	55.02	10.30	5.51	0.001*	20.3
	RC7	128	48.55	7.32	−2.23	0.027*	2.3
	RC8	128	50.50	8.02	0.71	0.482	5.5
	RC9	128	51.47	7.57	2.20	0.030*	4.7
Content Scales	ANX	128	50.54	6.60	0.92	0.357	12.5
	FRS	128	50.39	8.53	0.52	0.605	15.6
	OBS	128	48.34	8.13	−2.31	0.022*	8.6
	DEP	128	49.90	6.29	−0.18	0.855	4.7
	HEA	128	49.23	7.00	−1.25	0.214	10.2
	BIZ	128	51.06	8.40	1.43	0.155	14.8
	ANG	128	48.84	6.08	−2.16	0.032*	4.7
	CYN	128	56.95	8.38	9.37	0.001*	30.5
	ASP	128	49.71	5.97	−0.55	0.585	5.5
	TPA	128	49.75	7.71	−0.37	0.714	13.3
	LSE	128	48.25	7.58	−2.61	0.010*	7.0
	SOD	128	45.48	7.05	−7.25	0.001*	6.3
	FAM	128	46.34	8.47	−4.90	0.001*	7.8
	WRK	128	45.09	6.73	−8.24	0.001*	0.8
	TRT	128	49.88	8.68	−0.16	0.871	12.5

(continued)

Table 2 (continued)

	Scales	N	Mean	SD	t-test with Greek normative sample (Test value = 50)		Percent (%) $\geq 65_{(mean)}$ $\geq 60_{(mean)}$ (Content Scales)
					t value	p-value	
PSY-5 Scales	AGGR	128	50.73	7.12	1.15	0.251	2.3
	PSYC	128	51.16	8.57	1.53	0.129	10.2
	DISC	128	44.00	6.80	−9.98	0.001*	0.8
	NEGE	128	49.90	7.04	−0.16	0.871	3.9
	INTR	128	44.05	7.33	−9.17	0.001*	–
Supplementary Scales	A	128	46.71	6.90	−5.40	0.001*	1.6
	R	128	55.81	6.80	9.67	0.001*	14.8
	Es	128	51.48	7.28	2.31	0.023*	4.7
	Do	128	48.77	7.98	−1.74	0.085	1.6
	Re	128	53.73	7.73	5.46	0.001*	4.7
	Mt	128	47.54	6.20	−4.49	0.001*	0.8
	PK	128	46.55	7.31	−5.35	0.001*	3.9
	MDS	128	46.03	7.80	−5.76	0.001*	3.1
	Ho	128	52.54	7.05	4.07	0.001*	6.3
	O-H	128	53.36	9.24	4.11	0.001**	10.9
	MAC-R	128	49.20	8.40	−1.07	0.285	1.6
	AAS	128	42.70	5.37	−15.37	0.001*	–
	APS	128	42.91	8.61	−9.307	0.001*	1.6
	GM	128	50.20	7.85	0.28	0.779	1.6
	GF	128	51.46	6.89	2.40	0.018*	0.8

[a]Not included female, *$p < 0.05$

Notes L Lie, *F* Infrequency, *Fb* Infrequency back, *K* Correction, *S* Superlative Self-Presentation, *Hs(1)* Hypochondriasis, *D(2)* Depression, *Hy(3)* Hysteria, *Pd(4)* Psychopathic Deviate, *Mf(5)* Masculinity-Femininity, *Pa(6)* Paranoia, *Pt(7)* Psychasthenia, *Sc(8)* Schizophrenia, *Ma(9)* Hypomania, *Si(0)* Social Introversion-Extraversion, *RCD* Demoralization, *RC1* Somatic Complaints, *RC2* Low Positive Emotions, *RC3* Cynicism, *RC4* Antisocial Behavior, *RC6* Ideas of Persecution, *RC7* Dysfunctional Negative Emotions, *RC8* Aberrant Experiences, *RC9* Hypomanic Activation, *ANX* Anxiety, *FRS* Fears, *OBS* Obsessiveness, *DEP* Depression, *HEA* Health Concerns, *BIZ* Bizarre Mentation, *ANG* Anger, *CYN* Cynicism, *ASP* Antisocial Practices, *TPA* Type A, *LSE* Low Self-Esteem, *SOD* Social Discomfort, *FAM* Family Problems, *WRK* Negative Work Attitudes, *TRT* Negative Treatment Indicators, *AGGR* Aggressiveness, *PSYC* Psychoticism, *DISC* Disconstraint, *NEGE* Negative Emotionality/Neuroticism, *INTR* Introversion/Low Positive Emotionality, *A* Anxiety, *R* Repression, *Es* Ego Strength, *Do* Dominance, *Re* Social Responsibility, *Mt* College Maladjustment, *PK* Post-Traumatic Stress Disorder, *MDS* Marital Distress, *Ho* Hostility, *O-H* Overcontrolled Hostility, *MAC-R* MacAndrew Alcoholism, *AAS* Addiction Acknowledgment, *APS* Addiction Potential, *GM* Gender Role–Masculine, *GF* Gender Role–Feminine

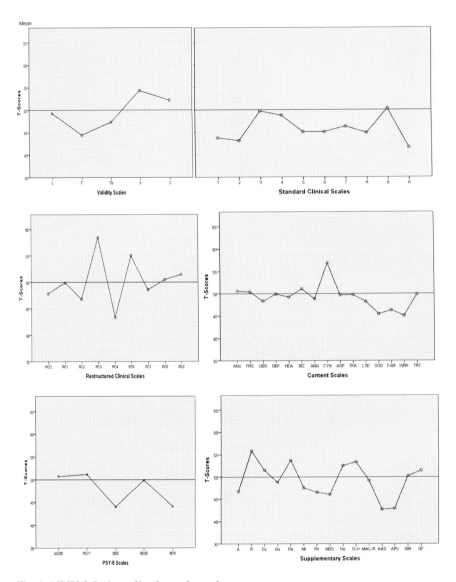

Fig. 1 MMPI-2 Scale profiles for total sample

Looking at significant differences on Restructured Clinical Scale between age groups, there are statistically significant differences on RCD ($F_{5,\ 128}$ = 2.53, p = 0.032), RC3 ($F_{5,\ 128}$ = 4.9, p = 0.001), RC4 ($F_{5,\ 128}$ = 2.6, p = 0.029) and RC7 ($F_{5,\ 128}$ = 2.9, p = 0.016) on age groups.

It seems that the younger and eldest groups present differences on T-Scores with the other age groups. The highest difference between means of T-Score appears in

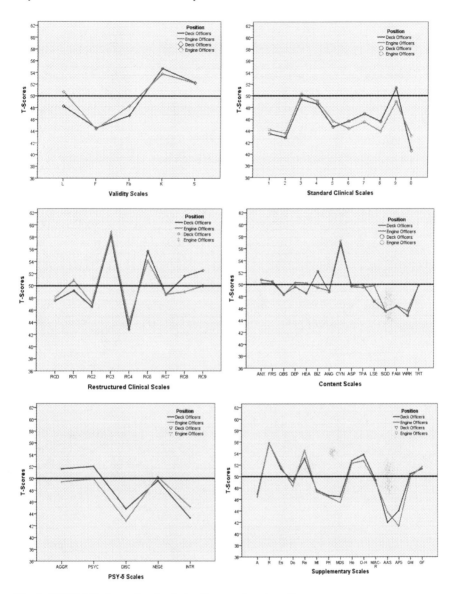

Fig. 2 MMPI-2 Scale profiles for deck officers and engine officers

the RC3 scale on 26–29 years and the >50 years group ($t = -9.913$, $p = 0.001$) (Table 3).

In addition, there seems to be statistically significant difference in T-Scores of some Content Scales and one from PSY-5 Scales on age groups. ANG, CYN, ASP, TPA and DISC T-Scores produce statistically significant differences ($p < 0.05$) between age groups, where in most profiles younger ages lead the differences

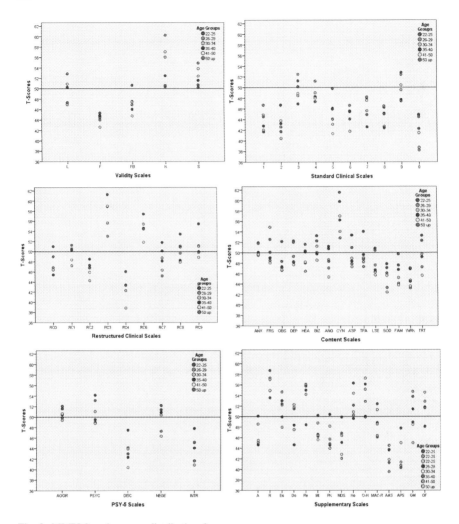

Fig. 3 MMPI-2 scale means distribution for age groups

(Table 3). The highest difference between mean of *T*-Score was indicated in the CYN scale for the >50 years group and 26–29 years ($t = -8.735$, $p = 0.004$) (Table 3).

Finally, in most *T*-Scores of Supplementary Scales can be seen a statistically significant difference between age groups ($p < 0.05$). The greatest difference between means of *T*-Scores can be seen in the GM scale for the >50 years group and 41–50 years ($t = -9.714$, $p = 0.003$) (Table 3).

Table 3 presents all the variations of *T*-Scores means on those age groups that seem to have a statistically significant difference.

Table 3 Comparison statistics with MMPI-2 scales and age groups of total sample and mean differences in statistically significant variables

Scales	ANOVA F (df = 5, 122) (df$_5$ = 5, 119)	p-value	Age groups	Age groups means	Age groups mean difference	p-value Multi comparisons Bonferroni
K	4.796	0.001*	22–25	50.34	−9.914*	0.001*
			26–29	60.26	9.659*	0.006*
			>50	50.60		
7	3.250	0.009*	22–25	48.07	−5.450*	0.019*
			35–40	42.62	−5.566*	0.018*
			26–29	48.19		
RCD	2.53	0.032*	22–25	51	5.571*	0.047*
			35–40	45.43		
RC3	4.9	0.001**	22–25	61.28	8.239*	0.003*
			26–29	53.04	−9.913	0.001*
			>50	62.95		
RC4	2.6	0.029*	22–25	46.07	7.212*	0.009*
			41–50	38.86		
RC7	2.9*	0.016*	22–25	51.80	6.571*	0.011*
			26–29	45.22		
ANG	2.905*	0.016*	22–25	51.21	5.850*	0.040*
			41–50	45.36		
CYN	4.055*	0.002*	22–25	59.79	6.978*	0.019*
			26–29	52.81	−8.735*	0.004*
			>50	61.55		
ASP	4.104*	0.002*	26–29	47.85	−5.493*	0.006*
			22–25	53.34	6.051*	0.009*
			30–34	47.29		
			22–25	53.34	4.964*	0.039*
			35–40	48.38		
TPA	2.719*	0.023*	22–25	54.03	6.701*	0.016*
			26–29	47.33		
DISC	2.826*	0.019*	22–25	47.48	7.054*	0.019*
			41–50	40.43		
A	2.895*	0.017*	22–25	50.10	5.474*	0.039*
			41–50	44.63		
Do	3.527*	0.005*	30–34	52.24	7.615*	0.021*
			22–25	44.62	−6.856*	0.032*
			35–40	51.48		

(continued)

Table 3 (continued)

Scales	ANOVA F (df = 5, 122) (df₅ = 5, 119)	p-value	Age groups	Age groups means	Age groups mean difference	p-value Multi comparisons Bonferroni
Re	4.149*	0.002*	26–29	55.00	6.586*	0.019*
			22–25	48.41	−7.351*	0.004*
			30–34	55.76		
			35–40	55.76	7.348*	0.009*
			22–25	48.41	−7.658*	0.024*
			41–50	56.07		
PK	3.131*	0.011*	26–29	44.59	−5.821*	0.036*
			22–25	50.41	6.414*	0.050*
			30–34	44.00		
MDS	3.091*	0.012*	30–34	42.82	−7.073*	0.037*
			22–25	49.90	7.825*	0.026*
			41–50	42.07		
Ho	3.70*	0.004*	22–25	56.31	6.681*	0.004*
			26–29	49.63		
APS	3.369*	0.007*	26–29	40.70	−7.055*	0.026*
			22–25	47.76	7.425*	0.031*
			35–40	40.33		
GM	4.566*	0.001*	35–40	53.76	8.762*	0.003*
			>50	45.00	−9.714*	0.003*
			41–50	54.71		
GF	2.449*	0.037*	22–25	48.10	−6.447*	0.018*
			>50	54.55		

$*p < 0.05$

Discussion—Concluding Remarks

In this section we compare the scale scores of our group of officers with the respective scores of the Greek general population (Karaminas et al. 2007). In this, we follow the interpretative suggestions by Friedman et al. (2015) and by Nichols (2011) unless otherwise stated.

The Validity Scales show us, as is usually the case in personnel assessment contexts, that a significant number of participants ($N = 55$, 27.8 %) approached the questionnaire with an *overtly defensive style of responding*, trying intentionally or unintentionally to present a positive picture of themselves (L and K). This percentage is close to those reported in other personnel assessment studies (Baer and Miller 2002). These protocols were excluded from the data analysis as invalid. Another Validity Scale (F) shows that our sample may be characterized by *conventionality*.

In relation to the Clinical Scales we see that the mean scores of our sample are significantly *lower* than those of the general population in most of the Clinical Scales (1, 2, 6, 7, 8, 5 and 0) and the percentage of participants having scores above the clinically significant level of 65T is small. It appears from the Clinical Scales and the number of participants who scored higher than 65T that our sample is *psychologically quite a well-adjusted group*. Our sample's scores are especially *low on introversion* (0) and the low score on scale 5 is *typical of occupations where a male-dominated culture prevails*—airline pilots (Butcher 1994), military federal agents (Funk 1997), police officers (Kauder and Thomas 2003) etc.

In the Restructured Clinical Scales we see that compared to the Greek normative sample our group have *lower* scores on scales measuring *general psychological distress (RCD and RC7), depression-spectrum symptoms (RC2) and anti-social or substance-related problems (RC4)*. On the other hand, they score *higher* on scales measuring *cynicism (RC3), mistrust towards others (RC6)* and, to a lesser degree, impulsivity and activation (RC9).

The higher scores in RC3 and RC6 have also been linked to *alienation*. As Sellbom et al. (2007) suggest: "... cynicism and unusual thinking ... have been linked to alienation—a construct that involves fear of victimization and questioning the loyalty of others (Tellegen and Waller 1992). Indeed, Sellbom and Ben-Porath (2005) found strong correlations between both RC3 and RC6 and Alienation, a primary trait scale from Tellegen's Multidimensional Personality Questionnaire".

Moving to the Content Scales with their obvious item content, we see the perception that the officers have of themselves, or the one they want to present. Our sample's scores are *higher* on the scale measuring *cynicism* (CYN) and *lower* on scales measuring *discomfort with social situations (SOD), problems related to their family and work (FAM and WRK)* and to a lesser degree indecision (OBS), poorly controlled anger (ANG) and low self-esteem, especially in the interpersonal context (LSE).

In the Personality Psychopathology Scales (PSY-5) we observe that the officers score significantly *higher* in scales measuring *conventionality, conformity and controlled behavior, which also imply high tolerance for boredom and routine and "relatively rigid adherence to traditional moral standards" (DISC) and sociability (INTR)*.

In the Supplementary Scales we see significantly *lower* scores in scales measuring *anxiety and worry (A), problems with current long-term relationships (MDS) and admittance to substance abuse (AAS)* and *higher* scores in scales measuring *repressed* ("suppressed" or "constricted") *emotionality with limited insight and avoidance of self-disclosure (R), dutifulness (Re), the tendency to perceive others as selfish, hostile and unsympathetic (Ho), the presence of a largely unconscious hostility and massive inhibitions around the expression of it (O-H)* and to a lesser degree stress tolerance, resourcefulness and self-reliance (Es). We are hesitant in interpreting certain scales which have produced, at least according to certain authors, equivocal research correlates (Mt, PK, APS, GM and GF).

There are no statistically significant differences in the profiles of deck and engine officers and this is interesting given the different work environments of each—it might suggest that the commonalities (living aboard ship) are greater than the differences for these two groups.

Considering the age group differences of our sample we observe the validity scales showing a significant *increase in defensiveness* when the officers officially acquire their professional role as junior officers at the age of 26 and a *decrease* after the age of 50—possibly because they have accepted and come to terms with who they are and what they do. In the Standard Clinical Scales the groups aged 22–25 and 26–29 have significantly *higher* (but still lower than the Greek normative sample) levels of *tension, worry, indecisiveness and obsessive behaviours* (Scale 7) than the 35–40 group. In almost all the other scales we see a trend of significant *decrease* in scores between the 22–25 group and some older age group(s), with the exception of two scales measuring the characteristics of *self-direction and dutifulness (Do and Re)*, where we see an *increase* in scores in older age group(s) compared to the 22–25 group. The other exception is with *cynicism (RC3 and CYN)*, where we see a significant *decrease* from the first to the second group and an *increase* in the last group. Taking as a reference point the younger group of apprentice officers it appears that, in general, *as age and/or job experience increase*, scores in some *occupationally "dysfunctional" behaviours are decreasing, or occasionally fluctuating* (7, RCD, RC3, RC4, RC7, ANG, CYN, ASP, TPA, A, MDS, Ho), and scores in some *"functional" behaviours* (Do, Re, -DISC) *are increasing*.

Two interesting and apparently inconsistent results are between a) the scores of Clinical Scale 6 and RC6 and b) the sociability and the cynicism that our group presents. We think that further research should clarify the relationship between the low score on Clinical Scale 6 and the high score on RC6, although some low Clinical Scale 6 scores may have equivalent clinical significance with high Scale 6 scores. "Ideas of persecution", the core construct of RC6, are measured by subscale Pa1 in Clinical Scale 6. The content of Pa1 has been described as *"externalization of blame for one's problems, frustrations [and] failures"* (Harris and Lingoes 1955, in Friedman et al. 2015). Friedman et al. (2015) suggest that *"low Pa scores appear to be associated with having low empathy for others and with low motivation for making relations with others easy and comfortable"*. Graham (1990, in Friedman et al. 2015) says that *"high [Pa1] scorers tend to blame others for their problems, feel that others have unfairly blamed or punished them, and feel misunderstood"*. In a study with nonclinical population Forbey and Ben-Porath (2008) found that RC6 is correlated with unusual thinking and more specifically with magical ideation and secondarily with depression. A factor we could bear in mind in future research considering the "magical ideation" of RC6, that is, the belief in supernatural causality, could be that seafaring is an occupation with a longstanding tradition and culture, part of which are the concepts of "superstition" and "luck". In law the term "Act of God" is an exception from liability for damages caused by overwhelming natural events "of an exceptional, inevitable and irresistible character" which are *beyond the control* of the seafarer (Tsimplis 2015, personal communication). The reference to the supernatural powers of God even where the notion concerns natural phenomena links well to the aforementioned tradition and culture.

In relation to the apparent contradiction between the *sociability and cynicism* of our sample a possible hypothesis would be that although our group is free from problems related to socializing, they perceive the motives of the people they come across with scepticism, if not distrust (or even mistrust). In this sense there is the possibility that a large part of their social relationships may be at a superficial level. Further research is also needed on this topic.

The overall picture shows a group of officers who may be quite well adjusted, sociable, with behavioural and emotional control (if not overcontrol). Cynicism, the distrust (or mistrust) of others' motives and alienation seem to be considerably present. Further research is needed to verify these preliminary results and clarify whether these characteristics are personality traits "attracted" by seafaring (Stokes 1994, in Obholzer and Roberts 1994), coping mechanisms occupationally and/or organizationally induced (Wanous et al. 2000), or both. A relative question is whether the apparent MMOs' cynicism is linked more to real-life occupational relationships than the less cynical attitude of the normative sample.

The characteristics portrayed in this study may correlate with multiple occupational targets aimed at by the maritime organizations, which optimally should be studied within a multidisciplinary perspective, like leadership, maritime human factors, communication and teamworking skills, emotional and social intelligence, team dynamics and team composition, safety management and culture, accountability, organizational commitment, performance, employee motivation for organizational change, job satisfaction, burnout and fatigue mitigation, improved retention rates, etc. Obviously they may also have an impact on individual, team and organizational learning and adaptation. Integration of these factors will require a systems approach (MacLachlan et al. 2013). Personality characteristics have also been correlated with health-related behaviours and cardiovascular morbidity and mortality (Arbisi and Butcher 2004; Almada et al. 1991; Friedman et al. 2015) and can inform organizational practices and appropriate occupational health campaigns.

Butcher has presented an impressive report of MMPI-2 scales combination linked to the measurement of competencies, which may be of particular interest in high-risk occupations as part of a more comprehensive assessment process. These competencies are *stress* tolerance and emotional control, acceptance of feedback and supervision, impulse control, positive attitudes, integrity, dependability and reliability, leadership, conformity to rules and regulations, anger control, adaptability and flexibility, vigilance and attention to detail, interpersonal interest and sensitivity and teamworking ability (Butcher et al. 2006).

Personality assessment tests cannot and should not be used on their own as evidence of the existence or absence of psychopathology in a select-out context—when screening for safety-critical occupations—or of other desirable or undesirable personality characteristics in a select-in screening context. A battery of appropriate tests should be used after a thorough job analysis concerning non-technical skills. In the case of the specific company's procedures, the results of the MMPI-2 were used as hypotheses of occupationally problematic or dysfunctional behaviours which had to be cross checked and validated, or rejected against other sources of data (clinical interview, interview by the crew manager, references, occupational history, performance appraisals, etc.) and when decided that it was necessary relevant administrative action was taken. The test results were also used to modify the methodology and the content of the non-technical skills/human element module of the company's training scheme and served as an instigator for a fruitful discussion related to organizational and managerial factors in the context of the company.

Conclusions

The data reported here are the first to describe the use of the MMPI-2 with merchant marine officers. Our data have a number of limitations: (a) the relatively small sample size and the very few female officers that were included in our study; (b) the fact that our sample comes from only one company; this may have an effect on test results, reflecting organizational factors and the culture of the specific company; (c) the limited access we had on demographic data. Variables like cultural factors, socioeconomic status of the family of origin, whether the officer's father was also a mariner, years of service with the current company, marital status and whether the officer has children may have an impact on various scale scores; (d) the tests were administered during a period of financial crisis in Greece. Although the Greek shipping industry has not been directly affected by this crisis, Greek society was undergoing major social and economic turmoil, which may also have had an impact on test results.

This chapter has, however, highlighted the potential value of psychometric assessment in personnel screening and assessment and in informing training and coaching programmes related to non-technical skills (human element). A prerequisite to all this is the use of psychometrically sound instruments with a strong research base. In our case the MMPI-2 revealed a well-adjusted group of officers characterized by conventionality, emotional and behavioural control, social ease, cynicism and alienation. The need for further research is evident as well as the potential correlations of these findings with desirable and undesirable occupational outcomes in seafaring.

Acknowledgments We would like to thank the officers and the Company for providing us with the data for this research. We would also like to thank Mr. Naoum Karaminas for his thought-provoking comments on an earlier draft of this chapter.

References

Aamodt, M. G. (2004). Special issue on using MMPI-2 scale configurations in law enforcement selection: Introduction and meta-analysis. *Applied H.R.M. Research, 9*, 41–52.

Almada, S. J., Zonderman, A. B., Shekelle, R. B., Dyer, A. R., Daviglus, M. L., Costa, P. T., et al. (1991). Neuroticism and cynicism and risk of death in middle-aged men: The Western Electric Study. *Psychosomatic Medicine, 53*, 165–175.

Arbisi, P. A., & Butcher, J. N. (2004). Relationship between personality and health symptoms: Use of the MMPI-2 in medical assessments. *International Journal of Clinical and Health Psychology, 4*(3), 571–595.

Baer, R. A., & Miller, J. (2002). Underreporting of psychopathology on the MMPI-2: A meta-analytic review. *Psychological Assessment, 14*(1), 16–26.

Bagby, R. M., Marshall, M. B., Bury, A. S., Bacchiochi, J. R., & Miller, L. S. (2006). Assessing underreporting and overreporting response styles on the MMPI-2. In J. N. Butcher (Ed.), *MMPI-2: A practitioner's guide* (pp. 39–69). Washington, DC: APA Press.

Branton, R. E. (2004). A multifaceted assessment protocol for successful international assignees. *Dissertation Abstracts International: Section B: The Sciences and Engineering, 64*, 4024.

Brewster, J., & Stoloff, M. L. (2004). Using MMPI special scale configurations to predict supervisor ratings of police officer performance. *Applied H.R.M. Research, 9*, 53–56.

Butcher, J. N. (1994). Psychological assessment of airline pilot applicants with the MMPI-2. *Journal of Personality Assessment, 62*(1), 31–44.

Butcher, J. N. (Ed.). (1996). *International adaptations of the MMPI-2.* Minneapolis, MN: University of Minnesota Press.

Butcher, J. N. (2012). References in personnel screening with the MMPI/MMPI-2. Retrieved from http://www1.umn.edu/mmpi/documents/PERSONNEL%20SCREENING%20WITH%20THE%20MMPI.pdf. Accessed June 17, 2015.

Butcher, J. N., Dahlstrom, W. G., Graham, J. R., Tellegen, A., & Kaemmer, B. (1989). *Minnesota Multiphasic Personality Inventory–2 (MMPI-2): Manual for administration and scoring.* Minneapolis, MN: University of Minnesota Press.

Butcher, J. N., Graham, J. R., Ben-Porath, Y. S., Tellegen, Y. S., Dahlstrom, W. G., & Kaemmer, B. (2001). *Minnesota Multiphasic Personality Inventory-2: Manual for administration and scoring* (Revised edition). Minneapolis, MN: University of Minnesota Press.

Butcher, J. N., Gucker, D. K., & Hellervik, L. W. (2009). Clinical personality assessment in the employment context. In J. N. Butcher (Ed.), *Oxford handbook of personality assessment* (pp. 582–598). New York: Oxford University Press.

Butcher, J. N., Ones, D. S., & Cullen, M. (2006). Personnel screening with the MMPI-2. In J. N. Butcher (Ed.), *MMPI-2: A practitioner's guide* (pp. 381–406). Washington, DC: American Psychological Association.

Caillouet, B. A., Boccaccini, M. T., Varela, J. G., Davis, R. D., & Rostow, C. D. (2010). Predictive validity of the MMPI-2 PSY-5 scales and facets for law enforcement officer employment outcomes. *Criminal Justice and Behavior, 37*, 217–238.

Campion, T. R. (2006). Predicting police aggression with the Psychopathic Deviant Scale on the MMPI-2. *Dissertation Abstracts International: Section B: The Sciences and Engineering, 66*, 5136.

Chibnall, J. T., & Detrick, P. (2003). The Neo PI-R Inwald Personality Inventory and MMPI-2 in the prediction of police academy performance: A case for incremental validity. *American Journal of Criminal Justice, 27*, 233–248.

Cigrang, J. A., & Staal, M. A. (2001). Re-administration of the MMPI-2 following defensive invalidation in a military job applicant sample. *Journal of Personality Assessment, 76*, 472–481.

Costa, P. T., & MacCrae, R. R. (1992). *Revised NEO personality inventory (NEO PI-R) and NEO five-factor inventory (NEO FFI): Professional manual.* Psychological Assessment Resources.

Dantzker, M. L. (2011). Psychological pre-employment screening for police candidates: Seeking consistency if not standardization. *Professional Psychology: Research and Practice, 42*, 276–283.

Davis, R. D., & Rostow, C. D. (2004). Using MMPI special scale configurations to predict law enforcement officers fired for cause. *Applied H.R.M. Research, 9*, 57–58.

Detrick, P., & Chibnall, J. T. (2008). Positive response distortion by police officer applicants: Association of Paulhus deception scales with MMPI-2 and Inwald Personality Inventory validity scales. *Assessment, 15*, 87–96.

Devan, J. L. (2004). A taxometric analysis of impression management and self-deception on the MMPI-2 among law enforcement applicants. *Dissertation Abstracts International: Section B: The Sciences and Engineering, 64*, 5777.

Dolmierski, R., Jeżewska, M., Leszczyska, I., & Nitka, J. (1990). Evaluation of psychic parameters in seamen and fishermen with a long employment period. Part 1. *Bulletin of the Institute of Maritime and Tropical Medicine in Gdynia, 41*(1–4), 115–121.

Dolmierski, R., Leszczyska, I., & Nitka, J. (1988). Evaluation of psychical state of the engine room crew members of a long period at sea. *Bulletin of the Institute of Maritime and Tropical Medicine in Gdynia, 39*(3–4), 149–154.

Elo, A. L. (1985). Health and stress of seafarers. *Scandinavian Journal of Work, Environment & Health, 11*(6), 427–432.

Enright, B. P. (2004). Personality measurement in the prediction of positive and negative police officer performance. *Dissertation Abstracts International: Section B: The Sciences and Engineering, 65*, 3154.

Equal Employment Opportunity Commission. (1995). The U.S. Equal Employment Opportunity Commission (EEOC) NOTICE Number 915.002 Date 10/10/95. Retrieved from http://www.eeoc.gov/policy/docs/preemp.html. Accessed June 8, 2015.

Federal Aviation Administration. (2008). Screening air traffic control specialists for psychopathology using the Minnesota Multiphasic Personality Inventory-2 (FAA Publication No. DOR/FAA/AM-08/13). Washington, DC: US Government Printing Office. Retrieved from http://libraryonline.erau.edu/online-full-text/faa-aviation-medicine-reports/AM08-13.pdf. Accessed May 19, 2015.

Federal Aviation Administration. (2010). The effects of testing circumstance and education level on MMPI-2 correction scale scores (FAA Publication No. DOT/FAA/AM-10/3). Washington, DC: US Government Printing Office. Retrieved from http://www.faa.gov/data_research/research/med_humanfacs/oamtechreports/2010s/media/201003.pdf. Accessed June 5, 2015.

Forbey, J. D., & Ben-Porath, Y. S. (2008). Empirical correlates of the MMPI-2 restructured clinical (RC) scales in a nonclinical setting. *Journal of Personality Assessment, 90*(2), 136–141.

French, L. (2002). Assessing law enforcement personnel: Comparative use of the MMPIs. *Forensic Examiner, 11*, 21–27.

Friedman, A. F., Bolinskey, P. K., Levak, R. W., & Nichols, D. S. (2015). *Psychological assessment with the MMPI-2/MMPI-2-RF*. New York: Routledge.

Funk, A. P. (1997). Psychological assessment of military federal agents using the MMPI-2: A look at employment selection and performance prediction. Master's thesis. Retrieved from http://oai.dtic.mil/oai/oai?verb=getRecord&metadataPrefix=html&identifier=ADA331909. Accessed June 19, 2015.

Gafford, J. S. (2001). Variations in psychological functioning among Roman Catholic religious professionals. *Dissertation Abstracts International: Section B: The Sciences and Engineering, 62*, 547.

Gamez, A. M. (2010). *The use of the Minnesota multiphasic personality inventory-II (MMPI-2) in pre-employment evaluations* (Doctoral dissertation). Retrieved from Dissertations and Theses database. (UMI No. 3424837).

Gamino, L. A., Sewell, K. W., Mason, S. L., & Crostley, J. T. (2007). Psychological profiles of Catholic deacon aspirants. *Pastoral Psychology, 55*, 283–296.

Goulielmos, A., & Tzannatos, E. (1997). The man-machine interface and its impact on shipping safety. *Disaster Prevention and Management: An International Journal, 6*(2), 107–117.

Graham, J. R. (1990). MMPI-2: Assessing personality and psychopathology. New York: Oxford University Press.

Haka, M., Borch, D. F., Jensen, C., & Leppin, A. (2011). Should I stay or should I go? Motivational profiles of Danish seafaring officers and non-officers. *International Maritime Health, 62*(1), 20–30.

Hamill, M. A. (2004). Cultural sensitivity of probation officers as a measure for pre-employment screening. *Dissertation Abstracts International: Section B: The Sciences and Engineering, 64*, 5217.

Harris, R. E., & Lingoes, J. C. (1955). Subscales for the minnesota multiphasic personality inventory: An aid to profile interpretation. (Mimeographed materials.) San Francisco, CA: University of California, Langley Porter Neuropsychiatric Institute.

Hathaway, S. R., & McKinley, J. C. (1943). *The Minnesota Multiphasic Personality Inventory Manual*. Minneapolis, MN: University of Minnesota Press.

International Maritime Organization. (2011). *Standards of training, certification and watchkeeping for seafarers—Including 2010 Manila amendments*. London: IMO.

Jeżewska, M. (2003). Psychological evaluation of seafarers. *International Maritime Health, 54*(1–4), 68–76.

Jeżewska, M., & Leszczyńska, I. (2004). A survey on the influence of personality on successful career development of the Maritime Academy students. *International Maritime Health, 55*(1–4), 39–51.

Jeżewska, M., Leszczyńska, I., & Grubman-Nowak, M. (2013). Personality and temperamental features vs. quality of life of Polish seafarers. *International Maritime Health, 64*(2), 101–105.

Karaminas, N., Georgakas, P., Kantas, A., Tsaousis, I., Marini, K., Karakosta, A., & Stalikas, A. (2007). The robustness of MMPI-2: The Greek standardization. *International Psychology Bulletin, 11*, 24–26.

Kauder, B. S., & Thomas, J. C. (2003). Relationship between MMPI-2 and Inwald Personality Inventory (IPI) scores and ratings of police officer probationary performance. *Applied H.R.M. Research, 8*(2), 81–84.

Kennedy, C. H., & Zillmer, E. A. (Eds.). (2006). *Military psychology: Clinical and operational applications*. New York: The Guildford Press.

King, R. E. (2014). Personality (and psychopathology) assessment in the selection of pilots. *The International Journal of Aviation Psychology, 24*(1), 61–73.

Laguna, L., Agliotta, J., & Mannon, S. (2013). Pre-employment screening of police officers: Limitations of the MMPI-2 K-scale as a useful predictor of performance. *Journal of Police and Criminal Psychology, 30*(1), 1–5.

Laguna, L., Linn, A., Ward, K., & Rusplaukyte, R. (2009). An examination of authoritarian personality traits among police officers: The role of experience. *Journal of Police and Criminal Psychology, 25*, 99–104.

Lijewski, A., MacDonald, D. A., & Panyard, C. M. (2013). Examination of the psychometric properties of the MMPI-2 restructured clinical (RC) scales with a sample of public safety officer candidates. *The International Journal of Educational and Psychological Assessment, 13*, 1–12.

Lipowski, M., Lipowska, M., Peplińska, A., & Jeżewska, M. (2014). Personality determinants of health behaviours of merchant navy officers. *International Maritime Health, 65*(3), 158–165.

Macintyre, S., Ronken, C., & Prenzler, T. (2005). Validity study: Relationship between MMPI-2 scores and police misconduct in Australia. *Applied H.R.M. Research, 10*, 35–38.

MacLachlan, M., Cromie, S., Liston, P., Kavanagh, B., & Kay, A. (2013). Psychosocial and organisational aspects of work at sea and their implications for health and performance. In T. Carter & A. Schreiner (Eds.), *Textbook of maritime medicine* (2nd ed.). Bergen: Norwegian Centre for Maritime Medicine.

Matyas, G. S. (2004). Using MMPI special scale configurations to predict police officer performance in New Jersey. *Applied H.R.M. Research, 9*, 63–66.

Morris, J. A., & Feldman, D. C. (1996). The dimensions, antecedents and consequences of emotional labor. *Academy of Management Review, 21*(4), 986–1010.

Nichols, D. S. (2011). *Essentials of MMPI-2 assessment* (2nd ed.). New Jersey: Wiley.

Obholzer, A., & Roberts, V. Z. (Eds.). (1994). *The unconscious at work. Individual and organizational stress in the human services*. London: Routledge.

Oil Companies International Marine Forum. (2008). *Tanker management and self assessment—A best practice guide for ship operators* (2nd ed.). London: OCIMF.

Perri, W. D. (2001). An analysis of psychologically evaluated Roman Catholic Priests and Brothers comparing vocation and lifestyle sexual orientation and age. *Dissertation Abstracts International: Section B: The Sciences and Engineering, 62*, 560.

Sanden, S., Johnsen, B. H., Jarle Eid, J., Sommerfelt-Pettersen, J., Koefoed, V., Størksen, R., et al. (2014). Mental readiness for maritime international operation: Procedures developed by Norwegian Navy. *International Maritime Health, 65*(2), 93–97.

Sellbom, M., & Ben-Porath, Y. S. (2005). Mapping the MMPI-2 restructured clinical (RC) scales onto normal personality traits: Evidence of construct validity. *Journal of Personality Assessment, 85*, 169–178.

Sellbom, M., Fischler, G. L., & Ben-Porath, Y. S. (2007). Identifying MMPI-2 predictors of police integrity and misconduct. *Criminal Justice and Behavior, 34*, 985–1004.

Sheneman, K. M. (2004). Traitors in the ranks: Understanding espionage-related offenses and considered implications for the use of personality assessment in personnel selection for federal law enforcement and intelligence candidates. *Dissertation Abstracts International: Section B: The Sciences and Engineering, 65*, 2683.

Stokes, J. (1994). The unconscious at work in groups and teams: Contributions from the work of Wilfred Bion. In A. Obholzer & V. Z. Roberts (Eds.), *The unconscious at work: Individual and organisational stress in the human services* (pp. 19–27). London: Routledge.

Tsimplis, Michael N. (2015). Professor of oceanography and maritime law, Institute of Maritime Law, University of Southampton.

Wanous, J. P., Reichers, A. E., & Austin, J. T. (2000). Cynicism about organizational change: Measurement, antecedents, and correlates. *Group Organization Management, 25*, 132.

Weiss, P. A., Vivian, J. E., Weiss, W. U., Davis, R. D., & Rostow, C. D. (2013). The MMPI-2 L scale, reporting uncommon virtue, and predicting police performance. *Psychological services, 10*, 123.

Weiss, P. A., & Weiss, W. U. (2010). Using the MMPI-2 in police psychological assessment. In P. A. Weiss (Ed.), *Personality assessment in police psychology: A 21st century perspective* (pp. 59–71). Springfield, IL: Charles C. Thomas.

Xiao, Z., Dacheng, C., Yuanli, Z., et al. (2006). Qingdao College of Ocean Seamen, Analysis of test result of Multiphasic Personality of ocean seamen. *China Journal of Health Psychology, 2*.

Zapata, A., Kreuch, T., Landers, R. N., Hoyt, T., & Butcher, J. N. (2009). Clinical personality assessment in personnel settings using the MMPI-2: A cross-cultural comparison. *International Journal of Clinical and Health Psychology, 9*, 287–298.

Sailing as an Intervention

Malcolm MacLachlan

Case Study

The Jubilee Sailing Trust (JST) registered as a charity in 1978 with the aim of integrating people with physical disabilities with non-disabled people in an enjoyable activity. JST's founder, Christopher Rudd, had experience of teaching children with disabilities and special needs to sail dinghies. Rudd believed that "the obstacles to sailing offshore were to a large extent artificial and could be overcome by thoughtful design and proper equipment. In addition, he believed that if physically disabled people were to sail alongside able-bodied people as part of the crew, it would help break down the prejudices and misunderstandings between people with different circumstances in life" (JST 2016).

In scoping the project with collaborator Tony Hicklin, they found that square-rigged ships were in fact ideal sailing vessels for people with disabilities as such ships require a large crew working together, and there are many different tasks involved, thus suiting different types of capabilities: "There was something for everyone—those who couldn't pull on ropes could ease them off, and those who could do neither could instead call out the 'two–six' hauling rhythm" (JST 2016).

Now with two purpose-designed square-rigged ships—*Lord Nelson* and *Tenacious*—participants in the Jubilee Sailing Trust have sailed hundreds of thousands of miles, mostly in European and North Atlantic waters, helping to change thousands of lives for those participating, and helping to change many more thousands of views of what people with disabilities can do.

Former Vice President of the Trust, the late Ian Shuttleworth, recalled:

M. MacLachlan (✉)
Centre for Global Health and School of Psychology, Trinity College, University of Dublin, Dublin, Ireland
e-mail: malcolm.maclachlan@tcd.ie

© Springer International Publishing Switzerland 2017 223
M. MacLachlan (ed.), *Maritime Psychology*, DOI 10.1007/978-3-319-45430-6_10

It was a complicated business bringing Lord Nelson into the world, but we never doubted it would work. Although the world has since advanced in its approach to inequality, we still feel we are proving something every day that is relevant and we are the only ships to offer what we do. Our voyage crew develop self-confidence, self-image and positive results. This is still relevant and important and is still learned on board. (JST 2016)

Introduction

There is a lot of psychology in sailing. There is a psychology of sailing, with an excellent example of this being Sadler's (1987) book of that title, subtitled "The sea's effects on mind and body". This remains an engaging and broad ranging review of sensory performance and sensory illusions at sea; seasickness, motivation and how to manage the "work" of sailing; and the crew as a social group— especially as regards living in close quarters with one another. There is also a psychology about achieving better performance at sailing. One of the initial descriptions of this is by Halliwell, who outlines how sport psychology contributed to the performance of the Canadian sailing team in the 1988 Olympics (Halliwell 1989). Indeed, along with sports medicine, Olympic sailing has been a stimulus to more evidence-based approaches to incorporating a psychological perspective into sailing (Allen and De Jong 2006).

The vast area of sport psychology can of course be applied to sailing, where many leisure sailors, but also some professional sailors, compete in yacht racing, from small dinghy sailing to the Volvo Ocean Race or America's Cup events. Yet at all levels these performances can be enhanced by psychological interventions to promote effective teamwork, positive imagery and attitudes, improved concentration and goal setting (see Brown 2011). Sailing has benefited not just from more evidence regarding sail performance at sea, but also in simulated environments to explore issues such as decision making in demanding situations (Araújo et al. 2005). This idea of developing a "winning mindset", as Brown (2011) calls it, not surprisingly can extend to other types of teamwork and performance, and therefore sailing can be used to simulate and stimulate the development of skills and attitudes that can extend into the corporate and government sectors. There are many companies offering sailing as a reward for, or for the development of, good teamwork in the corporate sector.

While each of the above uses of psychology in sailing is important, they are not the focus of this chapter. Here we are concerned with the self-development and therapeutic benefit of sailing, where the context of sailing and the maritime has been deliberately chosen as an intervention to be of personal benefit to its participants. However, there will hopefully always remain an unfathomable aspect to sailing. It is possible to have considerable expertise in the technical aspects of sailing and in the psychology of sailing, and yet for it to still retain its sublime existential value. Evans (2016), in his remarkable book "Thoughts, Tips, Techniques and Tactics for

Single-Handed Sailing", begins this authoritative volume with these enchanting lines:

> If I was the richest man in the world,
>
> I'd have a bigger boat and newer sails.
>
> But on a Saturday afternoon with only God and the wind,
>
> I wouldn't be any happier than I am right now.
>
> (2016, p. 1).

It is clear that there are many ways and levels at which psychology and sailing are interwoven. While some of these may indeed be relevant to the context of *sailing as an intervention*, these areas of research are not primarily concerned with the benefit of sailing to the participant, beyond of course its intrinsic enjoyment and the opportunity it offers to become absorbed in the "flow" of the activity. The enormous popularity of sailing as a hobby is testament to its intrinsic rewarding possibilities. However, this chapter instead places the benefit of sailing foreground, with the activity and indeed the maritime environment being somewhat back-grounded, as a sort of canvas on which interventions play themselves out. While such an intervention may be enjoyable, we are interested in those that seek to (and may or may not) stimulate a longer lasting, more profound and sustainable effect on the participant's well-being.

Sailing as an Educational Intervention

In the example of sail training in the above case study of the Jubilee Trust, sailing is not simply an enjoyable activity, but clearly also one that presents an environment that can be operated on in different ways to achieve different ends. McCulloch (2004) contrasts two case studies of UK sail training, considering the ethos of voyaging within each of them. The differences between them, McCulloch argues, can be understood in terms of different approaches to participation in decision making, and their associated and different interpretations of power. McCulloch argues that even the types of vessels used and the routes of voyages made are not neutral choices, but rather imbued with ideological significance.

In a subsequent multinational study of sail training for young people, McCulloch and colleagues (McCulloch et al. 2010) conclude that such opportunities allow for the development of social and emotional skills in self-confidence and the ability to work collaboratively, along with the acquiring of practical skills and knowledge. In fact, they argue that it is not necessarily the "seamanship dimension" of the experience that is crucial for such learning, but rather participation in a "structured purposeful programme", with the maritime environment providing a unique and stimulating learning environment in which to pursue it. McCulloch et al.'s study, using qualitative analysis of interviews with 25 participants across a range of different types of sail training vessels, states that

> There is clear evidence of various educational purposes and expectations in both sail training operators' accounts of purpose, and in participants' own stories. Our findings show that participation provides an opportunity for learning in the practical and cognitive domains in relation to skills and knowledge, and in the affective domain in relation to social confidence. (p. 675)

McCulloch et al. also found that the greater the extent to which structured and purposefully educational activities (and reviewing of learning from them) were used, the greater was the evidence of their association with increased self-confidence of the participants. They note that while on some vessels programmes are planned to explicitly facilitate trainees' learning, on others there was a greater emphasis on simply allowing the seafaring experience to "speak for itself", and for participants to draw their own learning from this. While the latter may be of value, some degree of structure and reflection seems to facilitate more learning and the building of more self-confidence.

In another paper, McCulloch (2013) has applied Erving Goffman's idea of total institutions to sail training, emphasizing the extent to which the physical boundaries of a boat, encapsulating its crew during its passage, help to create the sense of independence and self-sufficiency within the participants. This boundedness of the vessel and those within it may be one of the unique features of sailing as a context of intervention—individuals both bounded together and separated from all else—allowing for a particular type of environment, or culture, to develop on board, even during short durations at sea.

Others too have found the educative experience of seafaring to build certain desirable psychological characteristics. Hayhurst et al. (2015) explored the extent to which a "developmental voyage" for a group of youths was associated with increased resilience, both during the voyage and at follow-up 5 months later. They found that increased self-efficacy, social effectiveness, and less positive perceptions of the weather (!) were each individually associated with increased resilience.

These sorts of results for educational sail training chime with findings from other aspects of the "outdoors" being seen as fertile ground for the development of self, and self in relation to others. Cooley et al. (2015) investigated participants' perceptions of outdoor (ashore) groupwork skill programmes for undergraduate and postgraduate students, alumni and academic staff, over a 24-h period using video diary, one-to-one interview and focus group methods. Perceived benefits reported included increased social integration amongst peers, academic success, personal development and employability. Various factors felt to influence the extent of these benefits were elaborated in their "Model for Optimal Learning and Transfer".

This model has two broad domains that can each be broken down into several overlapping components. First there is the "Reaction & Learning" of the participant; this involves their preparation (needs analysis, priming and group formation), their own characteristics as learners (or learning styles, such as openness to and engagement with new experiences), and the learning context. The learning context incorporates the removal from familiar social norms, its experiential nature, the range of progressive challenges, the social and supportive elements, guided reflection and enjoyment. The second domain of the model, "Behaviour & Results", is seen to arise from the first. Here learner characteristics relate to the ability to generalize learning, mindful practice and self-reflection. Also included in this domain is transfer context, which relates to opportunity, challenge, informal prompting and follow-up, and peer support. Colley et al.'s model would seem to have relevance to the idea of sailing as an educational or self-development intervention. Its recognition of the preparation of participants and their learning styles also indicates awareness that there may be considerable individual differences in what constitutes an optimal outdoor learning environment, and we may assume that for some that would not be the maritime or sailing environment. Indeed, different people may perceive the same environment as threatening to quite different extents (Walsh-Daneshmandi and MacLachlan 2000) and there may be cultural differences in such perceptions (Walsh-Daneshmandi and MacLachlan 2006). In other words, people's background or group characteristics may determine the extent to which any type of intervention, especially an outdoor one, seems appropriate to them.

While "outdoor experiential learning", as it is referred to by Warren et al. (2014), may be of value for many, its social justice credentials have been questioned. Indeed, sailing is often seen as an elitist activity par excellence (Laurier 1999). Warren et al. concerned themselves with North American outdoor programmes, recognizing that cultural as well as contextual factors are likely to influence the meaning given to any such programmes. Social justice may be taken to refer to the promotion of equity in access to services and opportunity in society. So, equity in this context means providing different groups with the necessary means so that they can achieve similar outcomes (Amin et al. 2011). Outdoor activities—perhaps especially sailing—are often seen as rather privileged, well-off, middle-class, able-bodied, and (perhaps in the USA) white activities.

If such activities are the vehicle of privilege, then perhaps they can also be poignant symbols of inclusion, by more explicitly targeting social divides and social dominance (Pratto et al. 1994, Lee et al. 2011). Maybe outdoor experiential learning—outside conventional social norms—can offer a canvas on which to re-negotiate social difference and invigorate, or re-invigorate, shared identities and common purpose. Thus, taking social privilege and oppression outdoors, by engaging with race/ethnicity/culture, (dis)ability, gender, gender identity, religion and socioeconomic status, can be one way to embrace a social justice ethos.

For instance, in the case of people with disability, Warren et al. state,

> Any discussion of 'able bodied' is predicated on the assumption that there exists disabled 'others'. Rather than adopting this binary categorisation, ... [we] ... present the concepts of universal design, inclusion, and integration for all people engaged in OEE [outdoor experiential education] ... Integration is the act of combining individuals to make a unified whole, for example, wilderness experiences including persons with and without disabilities. (p. 92)

The Jubilee Trust ships can be seen as perhaps juxtaposing the idea of the inaccessibility of traditional sailing ships with the meaningful participation of people with disabilities in a very wide range of sailing activities. It is the disappearance of this apparent contradiction that is so empowering and causes us to reset our expectations and to be more open to unanticipated possibilities. Such efforts educate not just those viewing from the "inside" in regard to what people with disabilities can and cannot do, but they also educate and empower participants from the "outside" in terms of what they can expect.

In highlighting areas for future research and development that would promote social justice in outdoor experiences, Warren et al. (2014) suggest that fundamental challenges for learning in the outdoors include reconceptualization of the meanings of outdoor adventure; promoting the intersectionality of race, class, gender, and other identities; adoption of universal design principles and accessibility as the norm; and more attention to power relations and to how social justice theory can be used to promote constructive learning and practices. In this sense, sail training can therefore be a mechanism for cultivating pluralism (MacLachlan and O'Connell 2000). The ship at sea is therefore a potential new and bounded social culture, one that can reach beyond the extant social norms that constrain individual and group identities, and one that allows people to experience difference in a more constructive and empowering way, facilitating both educative and self-development goals.

Sailing as a Therapeutic Intervention

The maritime environment may also be able to contribute to therapeutic as well as educative experiences. "Adventure-based experiential therapy" (AET; Eckstein and Rüth 2015) has been used with child and adolescent psychiatry inpatients, often in the form of rock-climbing, caving or exploring a creek; these can provide considerably more stimulating environments than hospital settings for therapeutic work to be "worked out" in. Eckstein and Rüth (2015) call for more research and practice to explore this potential. Ewart (2014) has also reported benefits from "Outward Bound Program for Vets" (OB4V), used to complement other interventions for US soldiers experiencing various types of emotional reactions (such as PTSD and suicidal thoughts) to their soldiering experiences. The "macho" element of outdoors experiences may well suit the narrative of coping and building resilience common to military cultures.

There are a number of studies that have specifically used sailing for therapeutic benefit. Carta et al. (2014) explored the effects of sailing for 40 participants who had either a diagnosis of schizophrenia, affective psychoses, or severe personality disorder, who had been in treatment in a mental health care network for no less than 2 years, and who had reached clinical remission, but could nonetheless be considered to be experiencing chronic mental health problems. The researchers concluded that for those who participated in the "rehabilitation with sailing" programme—which included a series of cruises in the gulf of Cagliari (Sardinia)—there was a statistically significant improvement in their quality of life, as compared to a similar group who did not have such experiences. However, this study is very interesting, as much because of what did not change as what did change. They report that on the World Health Organisation Quality of Life Scale (Group 1998)—on which there are four sub-scales—there were positive changes for self-report scores on the physical and the environment components of quality of life, but only modest changes on the psychological scale and none at all on the social relations scale. Furthermore, even these benefits were not long-lasting and had disappeared at 12-month follow-up. This may suggest that clear psychological and social gains are required to maintain the benefits of shorter-lasting positive physical and environmental experiences.

du Moulin et al. (2013) describe their experience with Boston's "Community Boating Universal Access Program" (UAP): over a period of 6 years more than 1500 people, with a range of physical and cognitive disabilities, have participated in the programme, which is designed to promote therapeutic and recreational goals. They argue that the natural setting—particularly its unpredictability—allows for the development of motor skills, coordination and self-confidence, in a challenging, adventurous environment.

Perhaps one of the most innovative applications of sailing as an intervention is that being developed by Romero et al.'s (2014) Italian research group, comprising a team of designers and rehabilitation clinicians who are using a specially modified sailing boat as a rehabilitation strategy for people who have experienced a stroke. They argue that many people who experience a stroke are left with reduced muscle movement and/or some degree of mobility impairment. One of the challenges in the rehabilitation of people with such impairments is that post-stroke depression can disengage them from activities and the motivation necessary to gain functional recovery, participate in social activity and actively engage in effective problem solving. Romero et al. (2014) see sailing as an intervention that will facilitate better rehabilitation by helping to engage people more in the rehabilitative process through improving their quality of life, providing an enjoyable and relaxing intervention.

In this research, sailing is seen as providing both motor and cognitive challenges, and supporting the motivation of participants by giving them a (often new) life experience; perhaps something they had assumed they may no longer be able to have. However, sailing is also seen as having a very instrumental quality, with the authors describing the boat as "a floating rehab gymnasium", allowing participants to engage in a number of routine motor activities in a purposeful and sociable way, as opposed to simply repeating prescribed movement tasks, which may require much greater motivation. The yacht being used in this work takes a crew of six people, allowing the activity to be sociable and for people with stroke to support each other and see each other's success. This work is ongoing and will surely be important for informing the potential of sailing as a rehabilitative mechanism for stroke and other types of impairments.

We have already noted the perception that sailing is elitist. Recio et al. (2013) argue that many people view sailing not just as elitist and expensive, but also as dangerous, and that these perceptions, along with having no previous experience of sailing, act as a barrier to access, including for those without disabilities. For people with disabilities, physical access may be a further barrier. However, Recio et al. (2013) also claim that sailing has positive outcomes on self-esteem and general health for such participants. To address some of these access barriers Recio et al. trialled a real-time "ride-on" sailing simulator, to allow non-sailors to develop basic sailing skills before on-water experience. Following a 12-week therapeutic sailing programme using the VSail-Access sailing simulation system, they reported that participants with disabilities could gain both in technical sailing skills and in their psychological well-being. Importantly, participants were also able to participate in such activities with family members.

Koperski et al. (2015) describe "Adventure Therapy" as a modality of interaction which can augment other therapeutic approaches. They see its value in its ability to improve coping skills and so better manage stressful situations, with these effects being associated with a better therapeutic alliance. Sailing may be seen as one of the alternative forms of adventure experiences and as such connected with what has been referred to as ecopsychology. The realm of ecopsychology as a therapeutic or self-development intervention is well established.

According to the ethos of ecopsychology and ecotherapy it is human evolution —in particular our "moving away from nature"—that is at least in part responsible for some health, and particularly mental health, problems. The ecopsychology view is that living in urbanized environments is not optimal and disconnects people from the benefits of nature (Roszak 2001). An often-quoted study illustrating the power of nature to heal is by Ulrich (1984), who evaluated the post-operative recovery of hospital patients who had either a view from their hospital bed of a blank wall, or a view of trees. Records over a 10-year period showed that those with a view of the trees had shorter post-operative recovery times—being discharged earlier—than those with a view of the wall. This study was followed by a number of others with variations on the same theme, which can be summarized as indicating that patients who have some form of access to more natural environments (a window or even a picture) recover more quickly than those who do not. In fact this effect is now incorporated into the design of hospital environments.

The context of that work is the view that the industrialization of humanity has not only moved it away from nature but has also led it to destroy nature; in this sense ecopsychology can be seen as being about both getting back in contact with nature at an individual level, and at a species level, getting nature back into humanity's view of how as a species it should "develop", what it should value and how it can sustain itself and the planet on which it is dependent. Thus MIND (2013) defines ecotherapy as being about "building a relationship with nature, so that personal wellbeing is considered equally alongside the health of the environment" (p. 5).

Jordan (2013) discusses the relevance of the concept of the "frame" for under-standing the challenge that "taking therapy outside" constitutes to conventional therapy, where the space of the therapist's rooms frames the nature of the relationship between therapist and client, the sort of talk that is appropriate, and the roles—and status—of participants in the therapeutic encounter. By contrast, an encounter out-of-doors does not locate or confine the therapeutic space; it questions boundaries; it makes ambiguous the relative roles of the participants; it offers the potential for a more democratic and less status—and role—conscious encounter. It also allows for that encounter to be less hinged on specific personalized problems and more developed through the relationship between the participants.

The confidentiality, physical comfort and consistency of the therapy room is also often lost and these attributes need to be implicitly re-negotiated—in what is invariably a more fluid and dynamic context (Jordan 2013). Within this more complex, less rigid environment, there are opportunities for de-professionalizing of therapeutic encounters (with both the advantages and disadvantages this may involve). Importantly, Jordan (2013) found that therapists working outdoors felt that one of the values of their medium was to sometimes be able to "bypass language" (p. 169) and allow the sensory stimulation of natural environments to be at the forefront of experience. Jordan (2013) also stresses the need to develop a clearer understanding of what constitutes safe, ethical and professional practice, outdoors.

It is clear that the environment and indeed environmental threats are perceived and experienced differently by different people (Walsh-Daneshmandi and MacLachlan 2000), and both knowledge of, and attitudes towards, the environment may be culturally influenced (Walsh-Daneshmandi and MacLachlan 2006). Thus, while people will experience their exposure to the maritime context in different ways, there seems to be sufficient evidence to suggest that sailing in general as an intervention is at least worthy of further research.

Research Questions

This chapter has sought to review the idea of sailing as an intervention. Some questions for future research in the area are now briefly posed. What distinguishes sailing as an intervention compared to other types of outdoor interventions? And related to this, is sailing simply a variation in the outdoors that may be more attractive to some than to others, or is there an element of engaging with the maritime that makes it qualitatively different from other outdoor interventions? The research reviewed above also suggests that more structured interventions may be more beneficial and so, what is the optimal type of structure to bestow the greatest benefit for participants?

We have considered sailing as both an educational and therapeutic interventions. If there are benefits associated with sailing for such interventions, are they similar for the two types of interventions; are there commonalities, but also distinctive mechanisms in each case? In the case of corporate sailing interventions—on which there seems to be little systematic research—what are the possible mechanisms of benefit here?

We have also noted the challenges with sailing, for instance, its perception as an elitist activity, its cost, and the idea that therapy in the sailing context, like in other outdoor contexts, can remove many of the boundaries with which practitioners and therapists are familiar. A code of good practice and a mechanism to provide support and guidance to practitioners may be worthwhile developing. Norton et al. (2014) review the literature on adventure therapy with youth and call for training and professional development in adventure therapy and greater professionalization in practice, and through better research in the area (see also Gass et al. 2012).

We might also want to ask to what extent sailing can be offered more widely as an intervention. For instance, the excellent work done by Sail Training International is focused on "changing young people's lives". This is a very appropriate target, but with our changing demographics, surely there is scope for changing the lives of older people too! The innovative work on the rehabilitation of people with stroke could easily be extended to people with other types of rehabilitative needs. For instance, limb amputation and learning to use a prosthetic limb are challenges that are accompanied by many psychosocial issues (Desmond and MacLachlan 2002a, b). Learning how to use both upper and lower limb prostheses in purposive, enjoyable and often new experiences could be both motivating and empowering for participants. In all these situations, the potential for the intervention to be helpful will depend on being accurately able to assess the ability of the person to engage with and learn from such experiences, and so the development of assessment tools to help practitioners judge this would be another important area of future research.

Research in sailing as an intervention is in its infancy and so like many other innovative areas, initial research is often piecemeal, opportunistic and of modest scale. Despite this, some excellent research has already been undertaken and this should be built on through larger studies, and the collection of longitudinal data over longer time periods. The use of comparative or control groups through randomized controlled trials would provide a much more robust database on which to build future and further evidence-based practice. However, there is also a critical role for skilful qualitative research to pinpoint crucial experiential elements of sailing as an intervention, and to allow researchers to learn ideas from participants, as well as test their own ideas from theory or practice.

Conclusion

Art, drama and music are recognized as mediums of intervention that allow people to express themselves in ways that "talk" may not (MacLachlan 2004), and therefore to know and possibly define themselves in other and new ways. Similarly, the development of new sets of skills, such as carpentry, a new language or through hobbies, can be seen as a means of experiencing added aspects of the self and giving a greater—and often a more "rounded"—sense of self. Sailing is experienced variously as a skill, an art, an intellectual challenge, a connectedness to nature, as risk-taking, as calming. For the same person it may be all of these at different times. As an enjoyable realm of human activity sailing is certainly worth considering as a beneficial intervention, particularly with regard to its educative and therapeutic possibilities, but possibly also as a corporate intervention. There is already enough research to give us optimism regarding the benefits and possibilities of sailing as an intervention; however, to fully realize the potential of this medium will require several significant and complementary research programmes to be undertaken by different research consortia.

References

Allen, J. B., & De Jong, M. R. (2006). Sailing and sports medicine: A literature review. *British Journal of Sports Medicine, 40*(7), 587–593.

Amin, M., MacLachlan, M., Mannan, H., El Tayeb, S., El Khatim, A., Swartz, L., et al. (2011). EquiFrame: A framework for analysis of the inclusion of human rights and vulnerable groups in health policies. *Health & Human Rights, 13*(2), 1–20.

Araújo, D., Davids, K., & Serpa, S. (2005). An ecological approach to expertise effects in decision-making in a simulated sailing regatta. *Psychology of Sport and Exercise, 6*(6), 671–692.

Brown, I. (2011). *The psychology of sailing for dinghies and keelboats: How to develop a winning mindset.* London: Adlard Coles Nautical.

Carta, M. G., Maggiani, F., Pilutzu, L., Moro, M. F., Mura, G., Sancassiani, F., et al. (2014). Sailing can improve quality of life of people with severe mental disorders: Results of a cross over randomized controlled trial. *Clinical practice and Epidemiology in Mental Health: CP & EMH, 10*, 80.

Cooley, S. J., Cumming, J., Holland, M. J. G., & Burns, V. E. (2015). Developing the Model for Optimal Learning and Transfer (MOLT) following an evaluation of outdoor groupwork skills programmes. *European Journal of Training and Development, 39*(2), 104–121.

Desmond, D., & MacLachlan, M. (2002a). Psychosocial issues in prosthetic and orthotic practice: A 25 year review of psychology in Prosthetics & Orthotics International. *Prosthetics and Orthotics International, 26*, 182–189.

Desmond, D., & MacLachlan, M. (2002b). Psychosocial issues in the field of prosthetics and orthotics. *Journal of Prosthetics & Orthotics, 12*(2), 12–24.

du Moulin, G. C., Kunicki, M., & Zechel, C. (2013). Therapy on the water: Universal access sailing at Boston's Community Boating. *PALAESTRA, 27*(3), 9–17.

Eckstein, F., & Rüth, U. (2015). Adventure-based experiential therapy with inpatients in child and adolescent psychiatry: An approach to practicability and evaluation. *Journal of Adventure Education & Outdoor Learning, 15*(1), 53–63.

Evans, A. (2016). *Thoughts, tips, techniques and tactics for singlehanded sailors (Third Edition).* Singlehanded Sailors Society.

Ewert, A. (2014). Military veterans and the use of adventure education experiences in natural environments for therapeutic outcomes. *Ecopsychology, 6*(3), 155–164.

Gass, M. A., Gillis, L., & Russell, K. C. (2012). *Adventure therapy: Theory, research, and practice.* New York, London: Routledge.

Group, T. W. (1998). The World Health Organization quality of life assessment (WHOQOL): Development and general psychometric properties. *Social Science and Medicine, 46*(12), 1569–1585.

Halliwell, W. (1989). Delivering sport psychology services to the Canadian sailing team at the 1988 Summer Olympic Games. *The Sport Psychologist, 3*(4), 313–319.

Hayhurst, J., Hunter, J. A., Kafka, S., & Boyes, M. (2015). Enhancing resilience in youth through a 10-day developmental voyage. *Journal of Adventure Education & Outdoor Learning, 15*(1), 40–52.

Jordan, M. (2013). *Taking therapy outside-a narrative inquiry into counselling and psychotherapy in outdoor natural spaces.* Doctoral dissertation, University of Brighton.

Jubilee Sailing Trust (JST). (2016, June, 18). Downloaded from http://jst.org.uk/about-jubilee-sailing-trust/history/

Koperski, H., Tucker, A., Lung, M., & Gass, M. A. (2015). The impact of community based adventure therapy on stress and coping skills in adults. *The Practitioner Scholar: Journal of Counseling and Professional Psychology, 4*(1), 1–16.

Laurier, E. (1999). Elitism, working leisure and yachting. *Leisure/Tourism Geographies: Practices and Geographical Knowledge, 3*, 195–213.

Lee, I.C., Pratto, F. and Johnson, B.T., 2011. Intergroup consensus/disagreement in support of group-based hierarchy: an examination of socio-structural and psycho-cultural factors. *Psychological bulletin, 137*(6), 1029.

MacLachlan, M., & O'Connell, M. (Eds.). (2000). *Cultivating pluralism: Cultural, psychological and social perspectives on a changing Ireland.* Dublin: Oak Tree Press.

MacLachlan, M. (2004). *Embodiment: Clinical, critical & cultural perspectives on health & illness.* Milton Keynes: Open University Press.

McCulloch, K. H. (2004). Ideologies of adventure: Authority and decision making in sail training. *Journal of Adventure Education & Outdoor Learning, 4*(2), 185–197.

McCulloch, K. (2013). Erving Goffman: Sail training, interactionism and the 'total institution'. In E. C. J. Pike & S. Beames (Eds.), *Outdoor Adventure and Social Theory.* London: Routledge.

McCulloch, K., McLaughlin, P., Allison, P., Edwards, V., & Tett, L. (2010). Sail training as education: More than mere adventure. *Oxford Review of Education, 36*(6), 661–676.

Norton, C. L., Tucker, A., Russell, K. C., Bettmann, J. E., Gass, M. A., & Behrens, E. (2014). Adventure therapy with youth. *Journal of Experiential Education, 37*(1), 46–59.

Recio, A. C., Becker, D., Morgan, M., Saunders, N. R., Schramm, L. P., & McDonald, J. W., III. (2013). Use of a virtual reality physical ride-on sailing simulator as a rehabilitation tool for recreational sports and community reintegration: A pilot study. *American Journal of Physical Medicine and Rehabilitation, 92*(12), 1104–1109.

Roszak, T. (2001). *The voice of the earth: An exploration of ecopsychology.* Red Wheel/Weiser.

Pratto, F., Sidanius, J., Stallworth, L. M., & Malle, B. F. (1994). Social dominance orientation: A personality variable predicting social and political attitudes. *Journal of Personality and Social Psychology, 67*, 741–763.

Romero, M., Andreoni, G., Piardi, S., Ratti, A., Imamogullari, B. & Molteni, F. (2014). Sailing as stroke rehabilitation strategy. In T. Ahram, W. Karwowski, & T. Marek (Eds.), *Proceedings of the 5th International Conference on Applied Human Factors and Ergonomics AHFE 2014, Kraków, Poland* (pp. 19–23).

Sadler, M. (1987). *Psychology of sailing: The sea's effects on mind and body.* Camden, Maine: International Marine Publishing Company.

Ulrich, R. (1984). View through a window may influence recovery. *Science, 224*(4647), 224–225.

Walsh-Danishmandi, A., & MacLachlan, M. (2000). Environmental risk to the self: Factor analysis and development of sub-scales for the Environmental Appraisal Inventory (EAI) with an Irish sample. *Journal of Environmental Psychology, 20*, 141–149.

Walsh-Daneshmandi, A., & MacLachlan, M. (2006). Towards effective evaluation of environmental education: Validity of the CHEAKS using data from a sample of Irish adolescents. *Journal of Environmental Education, 37*, 13–23.

Warren, K., Roberts, N. S., Breunig, M., & Alvarez, M. A. T. G. (2014). Social justice in outdoor experiential education: A state of knowledge review. *Journal of Experiential Education, 37*(1), 89–103.

Index

Note: Page numbers followed by f and t indicate figures and tables, respectively

© Springer International Publishing Switzerland 2017
M. MacLachlan (ed.), *Maritime Psychology*, DOI 10.1007/978-3-319-45430-6

Printed in the United States
By Bookmasters